Phlebotomy Simplified

Diana Garza, EdD, MT(ASCP)ᶜᴹ

Health Care Consultant
Medical Writer/Editor
Houston, Texas

Kathleen Becan-McBride, EdD, MT(ASCP)ᶜᴹ

Director, Community and Educational Outreach
Coordinator, Texas-Mexico Border Health Services
Medical School Professor in the Department of Family & Community Medicine
The University of Texas Health Science Center at Houston
Texas Medical Center, Houston, Texas
Assistant Director for Academic Partnerships, Greater Houston AHEC

PEARSON
Prentice Hall

Upper Saddle River, NJ 07458

Library of Congress Cataloging-in-Publication Data

Garza, Diana.
  Phlebotomy simplified / Diana Garza, Kathleen
Becan-McBride.
        p. ; cm.
  Includes bibliographical references and index.
  ISBN 0-13-222478-x (alk. paper)
  1. Phlebotomy.
    [DNLM: 1. Phlebotomy—methods. QY 25 G245p 2008]
I. Becan-McBride, Kathleen (Date)– II. Title.

  RB45.15.G373 2008
  616.07'561—dc22

                                    2007011731

Notice: The authors and the publisher of this volume have taken care that the information and technical recommendations contained herein are based on research and expert consultation, and are accurate and compatible with the standards generally accepted at the time of publication. Nevertheless, as new information becomes available, changes in clinical and technical practices become necessary. The reader is advised to carefully consult manufacturers' instructions and information material for all supplies and equipment before use, and to consult with a healthcare professional as necessary. This advice is especially important when using new supplies or equipment for clinical purposes. The author[s] and publisher disclaim all responsibility for any liability, loss, injury, or damage incurred as a consequence, directly or indirectly, of the use and application of any of the contents of this volume.

Publisher: Julie Levin Alexander
Executive Editor: Mark Cohen
Associate Editor: Melissa Kerian
Editorial Assistant: Nicole Ragonese
Development Editor: Cathy Wein
Managing Editor for Production: Patrick Walsh
Production Liaison: Christina Zingone
Manufacturing Manager: Ilene Sanford
Manufacturing Buyer: Pat Brown
Media Editor: John J. Jordan
Media Project Manager: Stephen Hartner
Design Director: Maria Guglielmo
Interior Designer: Wanda Espana

Cover Designer: Anthony Gemmellaro
Production Editor: Carol Lallier
Compositor: Stratford/TexTech
Director of Marketing: Karen Allman
Senior Marketing Manager: Harper Coles
Marketing Specialist: Michael Sirinides
Marketing Assistant: Wayne Celia
Printer/Binder: Courier Kendallville
Cover Printer: Phoenix Color Corporation
Cover Image: Barry Rosenthal/Taxi/Getty, Images, Inc.
Chapter Opening Image: Jupiter Images–Picture Arts
      Corporation/Brand X Pictures Royalty Free
Photographer: Rocky Kneten Photography

Credits and acknowledgments borrowed from other sources and reproduced, with permission, in this textbook appear on appropriate pages within text.

Pearson Education LTD., London
Pearson Education Singapore, Pte. Ltd
Pearson Education Canada, Ltd.
Pearson Education—Japan
Pearson Education Australia PTY, Limited

Pearson Education North Asia Ltd
Pearson Educación de Mexico, S.A. de C.V.
Pearson Education Malaysia, Pte. Ltd
Pearson Education Inc., Upper Saddle River, New Jersey

1 0 9 8 7 6 5

ISBN-13: 978-0-13-222478-9
ISBN-10: 0-13-222478-X

"To my husband, Peter McLaughlin; my children, Lauren, Kaitlin, and Kevin; and my parents for their affection, patience, and constant support."

—*Diana Garza*

"To my husband, Mark; my sons, Patrick and Jonathan; my grandson, Finnaveir; my parents; my sister; and my parents-in-law for their support and devotion."

—*Kathleen Becan-McBride*

Brief Contents

Contents

Appendices

Procedures

Phlebotomy Simplified is designed for beginning health care students and practitioners who are responsible for blood and specimen collections (medical assistants, nurses, phlebotomists, clinical laboratory technicians and technologists, respiratory therapists, and others). The primary goal of the book is to link the novice phlebotomist (blood collector) to simplified, basic information, techniques, skills, and equipment for the provision of safe and effective blood collection procedures. It provides introductory competencies, including communication, clinical, technical, and safety skills, that all health care workers will use for the entry-level practice of phlebotomy. The book's format is an easy, step-by-step, practice-oriented approach of blood collection procedures to be used in a variety of settings, including hospitals, ambulatory clinics, and pediatric clinics.

The content is divided into 11 chapters. The order in which the material is presented generally follows the way in which a phlebotomist is educated and how he or she approaches the patient.

Chapter 1 Phlebotomy Practice and Quality Assessment Basics
Chapter 2 Ethical, Legal, and Regulatory Issues
Chapter 3 Basic Medical Terminology, the Human Body, and the Cardiovascular System
Chapter 4 Safety and Infection Control
Chapter 5 Documentation, Specimen Handling, and Transportation
Chapter 6 Blood Collection Equipment
Chapter 7 Preanalytical Complications in Blood Collection
Chapter 8 Venipuncture Procedures
Chapter 9 Capillary Blood Specimens
Chapter 10 Pediatric and Geriatric Procedures
Chapter 11 Special Collections

Problem-solving cases integrate the information into real-life situations. The glossary and appendices provide useful procedures and important terms, phrases, and symbols.

Key Features of Phlebotomy Simplified

- Colorful photographs show procedural steps and equipment.
- Flowcharts provide additional easy-to-follow procedures.
- Case studies encourage problem solving.
- The most recent safety features of phlebotomy supplies and equipment are reviewed.
- The medical terminology section and glossary terms are critical to effective communication.
- Key sections prepare the phlebotomist for age-related competencies and communication.
- Self-assessment exercises help the phlebotomist acclimate to the health care environment.
- Clinical alert symbols indicate procedures or concepts that have vitally important clinical consequences for the patient. The clinical alert indicates that extra caution should

be taken by the health care worker to comply with the procedure, thereby avoiding adverse outcomes for the patient.

■ Step-by-step procedural information is presented using an on-the-job perspective.

■ Key terms, objectives, and study questions are provided for each chapter.

■ A color chart of types of blood collection tubes relates appropriate color coding with additives.

■ Appendices contain essential elements for finding a job, Spanish phrases, symbols and units of measurement, military time, and NAACLS Competencies.

■ NAACLS Competencies are linked to the level of coverage and specific content in the text.

Companion CD-ROM

A companion CD-ROM was developed to integrate knowledge in a multisensory manner. It is organized to correlate with the textbook chapters and is a valuable tool for students and instructors. Features of this exciting ancillary include:

■ An audioglossary in which all key terms from the book are defined and pronounced.

■ A flashcard generator that allows students to customize their study of key terms.

■ A variety of interactive quizzes and games, such as word search and Beat the Clock, that can serve as ideal homework assignments and self-study applications.

Ancillary Resources

Phlebotomy Simplified has companion resources that are cross-referenced to the text. The Instructor's Resource Manual contains a wealth of material to help faculty plan and manage their course. It includes a detailed lecture outline, a complete test bank, teaching tips, and more for each chapter. An Instructor's Resource CD-ROM is available upon adoption (0-13-222483-6). The CD-ROM includes the complete test bank and PowerPoint lectures that contain discussion points with embedded color images from the book. Prentice Hall's *SUCCESS! in Phlebotomy,* 6th edition, is recommended reading to aid students and health care workers preparing for their certification examination. It also has an accompanying CD-ROM with a simulated board examination consisting of 100 multiple-choice questions and referenced explanatory answers. Students can practice taking the simulated examination in print or via computer. A diagnostic report identifies those topics that need further review and study and provides the score for each content area.

Phlebotomy Handbook: Blood Collection Essentials, 7th edition, is recommended for health care students and practitioners who need a book with an even greater in-depth comprehensive review of phlebotomy techniques, procedures, and regulatory guidelines.

In summary, the authors have created a book that health care professionals, instructors, and students will use as a basic introduction to blood collection practices.

Acknowledgments

We are grateful to many generous people, product suppliers, manufacturing companies, professional organizations, and health care organizations for their assistance in preparing this text. We are particularly indebted to BD Vacutainer Systems, Greiner Bio-One, the American Society for Clinical Pathology, the University of Texas M.D. Anderson Cancer Center, and the University of Texas Health Science Center at Houston for their support. We thank Estella Woodard, MT (ASCP), and Benjamin Lichtiger, MD, for their clinical expertise in coordination of the on-site photography, and Rocky Kneten, the photographer.

We greatly appreciate our working relationships with editors and copy editors who have encouraged us and improved our final version. Special thanks go to Cathy Wein, Melissa Kerian, and Mark Cohen.

Last, and most important, we are thankful to our families who have encouraged and supported us. They will always hold a special place in our hearts.

Diana Garza
Kathleen Becan-McBride

Reviewers

Cindy Abel, BS, CMA, PBT(ASCP)
Program Chair, Medical Assisting
Ivy Tech Community College
Lafayette, Indiana

Deborah J. Bedford, AS, CMA
Program Coordinator, Medical
    Assisting
North Seattle Community College
Seattle, Washington

Kim Boyd, MLT(ASCP), MT(AMT)
Education Coordinator and Instructor,
    Medical Laboratory Technology
Amarillo College
Amarillo, Texas

Konnie King Briggs, LVN
Instructor, Phlebotomy
Houston Community College
Houston, Texas

Cara L. Calvo, MS, MT(ASCP)SH
Program Director and Clinical
    Associate Professor, Clinical
    Laboratory Science
Ohio Northern University
Ada, Ohio

Donna Calvert, MEd, MT(ASCP)
Program Director and Assistant
    Professor, Clinical Laboratory
    Science
McNeese State University
Lake Charles, Louisiana

Patricia A. Chappell, MA, MT(ASCP)
Program Director, Clinical Laboratory
    Science
Camden County College
Blackwood, New Jersey

Andrea G. Gordon, MEd,
    MT(ASCP)SH
Professor and Program Director
    Clinical Laboratory Technician/
    Phlebotomy
New Hampshire Community
    Technical College
Claremont, New Hampshire

Sheri R. Greimes, CMA, PBT,
    RMA, RPT
Instructor, Phlebotomy Training
    Program
Everett Community College
Everett, Washington

Brenna D. Ildza, MT(ASCP)SH,
    PBT(ASCP)
Director, Phlebotomy Education
    Program
Saint Luke's Hospital
Kansas City, Missouri

Anna de Leon Harrison,
    MT(ASCP), MBA
Clinical Laboratory Manager
Coastal Bend College
Beeville, Texas

Cheryl Jackson-Harris,
    MS, MT(ASCP)SH
Professor and Program Coordinator,
    Clinical Sciences
California State University-
    Dominguez Hills
Carson, California

Frances Cassandra Johnson,
    MT, M(ASCP), BS, MHS
Program Director, Medical Laboratory
    Technician
Meridian Community College
Meridian, Mississippi

Bernice Lewis, RN, PBT, ASCP
Lead Instructor, Nursing Assisting
    and Phlebotomy
Brunswick Community College
Supply, North Carolina

Claudia Miller, PhD, MT(ASCP)
Professor, Health Studies
National-Louis University
Evanston, Illinois

Norma Moore, BS, MT(ASCP)
Department Chairperson, Allied
    Health
Laredo Community College
Laredo, Texas

Carole Mullins, MPA, CL Dir (NCA),
    BS, MT(ASCP)
Adjunct Faculty, Health and Human
    Services
Southwestern Michigan College
Dowagiac, Michigan

Angela Njoku, MS, MT(ASCP)
Assistant Professor, Clinical Laboratory
    Technician/Phlebotomy
St. Louis Community College
St. Louis, Missouri

Kathleen A. Park, MEd, BSMT
Program Director, Medical Laboratory
    Technician and Emergency Medical
    Services
Lamar State College-Orange
Orange, Texas

Evelyn Paxton, MS, MT(ASCP)
Program Director, Clinical Laboratory
    Technician/Phlebotomy
Rose State College
Midwest City, Oklahoma

Timothy Sandor, BS, CLS(NCA),
    MT(ASCP)
Instructor, Phlebotomy
Lake Superior College
Duluth, Minnesota

Julie H. Simmons, MPH,
    MT(ASCP)SBB
Program Director, Medical Technology
Wake Forest University Baptist Medical
    Center
Winston-Salem, North Carolina

Anh Strow, MPH, MT(ASCP),
    CLS(NCA)
Program Director and Associate
    Professor, Medical Laboratory
    Technician
Illinois Central College
Peoria, Illinois

Susan B. Thomasson, MEd,
    MT(ASCP)SH, LMBT
Program Coordinator, Phlebotomy
Carolinas College of Health Sciences
Charlotte, North Carolina

Chapter 1

Phlebotomy Practice and Quality Assessment Basics

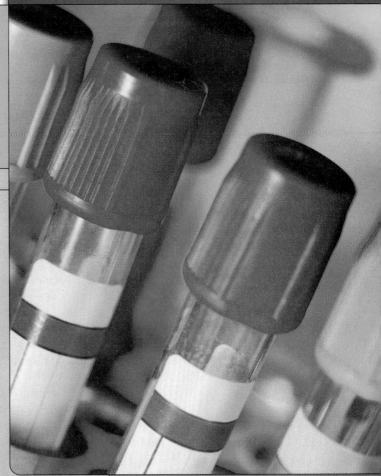

CHAPTER OBJECTIVES

Upon completion of Chapter 1, the learner should be able to do the following:

1. Define *phlebotomy* and describe phlebotomy services.

2. List professional competencies for phlebotomists.

3. List skills for effective communication.

4. Describe basic principles of quality and list examples of quality assessments for phlebotomy.

KEY TERMS

active listening
ambulatory care
American Society for Clinical
   Laboratory Science (ASCLS)
American Society for
   Clinical Pathology (ASCP)
competency statement
continuous quality improvement
   (CQI)
culture
expiration date
iatrogenic anemia
National Phlebotomy Association
   (NPA)

KEY TERMS *(continued)*

personal protective
   equipment (PPE)

phlebotomist

point-of-care

quality

standard operating
   procedure (SOP)

zone of comfort

Phlebotomy Practice, Definition, and Duties

The term *phlebotomy* is derived from the Greek words *phlebo*, which relates to veins, and *tomy*, which relates to cutting. Therefore, the definition can be summarized as the incision of a vein for the purpose of collecting blood.

The **phlebotomist**, or blood collector, is the individual who performs phlebotomy. Phlebotomists can also assist in the collection and transportation of specimens other than venous blood (e.g., arterial blood, urine, tissues, and sputum) and may also perform clinical, technical, or clerical functions. However, the primary function of the phlebotomist is to assist the health care team in the accurate, safe, and reliable collection and transportation of specimens for clinical laboratory analyses. The reliability and accuracy of *all* patient test results depend on the *preanalytical phase* of specimen collection—that is, the part of the process that occurs before the actual testing and analysis are performed. The preanalytical process is the fundamental and crucial domain of every phlebotomist (Figure 1-1 ■).

The requirement for a high-**quality** specimen that is correctly identified, collected, and transported is vital to the overall care of a patient. Phlebotomists' duties vary in scope depending on the setting. They may have duties related to all phases of laboratory analysis or may be assigned to only specimen collection duties in one area of a hospital. Technology has enabled laboratory testing to be performed closer to the **point-of-care** (e.g., at the patients' bedside, at ancillary or mobile sites, or even in the home). Phlebotomists' duties have become more coordinated with other health care processes. In some cases, health professionals—such as nurses, respiratory therapists, patient care technicians, and others—have been cross-trained to assume phlebotomy duties; in other cases, traditional laboratory-based phlebotomists have been cross-trained to assume expanded clerical or patient-care duties, such as electrocardiograms and low-risk laboratory procedures (Box 1-1).

Professional Competencies and Certifications

A high-school diploma or its equivalent is most often required to enter a phlebotomy training program in hospitals, community colleges, or technical schools. Typically, the length of training varies from a few weeks to months, depending on the location, the size

FIGURE ■ 1-1

Phases of Laboratory Testing: Preanalytical, Analytical, Postanalytical

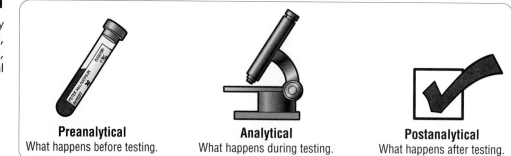

Preanalytical
What happens before testing.

Analytical
What happens during testing.

Postanalytical
What happens after testing.

BOX 1-1	Job Sites for Phlebotomists

HOSPITAL (INPATIENT) SETTINGS

Acute-care hospitals	Hospital-based clinics
Specialty hospitals (cancer centers, psychiatric, long-term care, pediatric)	Hospital-based emergency centers
Urban or rural hospitals	

AMBULATORY CARE (OUTPATIENT) SETTINGS

Health department clinics	Health maintenance organizations (HMOs)
Community health centers (CHCs)	Insurance companies
Rural health clinics	Physician group practices
Community-based mental health centers	Individual or solo medical practices
School-based clinics	Specialty practices
Prison health clinics	Rehabilitation centers
Dialysis centers	Mobile vans for blood donations
Multiphasic screening centers	Mobile vans for primary care delivery
Home health agencies	Mobile mammography units
Home hospice agencies	Free-standing surgical centers
Durable medical equipment suppliers	

of the facility, and the complexity of patients being served. Employers often require phlebotomy certification, which is accomplished by passing a national certification examination. Certification provides career advantages through job opportunities, career advancement, and portability (i.e., it is recognized from state to state).

Professional organizations that recognize phlebotomists are listed in Table 1-1 ■. Many of these organizations have developed **competency statements** to describe the entry-level

TABLE ■ 1-1

Professional Organizations for Phlebotomists

Organizations	Services Provided for Phlebotomists
American Society for Clinical Pathology (ASCP)	
ASCP Board of Registry 33 West Monroe Street, Suite 1600 Chicago, IL 60603-5617 (312) 541-4999 or (800) 621-4142 www.ascp.org	ASCP allows clinical laboratory personnel to gain associate membership status in the organization. ASCP offers many levels of certification, including a Phlebotomy Technician Examination, PBT (ASCP); an international certification examination for phlebotomists, PBT (ASCP)[i]; and educational programs for clinical laboratory personnel.
National Phlebotomy Association (NPA)	
1901 Brightseat Road Landover, MD 20785 (866) 329-9108 (301) 386-4203 (fax) www.nationalphlebotomy.org	NPA provides professional standards, a code of ethics, educational opportunities, and an annual phlebotomy certification examination resulting in a CPT (NPA).

(continued)

TABLE ■ 1-1

Professional Organizations for Phlebotomists *(continued)*

Organizations	Services Provided for Phlebotomists
American Society for Clinical Laboratory Science (ASCLS) and National Credentialing Agency for Laboratory Personnel (NCA)	
ASCLS 7910 Woodmont Avenue, Suite 530 Bethesda, MD 20814 (301) 657-2768 www.ascls.org NCA P.O. Box 15945-289 Lenexa, KS 66285 (913) 438-5110 www.nca-info.org	ASCLS offers educational programs and a phlebotomy certification examination through the NCA. The certification is a CLPlb (NCA).
American Medical Technologists (AMT)	
10700 West Higgins Road Rosemont, IL 60018 (847) 823-5169 or (800) 275-1268 (847) 823-0458 (fax) www.amt1.com	AMT offers a certification examination as a Registered Phlebotomy Technician (RPT).
American Society of Phlebotomy Technicians (ASPT)	
P.O. Box 1831 Hickory, NC 28603 (828) 294-0078 (message line) (828) 327-2969 (fax) www.aspt.org	ASPT offers a certification examination for phlebotomy that results in a CPT (ASPT) certification.
National Accrediting Agency for Clinical Laboratory Sciences (NAACLS)	
8410 West Bryn Mawr Avenue, Suite 670 Chicago, IL 60631 (773) 714-8880 (773) 714-8886 (fax) www.naacls.org	NAACLS accredits phlebotomy educational programs. No certification examinations are provided; however, accredited programs must teach students specified phlebotomy competencies. (Refer to Appendix 6.)
National Healthcareer Association (NHA)	
NHA-National Headquarters 7 Ridgedale Avenue, Suite 203 Cedar Knolls, NJ 07927 (800) 499-9092 (973) 605-1881 (973) 644-4797 (fax) www.nhanow.com	NHA offers a certification examination for phlebotomists, CPT (NHA).

skills, tasks, and roles performed by designated health care workers. In addition, some offer continuing educational opportunities via conferences, online course work, or correspondence courses. Professional organizations may provide guidelines for health care organizations to set **standard operating procedures (SOP)** covering the practices, conduct, behaviors, and courses of action that are acceptable in the field. The organizations listed in Table 1-1 have an interest in promoting and improving the practice of phlebotomy. They differ slightly in their membership requirements, fees, member benefits, continuing education courses, and whether or not they offer certification examinations specifically for phlebotomists. The eligibility requirements and documentation for each certification also differ among these groups. Before applying for one or more of the certification examinations, the phlebotomist should check to see which ones are most accepted in the local community or state. Sometimes health care organizations have preferences for specific certifications and will adjust salaries accordingly. Likewise, local community colleges and universities can also provide recommendations about which certification examination to take.

Box 1-2 lists typical examples of the duties of a phlebotomist. Table 1-2 ■ is an example of one organization's list of competencies for entry-level phlebotomy technicians. At minimum, these are the types of competencies that an employer might assess for the phlebotomist's performance evaluation. Refer to the appendices for a more detailed list of competencies from the National Accrediting Agency for Clinical Laboratory Sciences (NAACLS).

Competency statements describe the entry-level skills and tasks performed by phlebotomy technicians and measured on the certification examination. With regard to anatomy and physiology, specimen collection, specimen processing and handling, and laboratory operations related to phlebotomy, and in accordance with established procedures, the Phlebotomy Technician, PBT (ASCP), at career entry, should be able to accomplish the tasks listed in Table 1-2.

In addition to the competencies just discussed, those in Table 1-3 ■ encompass professional attributes, ability, and performance measures that employers might use for a phlebotomist's performance evaluation. Performance measures are observed through the phlebotomist's behavior, approach to the job, knowledge, and skills. There are many

---

BOX 1-2 **Typical Clinical, Technical, and Clerical Duties of Phlebotomists**

What are the clinical duties of phlebotomists?
- Identify the patient correctly
- Assess the patient before blood collection
- Prepare the patient accordingly
- Perform the puncture
- Withdraw blood into the correct containers/tubes
- Assess the degree of bleeding and pain
- Assess the patient after the phlebotomy procedure

What kind of technical duties do phlebotomists have to perform?
- Manipulate small objects, tubes, and needles
- Select and use appropriate equipment
- Perform quality control functions
- Transport the specimens correctly
- Prepare/process the sample(s) for testing/analysis
- Assist in laboratory testing procedures, washing glassware, and cleaning equipment

What clerical duties are expected of phlebotomists?
- Print/collate/distribute laboratory requisitions and reports
- Answer the telephone
- Answer all queries as appropriate
- Demonstrate courtesy in all patient encounters
- Respect privacy and confidentiality

TABLE ■ 1-2	
American Society for Clinical Pathology (ASCP) Board of Registry Competency Statements for the Phlebotomy Technician	**Apply knowledge of** • Principles of basic and special procedures • Potential sources of error • Standard operating procedures (SOPs) • Fundamental biological characteristics **Select appropriate** • Course of action • Equipment/methods/reagents **Prepare patient and equipment** **Evaluate** • Specimen and patient situation • Possible sources of error or inconsistencies • Quality control procedures • Common procedural/technical problems • Appropriate actions and methods • Corrective actions

Source: American Society for Clinical Pathology Board of Registry, www.ascp.org, 2006, with permission.

TABLE ■ 1-3	Attributes, Ability, Performance, Knowledge	Examples
Additional Measures of Phlebotomist's Performance	**Adherence to organizational policies** • Safety • Infection control • Fire and safety	• Attendance record • Dress code • Hand hygiene • Waste disposal • Gowning and gloving • Handling of fire extinguishers
	Communication skills • Verbal • Nonverbal • Listening skills	• Management of angry patients • Interactions with peers and coworkers • Telephone etiquette • Satisfaction of the patients • Courtesy • Use of appropriate medical and/or laboratory terminology
	Efficiency and quality • Productivity • Quality	• Waiting times • Complications during procedures • Number of uncomplicated blood draws in a specified period • Blood culture contamination rate • Number of unacceptable laboratory specimens

ways for supervisors to assess competency: for example, direct observation, videotaping, reviewing worksheets or log books, reviewing quality control records, providing simulations similar to real-life situations, and providing written examinations. Performance evaluations are important to both the employee and the employer, because they provide feedback, identify problems early, promote consistency in the evaluation process, encourage employees to stay abreast of policies and procedures, target improvement and high quality, and document that personnel are competent to perform tasks.[1]

PROFESSIONAL CHARACTER TRAITS

Within the health professions, organizations such as the ASCP and NPA have developed standards of ethical conduct and behavior for members, and members are expected to adhere to those standards of performance. The major points are as follows:

- Do no harm to anyone intentionally.
- Perform according to sound technical ability and good judgment.
- Respect patients' rights (which include patients' confidentiality, privacy, the right to know about their treatment, and the right to refuse treatment).
- Have regard for the dignity of all human beings.

Important character attributes for this career path include:

- **Sincerity and compassion**—Phlebotomists must possess an intense desire to serve people and a sincere interest in learning about blood and specimen collection practices.
- **Emotional stability and maturity**—Health care workers must be able to cope daily with seeing others in pain, handling blood and body fluids, facing injury and trauma, seeing disease sites, and the possibility of observing death. Responses to harsh situations must be prompt, professional, and reassuring to the patient, their families, and the health care team.
- **Accountability for doing things right**—Personal integrity, veracity (telling the truth), and "doing what is right when no one is looking" (e.g., washing hands between patient collections, observing precautions to gown and scrub in isolation, reporting one's own mistakes, and collecting timed tests at the proper time) reflect a health care worker's personal responsibility for his or her actions.
- **Dedication to high standards of performance and precision**—Health care workers must continually upgrade and maintain the quality of their skills. They must seek knowledge about new techniques and safety procedures, new supplies and equipment, and computer technology through continuing education. They should be willing to ask for assistance when dealing with a difficult patient or procedure and have the desire to follow rigid standards of performance. They should only collect the specimens ordered and only those that they have been trained to collect.
- **Respect for patients' dignity, privacy, confidentiality, and the right to know**—Phlebotomists have an obligation to respect all patients' rights, regardless of their personal opinions and biases. All patients must be treated with dignity and respect regardless of race, culture, religion, gender, age, or disabling conditions. Phlebotomists should have a full understanding of patients' rights to privacy, to confidentiality, and to knowing what procedures are being performed and by whom.
- **Propensity for cleanliness**—Phlebotomists must protect themselves and patients by accepting that sterile techniques, good personal hygiene, and cleanliness affect safety and the quality of health care. This is more important than saving time or cutting corners to save money.

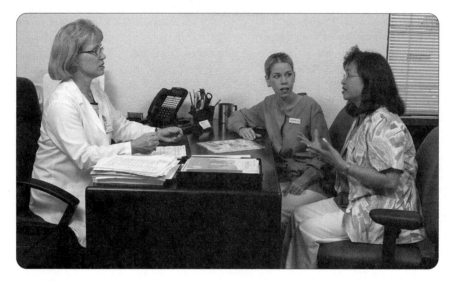

FIGURE ■ 1-2　Phlebotomists Are Part of the Health Care Team

■　**Pride, satisfaction, and self-fulfillment in the job**—Phlebotomists should attain professional satisfaction from continually improving their professional skills and knowledge, from knowing that others are dependent on the quality of their work, and from knowing that their skills contribute to the betterment of patients. The most successful, highly regarded phlebotomists are those who are most gratified with their work.

■　**Working with team members**—Phlebotomists are obliged to be flexible enough to work with a variety of health care professionals in a wide range of settings. Health care teams can improve skills (more talent, expertise, and technical competence), communication (more ideas, mutual respect, crossing departmental lines), participation (increased job satisfaction, combined efforts valued above individual efforts), and effectiveness (solutions likely to be implemented; the team has ownership of the shared decisions) (Figure 1-2 ■).[2]

■　**Take pleasure in communicating with patients**—The quality and ease of collecting blood specimens depends on both the technical skills of the health care worker and successful interactions with the patient. Phlebotomists should learn about transcultural communication strategies, communication barriers, and gender- or age-related issues that affect communication.

The decision to become a phlebotomist requires a special person with multiple talents and internal drive. The choice of this career path should not be taken lightly (Box 1-3).

Communication Strategies for Phlebotomists

Face-to-face communication is the most effective form of communication and is part of a phlebotomist's job every day. Verbal interactions can be depicted as a communication loop that starts when the message leaves the sender and reaches the receiver (Figure 1-3 ■). The receiver completes the loop by providing feedback to the sender. Without feedback, the sender has no way of knowing whether the message was accurately received or was somehow blocked by extraneous factors that can "filter out" meaning from a message.

BOX
1-3 **Phlebotomy Career Self-Assessment**

To consider a career in phlebotomy ask yourself the following questions. If there are doubts in your mind about your answers, think about whether you are willing to change or learn new skills.

1. Do I pay attention to details?
2. Do I like to work with small objects such as needles and test tubes?
3. Do I follow procedures exactly?
4. Does it bother me if I am closely watched or supervised?
5. Do I mind seeing blood, sick patients, body tissues, or fluids or smelling unpleasant odors?
6. What is my reaction to inflicting the pain of a needlestick on someone?
7. Am I willing to admit my own mistakes?
8. Do I like working with a team? Do I get along well with other people?
9. Am I willing to stand for long periods of time, walk extensively, reach, stoop, lift, or carry equipment?
10. Am I willing to work on holidays and weekends occasionally?

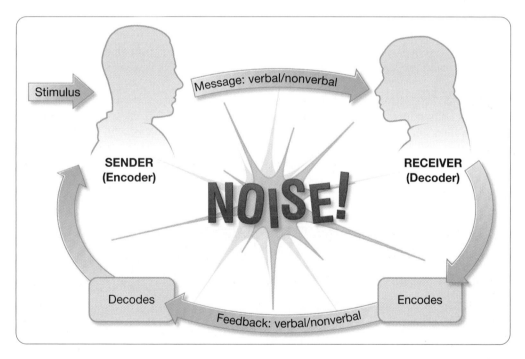

FIGURE ■ 1-3

Communication Loop

Filters can be damaging to effective communication because they do not allow the loop to be completed; thus, there is an increased risk that patients will not understand care instructions. Phlebotomists must be sure that the message they send is the same message received by the patient. In the following sections, communication is broken down into its three more detailed components:

Verbal communication—The actual words that are spoken, the tone of voice

Nonverbal communication—Body language, gestures

Active listening—Using verbal and nonverbal information to assess the situation

THE BASICS OF COMMUNICATION

Communication requires a sender, a receiver, and a message. The communication loop is complete when the sender receives feedback from the receiver about the intent of the message. Effective communication involves the following elements.[2]

- Show empathy (for waking up a patient, disturbing him or her, interrupting a meal) (Figure 1-4 ■)
- Show respect (for patient's privacy, for his or her condition, for family members)
- Build trust (maintain confidentiality, explain procedures clearly, tell the truth)
- Establish rapport (use common courtesy, show interest)
- Listen actively (face the patient, maintain a nonauthoritative posture, lean toward the patient, establish eye contact, do not interrupt, relax and listen intently)
- Provide specific feedback (about the patient's behavior, about a procedure)

VERBAL COMMUNICATION

Verbal communication involves conveying the right message in a professional tone of voice using language that is appropriate for the situation.

Language

Phlebotomists should use simple, everyday vocabulary, particularly with children. Complex medical jargon should be avoided. Patients must *not* be told, "This won't hurt." Most blood collection procedures are indeed slightly painful; therefore, it is important that the patient be forewarned and prepared (i.e., "This might hurt a little, but it will be over soon.").

Sensory Impairments

Deafness or blindness can have an impact on effective communication. A question such as, "Is there a step you would like me to repeat before we begin?" or "Do you want me to explain the procedure again?" yields better clues that the patient has understood than saying, "Do you understand?" If it is obvious that the patient did not hear, all efforts should be made to write down instructions for the patient. It is recommended that writing tools be kept at the bedside of these patients and also be accessible in ambulatory settings.

FIGURE ■ 1-4 Show Empathy for Patients

Note that the health care worker has a compassionate, caring look on her face. She is smiling and making eye contact with the patient in a pleasant and professional communication exchange.

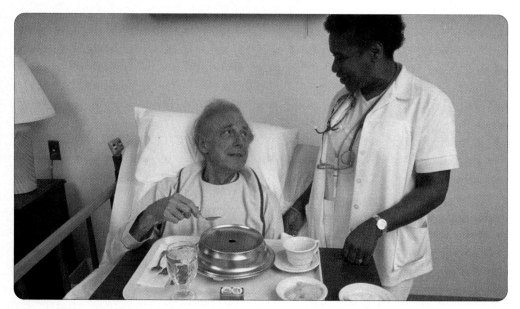

Languages Other than English

The diversity of languages spoken in this country is extensive. Patients who do not speak English can understand some basics from nonverbal cues, but the phlebotomist must know how to locate an interpreter or use translation services when possible. In the absence of a translator, written instructions in other languages may facilitate the process. Printed cards in different languages can be used to transmit information about the venipuncture procedures.

In many parts of the country, it is beneficial for phlebotomists to develop some skill in Spanish; however, it is recommended that the health care worker practice the phrases with someone who can speak the language before attempting to communicate with a patient, because mispronounced words may lead to confusion.

Another factor to consider in promoting effective communication is the setting. A busy, noisy environment distracts both the sender and receiver, often resulting in an unclear message. Box 1-4 offers tips for dealing with some common situations that may interfere with clear communication.

Clinical Alert !

In some states, children are not permitted to serve as translators for their parents when health care issues are discussed. Phlebotomists should check with their supervisors about the applicable laws in their states.

Age

The vocabulary of a teenager is different from that of an elderly person. Phlebotomists should be sensitive to word usage for each age.

Tone of Voice

The tone of one's voice and the inflection used can change a positive sentence into a negative-sounding statement. The tone of voice should match the words that are spoken.

BOX 1-4   **Communicating in a Noisy Environment**

A busy hallway, visitors, a television or radio in the room, or headphones can prevent the patient from hearing accurately. In these cases, the phlebotomist should take steps to reduce the sound level so that the patient can hear necessary instructions. Practice using the examples below:

To visitors: "Excuse me, please. It is important for me to explain this procedure to Mr. Jones. Would you mind if we have a quiet moment together? Thank you for your cooperation."

For the television: "Mr. Jones, I am sorry to disrupt your television show, but would you mind if we lower the volume for a few minutes so we can go over the procedure for collecting your blood sample? Thank you; this should only take a few minutes."

For headphones: "Mr. Jones, it is important that we discuss this procedure before beginning. Would you mind taking off your headphones for a few minutes? I will be brief. Thank you for your cooperation."

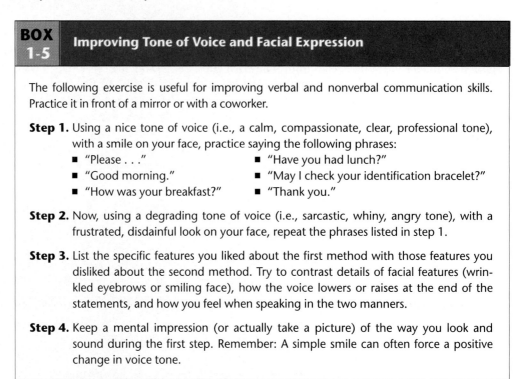

BOX 1-5 — Improving Tone of Voice and Facial Expression

The following exercise is useful for improving verbal and nonverbal communication skills. Practice it in front of a mirror or with a coworker.

Step 1. Using a nice tone of voice (i.e., a calm, compassionate, clear, professional tone), with a smile on your face, practice saying the following phrases:

- "Please . . ."
- "Good morning."
- "How was your breakfast?"
- "Have you had lunch?"
- "May I check your identification bracelet?"
- "Thank you."

Step 2. Now, using a degrading tone of voice (i.e., sarcastic, whiny, angry tone), with a frustrated, disdainful look on your face, repeat the phrases listed in step 1.

Step 3. List the specific features you liked about the first method with those features you disliked about the second method. Try to contrast details of facial features (wrinkled eyebrows or smiling face), how the voice lowers or raises at the end of the statements, and how you feel when speaking in the two manners.

Step 4. Keep a mental impression (or actually take a picture) of the way you look and sound during the first step. Remember: A simple smile can often force a positive change in voice tone.

Sarcasm is usually communicated just by tone of voice. Health care workers can avoid sending mixed messages to patients by practicing a calm, soothing, and confident tone of voice. Box 1-5 is a practice exercise for health care professionals to use in observing their own facial expressions and voice tones.

Emergency Situations

Emergency, or "STAT," blood collections are common in emergency rooms and in complicated medical cases. These phlebotomy procedures require extra speed and accuracy without jeopardizing the "personal touch." Patients in emergency rooms may not have identification information with them and/or may be unconscious. All facilities, however, should have documented procedures for the identification process with which phlebotomists should be familiar. Individual patients should be considered in terms of their privacy, dignity, and individual needs, not by nicknames such as "Mr. L down the hall" or "the broken leg in 3C." Each is entitled to professional, respectful care in all circumstances.

Bedside Manner

The climate established by a phlebotomist upon entering a patient's room affects the entire patient encounter. The feeling of confidence that comes from the knowledge that the blood collection tray is clean and well stocked is the first step in a good bedside manner. A pleasant facial expression, neat appearance, and professional manner set the stage for a positive interaction with the patient. The first 30 seconds after the phlebotomist enters the patient's room determine how that patient perceives the quality of patient care offered by that hospital. Most patients admit that the procedure they dread most is being "stuck" for blood collection, so phlebotomists should make every effort to minimize the negative effects of the situation.

THE PATIENT ENCOUNTER

When encountering the patient for the first time, there are some basic procedures to follow:

- Knock gently (do not pound) on the patient's hospital room door.

- Introduce yourself and state that you are from the hospital unit or laboratory staff, whichever is the case.

- Inform the patient that his or her specimen must be collected for a test ordered by the physician. (A statement indicating that this is routine hospital protocol often reassures the patient. A lengthy discussion of why a certain test was ordered is inappropriate. These questions should be referred to the patient's physician.)

- During all steps remain calm, compassionate, and professional and limit conversations to essential information.

- Let the patient know how the procedure is going (e.g., "this is going well," or "it is almost over").

- Do not be distracted from the phlebotomy procedure by excessive talk of unrelated issues.

- Before leaving the room, thank the patient for cooperating.

The following scenario is a typical one that might occur at the opening greeting between a phlebotomist and a hospitalized patient. Imagine both the verbal and nonverbal factors involved. The *wrong responses* are suggested in italics. They can be used as a discussion tool of how the phlebotomist can have a negative impact.

Phlebotomist:	Good morning. My name is Sally, and I am here to collect a blood sample for your laboratory tests. Could you please state your name and spell it? *Wrong response: Hi, are you Mrs. Betty Smith?*
Patient (softly):	My name is Betty Smith.
Phlebotomist:	Could you repeat that and spell it for me please? *Wrong response: Huh? What did you say?*
Patient:	My name is Betty Smith, B-E-T-T-Y S-M-I-T-H.
Phlebotomist:	Thank you, I think I have it now but I also need to check the identification number on your armband. I will be taking a blood sample from your arm so that the laboratory can perform tests that your doctor ordered. Have you had breakfast yet? *Wrong response: Okay, let's get on with it.*
Patient:	No breakfast yet; I just woke up.
Phlebotomist:	I need to look at your arms. Would you prefer your right side or left side?
Patient:	Nobody ever gets blood on the left side so we'd better try the right side.
Phlebotomist:	Thanks for that info; we can check the right side. Please hold out your arm so that I can feel for your veins. *Wrong response: Oh, don't worry about a thing. I'm pretty good at drawing from tough veins.*
Patient:	Okay, but will it hurt?

Phlebotomist: It will hurt a little, but I'll do my best to have it done quickly. Do you have any other questions?
Wrong response: No, it doesn't hurt.

Patient: Not really, just get it over with.

Phlebotomist: Thanks for your cooperation, Mrs. Smith.
Wrong response: Well, I'm just doing what I was told!

COMMUNICATION FOR PATIENT IDENTIFICATION

Clear communication practices for patient identification are essential. If the patient is hospitalized, identification should be accomplished by a match between the test requisition or labels and a unique identification number on the armband and by verbal confirmation from the patient. If a hospitalized patient does not have an armband, a positive confirmation must be made by a unit nurse who knows the patient. This process should be well documented by the phlebotomist. Special identification procedures should also be well documented for ambulatory patients, especially in cases of homebound patients, mobile vans, and other off-site locations. Armbands are not commonly used in ambulatory settings; however, an identification card usually is. It may include some demographic data and other identifying information, such as the patient's unique identification number, date of birth (DOB), a picture, address, or a combination of these. This information should be confirmed by the patient prior to blood collection.

Some health care facilities insist that the health care worker ask for the patient's complete address, whereas others require the mention of the patient's hometown, birth date, identification number, or street name to reinforce and confirm identity. Some prefer that patients spell out an unusual last name. This portion of the specimen collection procedure ensures that the remainder of the diagnostic testing protocol provides information on the correct person. Detailed identification procedures are covered in Chapter 8.

COMMUNICATION IN A CLINIC OR IN THE HOME

Phlebotomists who collect specimens in a clinic or home setting must take extra steps to assure the phlebotomy procedure is successful. These steps include the following:

- The phlebotomist introducing him- or herself and clearly explaining the purpose of the interaction.

- The patient should be directed to sit in a chair with sides and arms or recline during the procedure. This may involve walking to a private area, blood collection booth, or special recliner.

- If the phlebotomy procedure is taking place in an unfamiliar setting, such as the patient's home, the phlebotomist must take extra time to find the nearest bathroom (for handwashing or blood spillage) and the nearest bed, in case there are complications to the phlebotomy procedure (fainting).

- In a patient's home, the phlebotomist may need to find a phone or bring a cellular phone or computer to clarify laboratory orders or inquire about patient information.

- Information about the procedure should be fully explained (especially if it is a first-time blood collection for the patient or if it has been a long time since the last blood collection).

- Identifying the patient should be done meticulously and cautiously, using various methods to identify the patient positively (e.g., driver's license or identification card, confirmation of birthday and home address, or social security number, if available).

- The puncture site must be appropriately cared for, and it should be clear that the patient is physically fit to leave the area after the phlebotomy procedure. If the patient is homebound, the phlebotomist must be sure that the patient is no longer bleeding, that the puncture site has been appropriately bandaged, and that the patient is able to stay by him- or herself.

NONVERBAL COMMUNICATION

Some theories suggest that communication consists of 10 to 20 percent verbal and 80 to 90 percent nonverbal messages. Nonverbal cues, or body language, can be positive—and facilitate understanding—or negative—and hinder effective communication. (Table 1-4 ■ and Figure 1-5 ■.)

Positive Body Language

Smiling   A simple, compassionate smile can set the stage for open lines of communication. It can make each patient feel that he or she is the most important person at that moment. In addition, most people look better with smiles on their faces than they do with frowns. It takes fewer muscle movements to smile than it does to frown.

Clinical Alert !

The patient should always be asked, "What is your name?" not "Are you Ms. Smith?" The first question is a more reliable and direct way of confirming identity. The second question is inappropriate and less reliable because a patient who is heavily medicated will often agree with anything that he or she is asked.

TABLE ■ 1-4

Nonverbal Communication/ Body Language

Positive Body Language	Effects
Face-to-face positioning	Aids communication
Relaxed hands, arms, shoulders	Can make interactions more pleasant
Erect posture	
Eye contact, eye level (avoid looking down on someone)	
Smiling	
Appropriate zone of comfort	

Negative Body Language	Effects
Slouching, shrugged shoulders	Is distracting
Rolling eyes, wandering eyes	Prevents effective communication
Staring blankly or at ceiling	Causes discomfort, uneasiness
Rubbing eyes, excessive blinking	
Squirming, tapping foot, pencil, etc.	
Deep sighing, groaning	
Crossing arms, clenching fists	
Wrinkling forehead	
Thumbing through books or papers	
Stretching, yawning	
Peering over eyeglasses	
Pointing finger at someone	

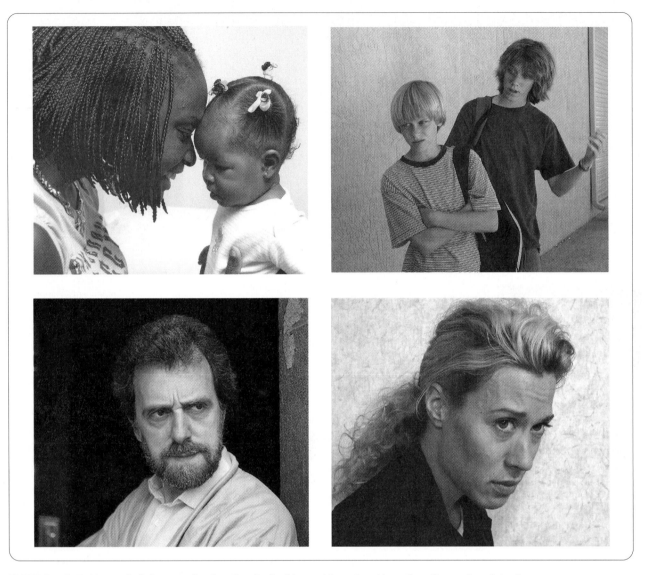

FIGURE ■ **1-5** Nonverbal Communication Can Be Positive or Negative. Note the effects of each look

Eye Contact and Eye Level Eye contact promotes a sense of trust and honesty between the patient and phlebotomist. It can make the entire procedure less traumatic for the patient if he or she sees a compassionate expression in the phlebotomist's eyes. There is an expression: "The eyes are the windows of the soul."

Eye level is also a consideration. Because bedridden patients must always "look up" to those in the room, it creates a feeling of intimidation, of being "looked down on," or of weakness. Most of the time, phlebotomists do not have the extra time to spend finding a chair to sit in so that they are at eye level; however, if a health care worker must explain a lengthy procedure or if it is noted that the patient is particularly nervous about the procedure, the explanation should be done while seated at eye level with the patient (Box 1-6).

A word of caution about eye contact is needed when dealing with patients of certain cultures. Generally speaking, Americans view eye contact as a positive aspect of human nature, and avoidance of eye contact might mean that someone is not being truthful. However, some Asian and Native American cultures believe that prolonged eye contact is rude and an inva-

BOX 1-6	**Practice Exercise for Developing Sensitivity to Bedridden Patients**

Health care workers should strive to be as compassionate as possible. Bedridden patients often feel intimidated because health care workers must repeatedly "look down" on them to provide care. Sometimes these patients are depressed because of their condition or prognosis. This exercise will help you imagine yourself in the patient's condition and can make you a more compassionate member of the health care team. Practice the exercise with a coworker whom you do not know very well.

1. Lie on a bed while your coworker stands directly over you, looking down.
2. Have the coworker go through the motions of a venipuncture procedure, including the greeting and identification process. Try to imagine the anticipation of the needle stick. Have the coworker maintain eye contact with you while conversing.
3. Repeat step 2, without eye contact.
4. List what you liked and disliked about this procedure.

sion of privacy. Muslim women may avoid eye contact because of modesty.[3] Patients may not appreciate direct eye contact with a health care provider because it may make them feel self-conscious; it may be unacceptable in their culture or may not be acceptable with the opposite sex. The health care worker should take cues from the patient. If the patient does not look at the health care worker when he or she is speaking, perhaps he or she would feel more comfortable with more space between them or less direct eye contact. The phlebotomist can take the interaction at a slower pace to monitor the patient's comfort level. The more secure and comfortable the patient feels, the easier the procedure will become for the phlebotomist.

Face-to-Face Communication Phlebotomists should face patients directly. Otherwise, the patient may feel neglected, that he or she is being avoided, or that information is being withheld. If a patient turns away from a phlebotomist, however, it should be taken as a cue that the patient is uncomfortable for some reason. The phlebotomist should do everything possible to make the patient feel more comfortable during the phlebotomy procedure.

Zone of Comfort Most individuals begin to feel uncomfortable when strangers get too close to them physically. A **zone of comfort** is the area of space around a patient that is private territory, so to speak, where they feel comfortable with an interaction. If that zone is crossed, feelings of uneasiness may occur.

For most Western cultures, there are four zones of interpersonal space:

■ **Intimate space (direct contact up to 18 inches)**—For close relationships and health care workers who bathe, feed, dress, and perform venipunctures

■ **Personal space (18 inches to 4 feet)**—For interactions among friends and for many patient encounters

■ **Social space (4 feet to 12 feet)**—For most interactions of everyday life

■ **Public space (more than 12 feet)**—For lectures, speeches, and so on

When a stranger gets too close, it can cause the patient to feel nervous, fearful, or anxious. Health care workers must be understanding and approach nervous patients slowly and gently, to avoid causing feelings of being threatened. This is particularly true with children, many of whom have a wide zone of comfort—that is, they do not like anyone to approach them except close relatives or friends. It is helpful to slowly approach the patient while crossing the zone of comfort, not to be too hasty, and to talk to patients during the process.

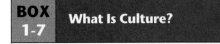

> ## BOX 1-7 — What Is Culture?
>
> Culture varies among groups of individuals, but it usually encompasses the following traits:
>
> **Values**—The accepted principles of a group: individualism versus socialism, importance of education and financial security, competition versus cooperation, sanctity of life, and so on
>
> **Beliefs**—Doctrine or faith of a person or group: spiritual orientation, family bonds, and so on
>
> **Traditions and practices**—Customs and behaviors associated with groups: holidays, foods, music, dance, health care practices, and so on

Cultural Sensitivity

Culture is a system of values, beliefs, and practices that stem from an individual's concept of reality (Box 1-7). Culture influences decisions and behaviors in many aspects of life. Learning about various ethnic groups and cultures is important for health care professionals to understand the reasons for patients' behaviors during times of health and illness.

Specific traits that vary among cultures have been addressed previously (e.g., eye contact and zone of comfort). However, with the changing demographics of the U.S. population, it is vital for all health care workers to become more sensitive and compassionate about accepting cultural practices that vary from our own. When a health care worker is unsure or unaware of acceptable patterns of behavior for a patient, the recommended action is to "follow the patient's lead." For example, if a patient speaks softly and slowly, speak the same way. If the patient turns to a family member when speaking to you, include the family member in the conversation. If a patient moves closer to you during the conversation, try not to back away from the patient's zone of comfort (Box 1-8). The best way to

> ## BOX 1-8 — My Space/Your Space Exercise—Finding Your Comfort Zone
>
> Having respect for an individual's personal space, or zone of comfort, is part of being a compassionate health care worker. The comfort zone of each person varies with gender, culture, and situation. However, most people feel uneasy when strangers are touching them or are "too close for comfort." An example of this uncomfortable sensation is standing in a crowded elevator. People take great measures to move so that they are not touching strangers, and, as people exit the elevator, the remaining people move and shift to provide more space around themselves. This same sense of uneasiness is felt by patients who are approached by unfamiliar health care workers.
>
> To simulate a real patient–health care worker interaction, practice the following exercise with a coworker who is not a close friend. Eye contact should be made during this exercise.
>
> 1. Lie on a bed as if you are a patient.
> 2. Have the coworker slowly approach you. He or she should begin 10 feet away and pause between steps.
> 3. Note at what distance you begin to feel awkward or uncomfortable. (Usually, this distance is about 2 to 4 feet from the bed.) This distance is the boundary of your zone of comfort.
> 4. Repeat the exercise with the same coworker. You will probably require a smaller zone of comfort because a person becomes a little more at ease after initial contact with an unfamiliar person.

become more culturally competent is to allow patients to teach us, to become active observers of how culturally diverse patients interact with each other and with health professionals. Becoming keen observers of mannerisms, gestures, and facial expressions of group members, reading about cultural groups, watching films and videos, reading novels that depict different cultures, and reading newspapers published by cultural groups will make health care workers better and more informed at what they do.[3]

Negative Body Language and Distracting Behaviors

Wandering Eyes   When people roll their eyes upward, they convey the sense of being bored, inattentive, or unwilling to perform a duty. The same can be said about gazing out the window or looking up at the ceiling. If a phlebotomist enters a patient's room and begins addressing the patient while looking out the window, the patient will feel neglected, and the phlebotomist will appear unconcerned. If the window is too tempting to avoid a glance at, the phlebotomist can include the patient in his or her observations. A friendly comment about the weather might be appropriate; then the phlebotomy procedure can be continued when full attention can be given to the patient. The objective is to make the patient feel at ease through good communication techniques so that the procedure can be successful.

Nervous Behaviors   Behaviors such as squirming or tapping a pencil or a foot can be very distracting. They can make a patient feel nervous, hurried, or anxious about the venipuncture. It is also helpful to recognize these behaviors in patients, especially children, so that efforts can be made to reduce fear. Allowing a few extra moments of conversation or preparation may help.

Breathing Pattern   A deep sigh can convey a feeling of being bored or a reluctance to do the job. Likewise, if a patient sighs deeply or moans at the mere sight of the phlebotomist, this should be a cue that a little extra attention, conversation, or a smile might ease the patient's reluctance for the procedure.

Other Distracting Behaviors   Many other actions can convey negative or defensive emotions. Among these are crossed arms, a wrinkled forehead, frequent glances at a clock or watch, rapid thumbing through papers, chewing gum, yawning, or stretching. Health care workers should realize that these behaviors can detract from their professional image when they are communicating with patients, families, visitors, coworkers, and supervisors. It is also important to realize what these cues mean if a patient exhibits them.

ACTIVE LISTENING

Another component of effective communication is the art of listening. **Active listening** helps close the communication loop by ensuring that the message sent can indeed be repeated and understood. Listening skills do not depend on intellect or educational background; they can be learned and practiced. Table 1-5 ■ provides tips for becoming an active listener. The steps presented in the table are a starting point for the development of listening skills. Because individuals can mentally process words faster than they can speak them, a good listener must concentrate and focus on the speaker to keep his or her mind from wandering. Development of these skills can help an individual in professional life as well as in personal life.

Listening carefully to the patient can have important ramifications in the test results. For example, the inpatient may have been instructed that he or she will be fasting or will have "nothing by mouth" until after the early morning blood collections. The phlebotomist should listen to patients' comments, such as, "I didn't have breakfast yet," and "they won't feed me." Even a question or comment about food may inspire a response to confirm that the patient was truly fasting. When in doubt, the phlebotomist can confirm

TABLE ■ 1-5		
Steps for Active Listening	Get ready	Concentrate on the speaker by "getting ready" to listen. Take a moment to clear your mind of distracting thoughts. Begin the interaction with an open, objective mind. Sometimes taking a deep breath can help clear your mind and prepare it to receive more information.
	Pause occasionally	Use silent pauses in the conversation wisely to mentally summarize what has been said.
	Verify that you are listening	Let the speaker know that someone is listening by using simple phrases, such as "I see," "Oh," "Very interesting," and "How about that," to reassure the speaker and communicate understanding and acceptance.
	Avoid making hasty judgments	Keep personal judgments to yourself until the speaker finishes relaying his or her idea. Listen for true meaning in the message, not just the literal words.
	Provide feedback	Verify the conversation with feedback. Make sure that everything was clear to the receiver. Ask for more explanation if necessary. Mentally review the key words to summarize the overall idea being communicated. Paraphrase the idea or conversation to ensure complete understanding.
	Notice body language	Pay attention to body language and ask for clarification. Simple prompts, such as "You look sad" and "You seem upset or nervous," can add more meaning to the conversation and encourage the speaker to verbalize feelings.
	Maintain eye contact	Eye contact communicates interest or concern.
	Use encouragement	Encourage the listener to expand his or her thoughts by using simple phrases, such as "Let's discuss it further," "Tell me more about it," and "Really?"
	Practice, practice, practice	Practice active listening at work and at home.

that the patient has been fasting by simply asking the patient if he or she has eaten or had anything to drink other than water.

Professional Appearance and Personal Health

APPEARANCE, GROOMING, AND PHYSICAL FITNESS
Posture

Phlebotomists usually perform their work while standing. There are occasions, however, particularly with ambulatory patients, when it is more effective to sit adjacent to the patient for the blood collection procedure. Erect posture conveys a sense of confidence and pride in job performance. Slouching conveys a sense of laziness and apathy. Good posture minimizes the health care worker's back and neck strain and eases the patient's mind about the confidence of the phlebotomist.

Grooming and Personal Hygiene

Physical appearance communicates a strong impression about an individual. Neatly combed hair; clean fingernails; a clean, pressed uniform; protective lab coat and gloves; and an overall tidy appearance communicate a commitment to cleanliness and infection control, and they instill confidence in a person. A daily bath or shower, followed by the use of deodorant, and appropriate dress are also recommended. Hygiene is particularly important in today's health care environment, where patients and employees are deeply concerned about the spread of infectious diseases. Employers of health care workers are legally required to provide **personal protective equipment (PPE)** or barrier protection for workers handling biohazardous, infectious substances. This includes gowns, gloves, masks, laboratory coats or aprons, and face shields. Because of latex sensitivities and allergies, employers must provide an array of sizes and styles of gloves and gowns to protect their employees. Table 1-6 ■ illustrates a dress code policy.

TABLE ■ 1-6

Sample of a Dress Code Policy

Purpose: Presenting a professional and positive image to all patients, customers, and members of the community is a goal of this health care organization. Professional dress, good grooming, and personal cleanliness are important aspects of the overall effectiveness and morale of all employees. To establish a standard appearance, the following guidelines will be enforced. Employees who appear inappropriately dressed or groomed will be sent home. Please note that these are minimum guidelines and that individual departments may have more rigid requirements because of safety, infection control, or patient preferences. Consult your supervisor regarding any questions you may have regarding these guidelines.

Identification	Name badges will be visibly worn at all times. Stickers, pins, or other types of tokens should not cover the employee or department name.
Daily hygiene	Having clean teeth, hair, clothes, and body are basic daily requirements. Clean, wrinkle-free clothes, scrubs, or uniforms that are in good condition should be worn.
Hair	Hair should be clean, neat, and trimmed. Moderate styles are recommended. Well-groomed, closely trimmed beards, sideburns, and mustaches are allowed. Shoulder-length hair should be pulled back and secured.
Nails	Nails should be clean, neatly manicured, and not more than 1/4 inch past the fingertip. Nail color and artificial nails are not recommended and are not allowed in many facilities in which there is direct patient contact (Figure 1-6 ■).
Fragrances/scents	Perfumes and fragrances can be offensive and/or nauseating to patients who are ill. It is recommended that the use of fragrances be minimized or eliminated.
Make-up	Make-up should be conservative and lightly applied. Extreme or excessive make-up is not allowed.
Clothing	Denim clothing is not usually allowed, except on special occasions announced by the hospital administration. Tight-fitting clothing or clothes that are revealing or distracting are not permitted. Shirts should be buttoned up to the second button. Shirttails should be tucked in, and T-shirts with logos or athletic prints will not be allowed. Proper undergarments should be worn at all times. Skirts and dresses should not be shorter than 3 inches above the knee. Shorts are not permitted. Pants/slacks should be worn with a belt if they have belt loops. Tight-fitting leggings are not permitted. It is recommended that male employees who are not involved in patient care wear ties.

(continued)

TABLE ■ 1-6

Sample of a Dress Code Policy *(continued)*

Shoes	Shoes should be comfortable, safe in the work environment, clean, and polished. Consideration should be made to minimizing noise when walking. Socks and/or proper hosiery should be worn. Sandals, flip-flops, and cloth shoes are not permitted.
Jewelry	Excessive jewelry is not allowed. Because safety is a major concern, chains must be worn inside the collar, and long dangling earrings are not acceptable. Other types of exposed jewelry (facial piercings) may also pose hazards and/or may become irritated with the use of personal protective equipment; therefore, they are not recommended.

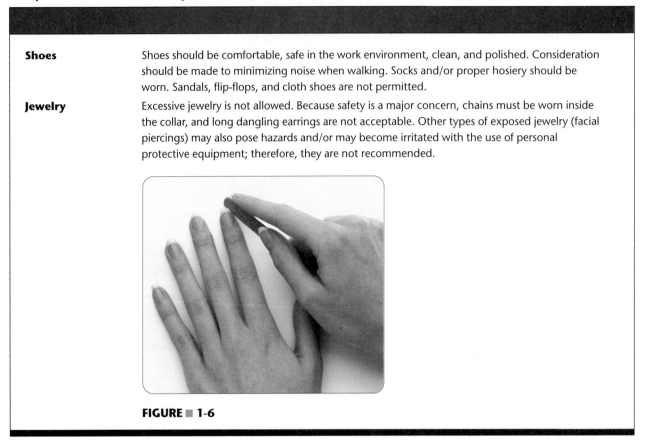

FIGURE ■ 1-6

NUTRITION, REST, AND EXERCISE

The role of a health care worker requires physical stamina because the pace is often hectic, and overtime work is common. Good health improves the health care worker's appearance, attitude, job performance, and ability to cope with stress (Box 1-9). Appropriate eating habits, rest during lunch and break periods, and off-duty exercising are essential to an individual's well-being and stress reduction. Practicing a healthy lifestyle while on and off duty will facilitate a return to work with a refreshed and more productive attitude.

ROLE OF FAMILY, VISITORS, AND SIGNIFICANT OTHERS

Family members and friends of patients are often present when phlebotomists need to acquire specimens. It is important to realize that their presence can make the patient more secure and comfortable. Sometimes, however, families and visitors are much more difficult to deal with than the patients. They may make requests that are beyond the phlebotomist's scope of acceptable or authorized responsibilities, and it is better then to inform the appropriate health care team member of the family member's request. If several visitors are in the hospital room with the patient, they may be asked to step into the hall while the blood specimen is being drawn. If the health care worker believes that assistance is required (to give emotional support, etc.) and the patient agrees, a family member may be asked to

BOX 1-9	Tips for Dealing with Stress

Find time for privacy.

Plan rest/relaxation periods (take short naps, meditate, listen to relaxing music, read poetry, practice yoga).

Associate with gentle people and share feelings with them.

Devote time to physical exercise (10 minutes at three different times a day is better than none).

Eat more nutritious foods (imagine your plate with 50% vegetables/fruits, 25% protein, and 25% carbohydrates).

Engage in satisfying hobbies and social activities.

Rearrange your schedule to make it work more effectively.

Keep a journal.

Read interesting books and articles to get new ideas.

stay during the procedure. Children should be accompanied by a parent or guardian. This can make the family members feel helpful and provide reassurance to patients.

Physicians, priests, and chaplains have the right to visit privately with patients. Unless the blood specimen is "timed," the health care worker should respect that privacy and return to the patient after completing the other draws in the unit or area. If the procedure is timed or STAT, the health care worker can apologize for the interruption, explain the nature of the request, and ask permission to collect the specimen.

Families and visitors of patients except for parents of pediatric patients should not be permitted in the clinical laboratory or provided with patient information, except by prior arrangement and permission of the patient. The patient's privacy and safety and the confidentiality of patient records must be considered.

TELEPHONE COMMUNICATIONS

Because the telephone is a vital communication tool for all health care facilities, it is important to follow the rules of good communication for incoming or outgoing calls.

Guidelines for Telephone Communications

Incoming calls

1. Answer on the first ring if possible and no later than the third ring.
2. Try to smile as you answer, to reflect a positive tone of voice.
3. Speak clearly and courteously.
4. Identify the department or doctor's office: "Good morning, Dr. Jones's office."
5. Identify yourself by stating your name and title: "This is Ann, the phlebotomist."
6. Ask how you may help the caller: "How may I help you?" (Always use the word *may* instead of *can*.)
7. Acquire information from the caller using proper etiquette and record the date and time:
   a. May I have your name, please?
   b. Could you please spell that?
   c. Could you repeat that, please?
8. If you cannot provide the proper response, ask for assistance.

9. Before putting the caller on hold, give the caller an option to hold or leave a message. Ask the caller, "May I put you on hold for a few moments while I get the information?"

10. Do not keep the caller on hold for more than 30 seconds, or check back with the caller to see if he or she wants to continue holding.

11. Read the message back to the caller to ensure that you have the correct information. Double-check spellings, phone numbers (with area codes), and other pertinent information.

12. Allow the caller to hang up first, just in case he or she may want to add something at the last minute.

Outgoing calls

1. Be prepared: have pencils, message pads, telephone set-up, and all information available prior to calling.

2. Do not call to socialize, and remember to use discretion with confidential information.

3. State your name, where you are calling from, and the purpose of your call.

4. Leave preferred times and phone numbers where you can be reached if a follow-up call is necessary.

5. Thank the receiver for taking your message.

Quality Assessment

QUALITY BASICS

The quality of phlebotomy services can encompass many factors that involve organizational structures, processes, outcomes, and customer satisfaction. The area where individual phlebotomists have the greatest impact is on constantly improving the services that are provided to stakeholders or customers. Quality improvement efforts for phlebotomy services often involve evaluating the following:

- The health care worker's technique
- Complications, such as hematomas
- Recollection rates resulting from contamination
- Multiple sticks on the same patient

All these issues have the potential to result in a negative outcome for the patient. Thus, continuous improvement in minimizing these problems would be most beneficial to the patient and the health care worker.

EXAMPLES OF STAKEHOLDERS (CUSTOMERS) IN HEALTH CARE

Stakeholders are also considered to be "customers." External stakeholders are individuals or groups outside the organization; internal stakeholders are individuals or groups within a health care organization itself.

External stakeholders include the following:

- Local community
- Insurance companies that pay for services
- Employers who pay for services for their employees
- Grant agencies and/or foundations that provide funding
- Federal or state agencies—OSHA, CDC, and so on

- Accrediting agencies—The Joint Commission (formerly the Joint Commission for the Accreditation of Healthcare Organizations, or JCAHO), CAP
- Advocacy groups—AARP

Internal stakeholders (within the health care organization and/or specimen collection services) include the following:

- Inpatients and outpatients
- Patient's families and friends
- Patient support groups
- Clinical laboratory staff
- Pathologists and other medical doctors
- Students
- Research staff
- Volunteers

A QUALITY PLAN FOR PHLEBOTOMY SERVICES

Quality assessment for phlebotomy involves reviewing structures, processes, outcomes, and customer satisfaction.

Factors related to structure—Physical or organizational properties of the settings where care is provided. Assessments of structural components include:

- **Physical structure**—Facilities where services are provided, adequacy of supplies and equipment, safety devices, safety procedures, and availability and condition of equipment, such as computers, sterilizers, refrigerators, thermometers, centrifuges, autoclaves, and glucose-monitoring devices.
- **Personnel structure**—Adequate numbers of personnel and support staff, ratios of staff to patients, qualifications of staff, and availability of the medical director or supervisors.
- **Management or administrative structure**—Updated, available procedure manuals, adequacy of systems for secure record keeping, and open lines of communication throughout the organization.

Quality assessments of structural components may reveal potential problems that other assessments cannot. For example, the use of outdated blood collection tubes may cause faulty laboratory test results, even though the blood collection, testing, and reporting processes are perfect and the treatment plan for the patient is appropriate.

Assessment of processes—What is done to the patient or client. Process assessments are common throughout the specimen collection and clinical testing arenas and include procedures and skill assessment. This is where traditional quality control (QC) measures are applicable. In addition to the normal laboratory data collection routines, however, other methods are effective for monitoring processes. These include evaluation of patient records for complications, correct technical skills, and correct documentation procedures; direct observation of practices; videotaping of health care interactions and practices; patient interviews; and questionnaires.

Assessments of outcomes—What is accomplished for the patient. Most outcomes assessments rely on information in the patient's medical record. Chart reviews usually evaluate the health status after services are provided. Timing is usually an important component of these measures. Outcomes assessments are typically the most difficult to measure and often relate to recovery rates, infection rates, incidence of **iatrogenic anemia**, return to normal functions, and so on. Poor patient outcomes have been described as the "5 Ds": death, disease, disability, discomfort, and dissatisfaction.

Customer satisfaction—Knowing why customers are dissatisfied and which customers are unhappy. The study of satisfaction among patients is accomplished by using questionnaires, mail-outs, and telephone or personal interviews.

Clinical Alert ❗

Unfortunately, phlebotomists can have a negative impact on quality. For example, misidentification of a patient can result in an erroneous cross-match and blood transfusion, which could be fatal to a patient (death). Inappropriate cleansing techniques or hand hygiene could result in transmitting nosocomial infections (hospital-acquired disease). Repeated blood collections or drawing too much blood at one time can result in iatrogenic anemia. Poor venipuncture techniques, such as improper needle insertion or excessive probing, could result in nerve damage (disability) or severe pain (discomfort). Lengthy waiting times, rude behavior, or messy work sites can contribute to an overall feeling of patient dissatisfaction.

TOOLS AND PRACTICE EXERCISE FOR PERFORMANCE ASSESSMENT

In a laboratory, check sheets, run charts, and statistical tests can be used to review both the analytic and nonanalytic parts of the laboratory. The phlebotomist should be a routine part of quality and performance assessments.

Tools for implementing **continuous quality improvement (CQI)** include the following:[4]

- **Flow charts.** Useful for breaking a process into its components so that people can understand how it works (Figure 1-7 ■).
- **Pareto charts.** Bar charts that show the frequency of problematic events; the Pareto principle says that "80 percent of the trouble comes from 20 percent of the problems" (Figure 1-8 ■).
- **Cause-and-effect (Ishikawa) diagrams.** Diagrams that identify interactions between equipment, methods, people, supplies, and reagents (Figure 1-9 ■).
- **Plan-Do-Check-Act cycle (PDCA).** A cycle for assessing and making positive changes, then reassessing.
- **Line graphs, histograms, scatter diagrams.** Pictorial images representing performance trends.
- **Brainstorming.** Method used to stimulate creative solutions in a group (Box 1-10).

BOX 1-10   Brainstorming Exercise

This exercise can be used in groups of no more than three or four people or by individuals. Groups are preferred because they tend to come up with a greater number and more creative ideas.

One group should take the viewpoint of a new phlebotomist, and the other group should take the viewpoint of the patient. (There are no "wrong" answers!)

Consider the idea of "excellence" or "perfection" in a phlebotomy encounter. What quality factors are important from your point of view? List/discuss as many and all ideas as you can in about 10 minutes. Next, come to a consensus about the order of importance of the factors. Make sure everyone in the group has a chance to participate and give their opinions about the order of importance. Compare and discuss the lists from each group's viewpoint.

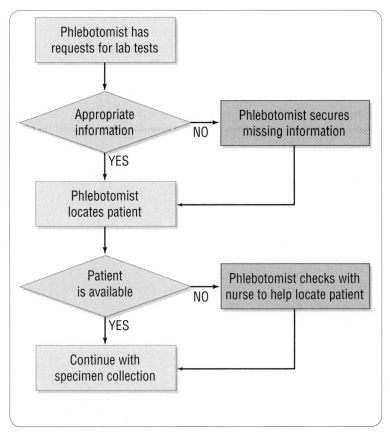

FIGURE ■ 1-7 Flow Chart

Flow charts demonstrate steps in a process

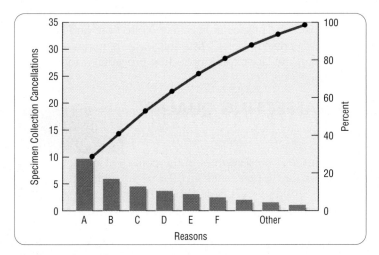

FIGURE ■ 1-8 Pareto Chart

Pareto charts tally the number of times each specified problem occurs. Letters across the bottom indicate reasons for cancellations (e.g., the patient was unavailable, supplies were not accessible, documentation was incomplete)

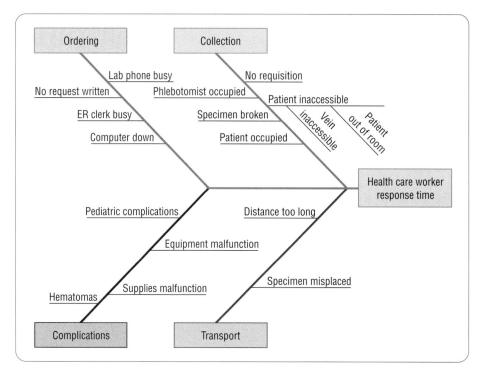

FIGURE ■ 1-9 Cause-and-Effect Diagram

Cause-and-effect diagrams demonstrate interactions or factors that influence an outcome. For example, this cause-and-effect diagram demonstrates the issues affecting response time

QUALITY IN SPECIMEN COLLECTION SERVICES

Phlebotomists can consider the clinical laboratory testing process in several phases, such as preanalytical, analytical, and postanalytical. These phases in specimen collection, processing, and testing are part of every laboratory's operation. For purposes of this text, the quality assessment discussion focuses on the preanalytical phases, where the phlebotomist has the most impact. Box 1-11 summarizes the phases in specimen collection, and Box 1-12 indicates examples of quality assessments. Box 1-13 lists the basic requirements for a quality specimen. A periodic review of the laboratory's collection procedures and policies is recommended to reduce collection errors.

IMPORTANT FACTORS AFFECTING QUALITY

Anticoagulants and preservatives

- Phlebotomists use anticoagulants and preservatives in the collection of blood specimens. (A more thorough discussion is presented in Chapter 6.) Phlebotomists are responsible for filling the tubes in the correct order, so that carryover of anticoagulants to other tubes will not occur, and for mixing the specimens with the anticoagulant promptly after blood is drawn.

- When restocking the supply of collection tubes, phlebotomists should place the tubes with a shelf life (**expiration date**) nearest the current date at the front of the shelf so that these tubes are used first. The phlebotomist should be cognizant of expiration dates on any item used in specimen collection.

- Phlebotomists should know how to store or preserve specimen tubes if the blood specimen is not to be tested immediately.

BOX 1-11 **Examples of Preanalytical, Analytical, and Postanalytical Factors in the Phases of Specimen Collection, Processing, Testing, and Reporting**

Even though clinical laboratories differ in their operating procedures, the nature of their services includes the phases listed below. Phlebotomists have the greatest impact on laboratory testing in the preanalytical phases.

Preanalytical Phase Outside the Laboratory

Patient identification and information

Isolation techniques

Standard precautions

Correct venipuncture or skin puncture technique

Appropriate use of supplies and equipment

Appropriate transportation and handling

Preanalytical Phase Inside the Laboratory

Sample treatment
Specimen registration and distribution
Centrifugation

Identification of aliquots
Appropriate storage

Analytical Phase

Testing the specimen

Postanalytical Phase

Reporting results

Appropriate follow-up or repeat testing

BOX 1-12 **Quality Assessments for Specimen Collection Services**

- Worker response time (for inpatients)
- Patient waiting time (for outpatients)
- Time required for completion of the phlebotomy procedure
- Percentage of successful blood collections on the first attempt
- Number of successful blood collections on the second attempt
- Daily blood loss per patient due to venipunctures
- Number and size of hematomas
- Number of patients who faint
- Amount of time spent and number of telephone calls needed to acquire appropriate identification
- Number of redraws due to inadequate specimens
- Turnaround times of designated laboratory tests
- Number of incomplete forms, documents, logs, and so forth
- Number of therapeutic drug-monitoring tests with incorrect timing documentation
- Number of specimens received in incorrect tubes
- Contamination rate for blood cultures
- Patient satisfaction questionnaires
- Frequency of complaints

BOX 1-13 **Basic Requirements for a Quality Specimen**

Aspire to provide the highest quality patient specimens in a professional and safe environment 100 percent of the time. Be familiar with the following requirements:

1. Using universal standard precautions, identify, assess, and properly prepare the patient, and avoid medication interference if possible.
2. Collect specimens from the correct patients and label appropriately.
3. Use correct anticoagulants and preservatives and collect a sufficient amount of blood. Use devices that minimize accidental needle sticks.
4. Handle specimens carefully to prevent damage and/or hemolysis.
5. Collect fasting specimens in a timely fashion and verify that they are actually fasting samples. If they are not, note the condition.
6. Correctly time and document timed specimens.
7. Allow specimens without anticoagulants to stand a minimum of 30 minutes, so that clot formation can be completed. (Gel separator tubes, depending on the manufacturer, may shorten the time of clot formation.)
8. Transport specimens to the clinical laboratory in a timely fashion (within 45 minutes), and it is recommended that the blood cells be separated from serum or plasma within 2 hours. Document a list of the specimens that are delivered after the designated time limits, to help detect the source of the problem if necessary.

Number of blood collection attempts

- Many laboratories periodically monitor the number of unsuccessful blood collection attempts (i.e., the number of times a patient is stuck unsuccessfully). If a phlebotomist has had consecutively unsuccessful phlebotomy attempts on different patients, his or her blood collection technique must be reviewed, modified, and improved.

Blood loss due to phlebotomy

- For adults, blood loss due to venipuncture is usually well tolerated physiologically because the volume constitutes a small percentage of the total blood volume in the body. However, in some cases, if patients are very ill, more laboratory tests are ordered, which results in more total blood collected. The same is true for neonates and infants. When too much blood is taken for laboratory analysis, the patient may become anemic, so blood conservation becomes a priority.

Clinical Alert ❗

If too much blood is withdrawn in a short period of time, a patient may become anemic and require a blood transfusion. This type of induced blood-loss resulting in anemia is called iatrogenic anemia. It is important to monitor daily blood loss if patients are neonates, have poor prognoses, or are being tested frequently. In these cases, the use of smaller test tubes and/or microcollection techniques is warranted.[5]

EQUIPMENT AND PREVENTIVE MAINTENANCE

Phlebotomists also participate in quality control checks and preventive maintenance of laboratory instruments, including thermometers, sphygmomanometers (blood pressure cuffs), and centrifuges. For example, a centrifuge that is used to "spin down" the blood must be checked for accurate speed.

Self Study

Study Questions

The following questions may have more than one answer.

1. Examples of nonverbal, distracting behaviors include which of the following:

   a. tapping a pencil
   b. gazing outside the window
   c. direct eye contact
   d. glancing at the clock

2. Which of the following statement(s) is inappropriate during a phlebotomy procedure?

   a. "This won't hurt a bit!"
   b. "Your name is Mrs. Jones, isn't it?"
   c. "You are required to cooperate with this."
   d. "Could you please spell your last name for me?"

3. Which of the following are key elements in effective communication?

   a. active listening
   b. nonverbal cues
   c. verbal skills
   d. point-of-care procedures

4. Which of the following is the main area of responsibility for every phlebotomist?

   a. analytical testing
   b. data collection
   c. reporting results
   d. preanalytical processes

5. What feelings does one experience when a stranger gets "too close for comfort"?

   a. anxiety
   b. fear
   c. confidence
   d. security

For the following questions, select the one best answer.

6. What are "competency statements" for phlebotomists?

   a. verbal cues for patients
   b. entry-level skills, tasks, roles
   c. identification policies
   d. certification exam questions

7. Veracity is an essential character trait for a phlebotomist. Select the most appropriate example of what it means.

   a. being an impeccable dresser
   b. ability to tell a good story
   c. telling the truth
   d. performing well in harsh situations

8. How should a phlebotomist treat a patient who may have deafness?

   a. speak in a very loud voice
   b. ask the patient whether you should repeat the steps before proceeding
   c. tell the patient not to worry about anything
   d. assure the patient that "it won't hurt"

9. Why is eye contact helpful during a phlebotomist–patient interaction?

   a. it promotes a sense of trust
   b. it is an expression of authority
   c. it helps them focus on the phlebotomist's instructions
   d. it helps the phlebotomist read the patient's lips

10. Select the best example of internal stakeholders for clinical laboratory services.

    a. doctors and nurses
    b. health insurance companies
    c. advocacy groups
    d. accrediting agencies

Case Study

Mrs. Gonzales is an alert, ambulatory, 84-year-old patient who speaks English with a heavy Spanish accent. You observe that she argues about everything and does not seem to like anyone. Many of your coworkers are afraid to approach her, and you are assigned to collect her blood for laboratory analysis.

Questions

1. Describe what you would do or say to communicate with Mrs. Gonzales.

2. Identify factors that may be contributing to her anger or anxiety.

3. Describe what you might tell your coworkers about cultural issues affecting communication with Mrs. Gonzales.

Self Assessment

Check Yourself

Readiness for Phlebotomy Practice

1. Examine your lifestyle and character traits. List the values, beliefs, and traditions that are important to you. Think about how these might relate to your work as a phlebotomist. Which traits might be most beneficial in the work place (e.g., compassion, integrity)?

2. Based on your own experiences having blood specimens collected, can you think of ways to help improve the phlebotomy experience? Describe your impressions during a phlebotomy procedure.

3. Imagine yourself in 5 years. What do you expect to learn from being a phlebotomist?

4. Describe examples of communication styles that you like and dislike. Think about how you would change the negative styles to make them more positive.

Competency Checklist: Communication

This checklist can be completed in a classroom setting using a make-believe scenario or in the clinical setting during a patient interaction. The phlebotomist should do the following:

(1) Completed (2) Needs to improve

_____ 1. Demonstrate empathy for the patient.

_____ 2. Demonstrate respect for the patient's privacy, for their condition, for their family members.

_____ 3. Build trust by maintaining confidentiality and telling the truth.

_____ 4. Explain procedures clearly using simple terms appropriate to the age of the patient.

_____ 5. Establish rapport by being courteous and showing interest.

_____ 6. Listen actively by facing the patient, maintaining non-authoritative posture, establishing eye contact, and listening intently.

_____ 7. Provide specific feedback to the patient when appropriate.

Competency Checklist: Quality Basics

The phlebotomist should have an understanding of some fundamental factors related to providing quality services. The phlebotomist should do the following:

(1) Completed (2) Needs to improve:

_____ 1. Provide 5 examples of stakeholders (customers).

_____ 2. Give one example of how a phlebotomist may have a negative effect on quality.

_____ 3. List 5 examples of quality improvement assessments that could be monitored for phlebotomy services.

_____ 4. Describe at least 3 examples of preanalytical factors that affect phlebotomy services.

References

1. Wright D: *The Ultimate Guide to Competency Assessment in Healthcare*, 2nd ed. Minneapolis, MN: Creative Healthcare Management, 1998.

2. Johnson DW, Johnson RT: *Joining Together, Group Theory and Group Skills*, 6th ed. Boston, MA: Allyn & Bacon, 2000.

3. Luckman J: *Transcultural Communication in Health Care*. Albany, NY: Delmar, 2000.

4. Graham NO: *Quality in Health Care: Theory, Applications, and Evolution*. Gaithersburg, MD: Aspen Publishers, 1995.

5. McPherson RA: Blood sample volumes: Emerging trends in clinical practice and laboratory medicine. *Clin Leader Manage Rev*, Jan/Feb 2001: 3–10.

Chapter 2

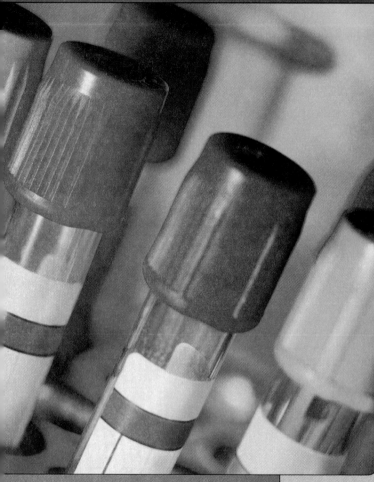

Ethical, Legal, and Regulatory Issues

CHAPTER OBJECTIVES

Upon completion of Chapter 2, the learner should be able to do the following:

1. Explain why ethics and laws are important to health care providers.

2. Describe the basic functions of the medical record.

3. Define *informed consent*.

4. Describe how to avoid blood collection lawsuits.

5. Identify two reasons for HIPAA and CLIA.

6. Identify methods to maintain confidentiality of privileged information on patients.

7. Define the medicolegal terms related to phlebotomy procedures, policies, and protocols designed to avoid medicolegal problems.

KEY TERMS

assault

battery

Clinical Laboratory Improvement
  Amendments (CLIA)

ethics

Health Insurance Portability and
  Accountability Act (HIPAA)

informed consent

liable

litigation process

malpractice

medical records

negligence

patient's confidentiality

Ethics and Laws

All health care workers are faced with ethical decisions at one time or another. **Ethics** are a set of principles or values based on religious and moral teachings. These ethics provide a standard of conduct by which a health care worker involved in blood collection guides his or her own actions and judges those of others (refer to Box 2-1). Fairness and honesty are linked closely to ethical values needed in the phlebotomy profession. But how do ethics and laws compare? Laws are a collection of rules to enforce order in a community, state, or other group. Laws have been developed for the community and society. An action can be moral but not legal, and vice versa. For example, an elderly paralyzed woman who is in a rehabilitation center stops breathing, and the health care professional does not attempt to take action so that the patient will start breathing again. This action is probably ethical if, on previous occasions, the patient had expressed a desire to die, but it could be questioned whether the action is legal.

To evaluate a difficult situation as a health care professional, the following questions should come to mind:

- Is this action legal?
- Does it foster a "win-win" situation with the patient and my supervisor?
- How would I feel about myself if I read this decision in the newspaper?
- Can I live with myself after making this decision, and is it right?

Basic Legal Issues

Patients know more about health care these days because of the Internet, the newspaper, and other sources. Thus, they are much more willing to sue anyone whom their lawyer believes has caused them harm in providing health care, including health care workers who are collecting blood specimens. Consider the following scenarios and ask yourself whether the health care worker has truly made an error and should be sued for the error due to malpractice.

> **Scenario 1:** When a child refused to have his blood collection, the health care worker locked the child in the blood collection room, and the child was forced to have his blood collected.

BOX 2-1 **Example of Ethical Behavior for a Health Care Worker**

If the health care worker realizes that he or she has made a mistake in identifying a patient and specimens, he or she faces an ethical decision about whether to report the mistake. Reporting it may result in disciplinary action against him or her.

- Each health care worker should go through the ethics check questions to see that the right ethical decision is to report his or her own mistake as soon as possible in order to avoid any medical treatment based on the wrong test results.

- This is the right decision because it creates a "win-win" situation for the patient and doctor, and, above all, it is just the right thing to do. In addition, a lawsuit is less likely for the phlebotomist and the health care facility if the error is corrected and documented.

Scenario 2: Two health care workers discuss a patient's medical condition on the elevator as they are going back to the laboratory with the blood specimens.

Scenario 3: A health care worker performing bedside glucose testing misread the Glucometer and wrote the wrong glucose results on the test reporting slip.

LEGAL TERMINOLOGY

If a health care worker understands words used for legal activities, this understanding can help to determine whether he or she is legally in trouble for activities that may occur in this field of health care. Such understanding can reduce the risk of legal action in health care activities.

Liability for causing harm or loss due to the lack of proper health care may be enforced on any health care worker, including health care institutions, physicians, nurses, laboratorians, patient care technicians, and phlebotomists. The number of lawsuits against health care workers as a result of improper care has grown in recent years as patients have become more sensitive to possible harmful effects of health care treatments.

Because the legal system is becoming more involved in health care, the health care worker should have some knowledge of basic legal terminology. A few major definitions with health care examples can be found in Box 2-2.

NEGLIGENCE

In the past decade, the number of legal cases in which blood collectors have been directly or indirectly involved has increased noticeably and related to **negligence**.[1] Negligence is "failure to provide proper care, resulting in injury to others."

Many things could be considered negligence if health care workers are not extremely careful. For example, there have been legal cases in which the confusion of patient samples led to a patient's death.[2]

BOX 2-2 Legal Terminology

■ **Assault.** Without permission, the attempt to touch a person or the threat to do so in such circumstances as to cause the other to believe that it will be carried out or to cause fear. An assault may be permissible if proper consent has been given (e.g., consent to obtain a blood specimen).

■ **Battery.** The intentional touching of another person without permission (consent); also, the unlawful beating of another or carrying out of threatened physical harm. Because battery always includes an assault, the two are commonly combined in the phrase assault and battery. Liability of hospitals, physicians, and other health care workers for acts of battery is most common in situations involving lack of or improper consent to medical procedures, such as blood collection. For example, a small boy who refused to have his blood collected was locked in the blood collection room by the health care worker and was forced to have his blood collected by the health care worker. The patient's parents sued and won the lawsuit against the phlebotomist for this assault and battery.

■ **Litigation process.** The process of legal action to determine a decision in court. Many malpractice cases are settled out of court.

■ **Standard of care.** All health care workers must conform to a specific standard of care to protect patients. It is a measuring stick that represents the conduct of the average health care worker in the community. The community has become a "national" standard.

MALPRACTICE

Malpractice, or professional negligence, is defined as improper care of a patient by a health care professional, resulting in injury to the patient. If the physician is the medical director overseeing clinical laboratory testing, in most cases he or she is responsible under the law for all aspects of laboratory testing. Therefore, the health care worker collecting blood for laboratory tests could place both the physician and him- or herself at risk.

PATIENT'S CONFIDENTIALITY

Negligence cases can also occur when a health care worker abuses a **patient's confidentiality**. "No one except the patient may release patient results without a clinical need to know." Patient or employee laboratory test results must be considered strictly confidential. For example, negligence can be claimed if employees' or patients' drug abuse test results are released to anyone other than the attending physician or other authorized individuals. This is particularly true regarding employee or athlete drug or alcohol abuse screening and human immunodeficiency virus (HIV) testing. Confidential materials include communications between the physician and the patient, the patient's verbal statements, medical computer entries on patients, and nonverbal communications, such as laboratory test results.

CONFIDENTIALITY AND HIV EXPOSURE

An increasing concern for health care workers collecting blood from patients who are homebound is the health care worker's rights in relation to accidental exposure to blood or body fluids, whether by a needlestick or some other means. In some states, laws allow health care workers to know the identity of a patient who has acquired immunodeficiency syndrome (AIDS) or who is HIV positive. Many states, however, do not allow this sensitive patient information. A home health care worker who routinely collects blood specimens from homebound patients should obtain information about the state's law regarding confidentiality and HIV status.[3] It can be obtained from the health care worker's employer, from lawyers, or from a national or state health professional organization.

It is important to use the proper blood collection techniques with safety steps and required infection control procedures for homebound patients. If exposure to the blood occurs through a needlestick, a lancet, or another means, the home health care worker needs to obtain the patient's HIV status and other potential infectious diseases (e.g., hepatitis C), to ensure that the proper immediate and long-term self-protective procedural steps can be taken.

If employed by a health care facility, the health care worker should follow the guidelines established by the facility. If self-employed, it is important to see a health care provider for a postexposure protocol and follow-up. Also, counseling should be sought to obtain emotional support during this stressful time.

INFORMED CONSENT

Informed consent is voluntary permission by a patient to allow touching, examination, and/or treatment by health care providers. It allows patients to decide what will be performed on or to their bodies. Without informed consent, intentional touching can be considered a criminal offense. Patients must be told about the possible positive and negative outcomes of having or not having particular medical treatments. An informed consent form is then signed by the patient to approve the medical treatment(s), including blood collection. Essential to consent is the patient's belief that the health care worker to whom the consent is given has the knowledge and technical ability to properly perform the tasks.

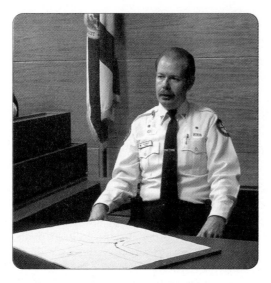

FIGURE ■ 2-1 Giving Testimony in a Lawsuit

Being involved in a lawsuit can be very
unsettling for both the plaintiff and defendant

Thus, the patient can expect the blood collector to know the proper blood collection
techniques and procedures.

Clinical Alert ❗

- Children must have the informed consent of their parents or legal guardians for medical
  care, including blood collection.
- If a patient does not speak English, an interpreter may be necessary so that information
  for consent may be given in the patient's native language.
- States have laws requiring that informed consent be obtained before most HIV specimen
  collection and testing is performed. The laws state the type of information that must be
  given for the patient to be considered informed. This information includes:

  - A description of the laboratory test;
  - Possible uses of the HIV test; and
  - The meaning of the test results.

ADVICE TO AVOID LAWSUITS

Lawsuits are very expensive. Lawyers' fees typically range from $300 to $800 per hour,
and other costs can lead to thousands of dollars in legal fees. In addition, lawsuits are time
consuming and, most of all, emotionally draining (Figure 2-1 ■). Thus, to avoid a malpractice lawsuit, the health care provider should heed the advice in Box 2-3.

Medical Records

Medical records are necessary for every patient. A health care worker cannot be
expected to remember a patient from whom blood was collected 3 to 4 years ago. The
medical records must be neat, legible, and accurate. They are extremely important if a
medical malpractice case goes to court (Box 2-4).

Medical records are also used for nonmedical reasons that are not directly tied to
medical services, such as billing, utilization review, quality improvement, and so on.

BOX 2-3	**Lawsuit Prevention Tips for Minimizing Risks**

Common Issues in Lawsuits Against Health Care Providers	**Prevention Tips for Health Care Providers Involved in Blood Collection**
Documentation	Always document the time, date, and blood collector's initials on the blood collection containers.
Reporting of incidents	Document the information legibly and spell correctly. If an injury occurs to the patient and/or the blood collector before, during, or after blood collection, report the incident to your immediate supervisor and complete the appropriate documentation.
Failure to follow health care facility's procedure	Be knowledgeable about the policies and procedures in the health care facility.
Failure to ensure patient's safety	Check to see that the patient is okay during and after blood collection. Return bed rails to the raised position if the bed rails were raised before blood collection.
	Secure the patient in the blood collection chair for the complete blood collection procedure.
	If an outpatient says that he or she faints during blood collection, have the patient lie down to collect blood and make the patient stay in that position for at least 20 minutes after collection before letting him or her stand up and leave the facility.
	Remove all supplies and equipment after the procedure.
Improper treatment and performance of treatment	Use proper techniques and equipment (e.g., gloves) when performing procedures.
	Update your collection skills and techniques through continuing education classes.
Failure to monitor and to report	Report any changes in a patient's condition (e.g., patient continues to bleed from the puncture site after blood collection).
Equipment use	Learn how to use blood collection equipment as designed.
	Use biohazardous waste containers as indicated in procedures.
	If involved in off-site blood collections, carry biohazardous waste containers.
	If involved in off-site collections, have the correct types and amounts of insurance coverage.

BOX 2-4	**Purpose of Medical Records**

Medical records have four basic purposes:

1. To monitor for continuous patient care;
2. To provide a record of the patient's illness and treatment;
3. To provide a method of communication between the physician and the health care team; and
4. To provide a legal document that can be used by patients and hospital or health care workers to protect them in a possible lawsuit and for regulatory agency compliance.

Health care workers and their supervisors have a legal duty to keep records, documentation, and laboratory test results confidential. Medical record documentation is covered in more detail in Chapter 5.

HIPAA

The federal **Health Insurance Portability and Accountability Act (HIPAA)** (Figure 2-2 ■) was created in 1996 to protect the privacy and confidentiality of every patient's medical information.[4] HIPAA requires that health care providers obtain a patient's written consent before transferring the patient's medical information for routine uses that include diagnosis, treatment, and payment. Thus, each laboratory must give patients information about their rights and about the ways in which their laboratory test results will be used.[5] Health care workers involved in blood collection must have HIPAA training and then sign an agreement that indicates that they know that privacy and confidentiality are basic rights in our society and that these rights must be protected for all patients.

This signature verifies that they will:

- keep the confidentiality of all patients' information, including lab tests to be performed;
- keep the computer password for entering the laboratory patients' database secure from others' knowledge; and
- maintain the confidentiality of patients' information when looking at the computer database of patients' medical record information.

Some examples of seemingly innocent activities that can lead to lawsuits include:

- Discussing patient information with a patient's family member without the patient's permission.
- Throwing laboratory test requests into the regular trash.
- Not logging off the computer after entering blood collection updates.
- Sending a patient's laboratory test requests to be printed and forgetting to take it off the printer.

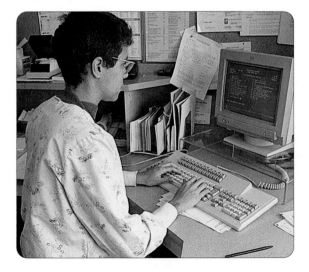

FIGURE ■ 2-2 Proper Documentation

Proper electronic or written documentation of laboratory test results into medical records is extremely important

Legal Cases Related to Clinical Laboratory Activities

Most phlebotomy cases are settled after a lawsuit is filed but before the court passes down a judgment. The following sections discuss cases that are of interest to health care workers involved in blood collection.

SCHMERBER V. STATE OF CALIFORNIA

Nurses, technologists, and health care workers are concerned about drawing a blood sample from an unconscious patient or from a patient who has not given consent but whose sample has been requested by police. The U.S. Supreme Court ruled in *Schmerber* v. *State of California* that tests performed on a blood sample drawn by a hospital physician from a person arrested by the police were admissible in a court action. This may vary by state.

LAZERNICK V. GENERAL HOSPITAL OF MONROE COUNTY (PA 1977)

A patient who was pregnant for the first time had her blood typed in January 1971. The report sent to her physician indicated that her blood type was A positive. The patient gave birth to her second child in June 1977. The child was brain damaged and paralyzed on the right side of the body as a result of hemolytic blood disease. The laboratory records in 1971 and 1977 showed that the mother's blood type was O negative. In a malpractice suit, the parents charged that the physician's and his employee's negligence caused the child's injuries. The physician, who was chief of the laboratory when the blood test was performed, was found **liable**, as was the health care worker.

HELMANN V. SACRED HEART HOSPITAL

Failure to follow proper isolation techniques, such as proper handwashing and prevention of cross-contamination, is a major area of concern for hospitals. The patient in *Helmann* v. *Sacred Heart Hospital* (62 Wash. 2d 136, 381 P. 2d 605 [1963]) had multiple fractures in the area of the left hip socket. After surgery on his hip, he was returned to a semiprivate room. His roommate complained of a sore under his right arm. After 11 days in the same room, it was determined that the roommate had a highly contagious wound infection caused by *Staphylococcus aureus*. The infected roommate was immediately placed in an isolation unit. For the preceding 11 days, however, the hospital attendants had administered care to both patients without washing their hands between patient care.

The patient with the hip injury developed a *Staphylococcus aureus* infection at the site of his hip incision. The infection penetrated into the hip socket, destroying tissue and leading to additional surgery and the hip being fused into a nearly immovable position. The patient with the hip injury won a malpractice lawsuit against the health care workers and the hospital for negligent care.

Cases Resulting from Improper Technique and Negligence

Health care workers who collect blood by venipuncture must be thoroughly trained and skilled in proper techniques, safety, and the use of collection equipment. Problems that can arise include:

- Wristband or identification error
- Hematoma

- Abscess at the puncture site
- Patient falling
- Fainting
- Nerve damage
- Emotional distress

In one case settled out of court, a health care worker had not received proper blood collection training. She performed a venipuncture by inserting the needle approximately 2 inches above the antecubital fold. The needle went through the vein, through muscle, and into the nerve, severely injuring the patient's arm, which remained permanently damaged even after three surgeries to repair the damage caused by the resultant hematoma and nerve injury.

Another case involved a medical technologist under pressure to collect specimens from ambulatory patients as quickly as possible. One of the patients stated before blood collection that she had fainted during blood collection at a previous time. The phlebotomist, however, took no precautions to avoid syncope, collected the patient's blood, and allowed the patient to leave immediately. The patient fainted at the elevator and suffered a permanent loss of smell and a permanent "ringing sound" in her ears.

In another case, a health care worker collecting bedside glucose results misread the Glucometer and caused the deaths of three patients with diabetes. The errors might have been avoided with better training, supervision, and quality monitoring.

In yet another case, a phlebotomist collected blood at an excessive angle of needle insertion from the patient's basilic vein when the median cubital vein was clearly an option for collection. The blood collection resulted in injury to the patient's median nerve and a malpractice lawsuit. In addition, documentation errors were evident for the collection. In all, the patient was awarded thousands of dollars for the health care worker's violations regarding proper standards of care.[6]

HIV-Related Issues

If a health care worker becomes infected with HIV during employment at a health care facility, workers' compensation benefits are usually available. The health care worker must, however, demonstrate a causal connection between his or her HIV infection and his or her employment. This causal connection includes having a documented incident report at the health care facility involving a needlestick injury, a puncture wound, or other exposure to HIV-contaminated blood or body fluids. In addition, the health care worker's lifestyle will be investigated to determine whether the exposure occurred elsewhere. Pre-employment health evaluations may prove to be useful later should the health care worker allege contraction of infection during the time of employment. Employers are legally responsible for monitoring postexposure follow-up.

If a health care worker resigns because of contracting AIDS, unemployment benefits may be available if the worker can show that he or she believed in good faith that continued employment would jeopardize his or her health.

Malpractice Insurance

Because hospitals are places where seriously ill patients are admitted and treated with highly sophisticated medical technology, the likelihood for problems is greater there than in other health care settings. Often, the health care staff in the hospital or clinical laboratory is covered by a blanket malpractice insurance policy. If, however, the health care worker is

BOX 2-5	Purchasing Malpractice Insurance

If the health care worker decides to purchase malpractice insurance, the following factors should be carefully considered:[8]

1. Does the health care facility carry liability insurance for the health care worker?
2. Is adequate dollar value coverage provided? In recent lawsuits, total damages of $1 million or more have been awarded against physicians.
3. What are the coverage limitations? How much does one have to lose if sued?
4. What are the procedures that must be followed for the policy to provide coverage? The health care worker should not assume that the lawyers representing the hospital, laboratory, or clinic will have his or her best interests at heart. The attorney's first obligation is to serve those who have hired him or her. There have been cases in which the hospital was cleared of all charges but the health care professional was held liable for damages.
5. Is a job change expected soon?
6. Are specimen collecting services provided off-site or in patients' homes?

employed by a physician who has a contract with an institution or owns a clinic, the staff may be protected by the physician's malpractice insurance policy.

Health care workers, in the past, have not been the targets of lawsuits because they do not carry malpractice insurance and do not have as much money as hospitals have. The advances in technology and increased complexity of health care, however, have increased legal exposure for allied health and nursing professionals. The health care worker who routinely deals with the public in patient–health care worker relationships is indeed liable. Therefore, each individual should examine the possibility of malpractice suits and the need for malpractice insurance from a personal standpoint (Box 2-5).[7]

The lawyer's fee and court costs are usually covered if professional liability insurance is bought. Some professional organizations offer professional liability insurance at a reduced rate. A record of continuing education courses, seminars, workshops, and academic credits should be a part of each health care worker's personal file.

Clinical Laboratory Improvement Amendments (CLIA)

In October 1988, the U.S. Congress passed Public Law 100-578, **Clinical Laboratory Improvement Amendments (CLIA)**.[9] These regulations are enforced to ensure the quality and accuracy of laboratory testing. CLIA '88 essentially applies to every clinical laboratory testing facility in the United States and requires laboratory certification by the federal government. The certification requires an inspection by federal and/or state agencies to determine whether the laboratory testing facility uses methods to test patients' specimens that lead to accurate, reliable, and good-quality test results. The blood collection procedures area is a major part of CLIA inspections, because it has been found that most laboratory errors occur during the preanalytical (specimen collection and handling) phase of testing.

Self Study

Study Questions

For the following questions, select the one best answer.

1. A nurse just came out of a patient's room stating that the patient threw his arm up when she was performing a venipuncture and that the needle jabbed her as it flew out of his arm. When should the nurse report this incident?

   a. after seeing the employee health physician
   b. after 24 hours to see whether the needlestick is healing
   c. immediately
   d. at the end of the work shift

2. A health care worker is given voluntary permission to touch a patient for blood collection under what legal term?

   a. assault and battery
   b. battery
   c. informed consent
   d. ethics

3. Specimen collection and handling is referred to as

   a. analytical phase
   b. preanalytical phase
   c. postanalytical phase
   d. analytical prephase

4. The federal law that regulates the quality and accuracy of laboratory testing (including blood collection) through certification inspections is referred to as

   a. CLIA '88
   b. FDA
   c. EPA
   d. HCFA

5. Malpractice in blood collection is the same as

   a. professional negligence
   b. informed consent
   c. battery
   d. criminal action

6. The measuring stick representing the conduct of the average health care worker is the

   a. community where the health care provider works
   b. community where the health care provider lives

   c. national community
   d. international community

7. A phlebotomist forgot her password for the laboratory computer and used a colleague's password to enter the laboratory access files to check on a patient's blood work to be performed. What law has she violated?

   a. OSHA
   b. HIPAA
   c. no law has been violated, because she was checking on blood tests for a patient
   d. CLIA

8. For potential lawsuits that may occur in the health care facility, which of the following must be maintained in the health care worker's employee file?

   a. number of patients from whom the health care worker has collected blood during the preceding year
   b. names of patients from whom the health care worker has collected blood during the preceding year
   c. record of continuing education courses
   d. whether the health care worker has additional jobs other than the one at the health care facility

9. The intentional touching of another person without permission is considered to be

   a. assault
   b. battery
   c. malpractice
   d. negligence

10. Before a patient's laboratory test results can legally be released, the patient must

    a. tell his or her physician that it is okay
    b. express verbal permission to the laboratory receptionist
    c. provide written consent
    d. provide written consent from his or her lawyer

Case Study

The health care worker, Mr. Riley, was in the outpatient clinic and was going to collect blood from Ms. Emily Dickinson for a complete blood count (CBC) and chemistry profile. After Mr. Riley prepped the arm for the venipuncture, he inserted the needle into the arm; as he did, Ms. Dickinson jumped with apparent pain. Apparently, because of the needle insertion at the time of the patient's jump, the needle went through the vein and deeper into the arm. The patient screamed, and then Mr. Riley pulled the needle back out of the arm. He placed gauze on the venipuncture site and also applied pressure with his fingers to the site as he raised her arm. After a few minutes, he checked the venipuncture site and a large hematoma had developed.

Questions

1. What should Mr. Riley do next?

2. What corrective actions, if any, should be taken?

3. What legal situations might arise from this situation?

Self Assessment

Check Yourself

Ready to Collect Blood

1. Examine your steps thoroughly each time you approach a patient to collect blood, and recall the prevention tips for minimizing risks for patient injury and lawsuits as you prepare for another blood collection.

2. You are having lunch with your new coworker in the cafeteria at Sacred Heart Hospital, where both of you work. Your coworker starts the conversation with the topic of the pregnant patient on Floor 15 whom he heard has AIDS. Describe what you should say at this point in the conversation.

Competency Checklist: Ethical, Legal, and Regulatory Issues

This checklist can be completed as a group or individually.

(1) Completed (2) Needs to improve

_____ 1. List four common issues in lawsuits against health care providers.

_____ 2. List four problems that have occurred in patients as a result of negligence on the part of the phlebotomist.

References

1. Kozier B, Erb G, Berman A, Snyder S: *Fundamentals of Nursing–Chapter Four: Legal Aspects of Nursing.* Upper Saddle River, NJ: Prentice Hall Publishers, 2004.

2. *Parker v. Port Huron Hospital,* 105, N.W. 2d 854, 1981.

3. Brent NJ: Confidentiality and HIV status: The nurse's right to know. *Home Healthcare Nurse* 1990; 8(3): 6–8.

4. U.S. Congress. *Health Insurance Portability and Accountability Act of 1996,* 18th Cong., 2nd sess. Rep. 64.

5. Travis J: Complying with HIPAA: Are you ready? *ADVANCE Med Lab Professionals* 2003; 15(4): 16–18, 25.

6. Ernst D: Phlebotomy on trial. *MLO* April 1999: 46–50.

7. Pozgar GD: *Legal Aspects of Health Care Administration.* Gaithersburg, MD: Aspen Publishers, 1993.

8. Markus K: Your legal risk in giving advice or care. *Healthweek* October 6, 1997: 5.

9. Clinical Laboratory Improvement Amendments of 1988 (CLIA): Final Rule for the Centers for Medicare & Medicaid Services CMS-2226F. *Fed. Register* January 24, 2003. Available at: http://www.cms.hhs.gov/CLIA.

Chapter 3

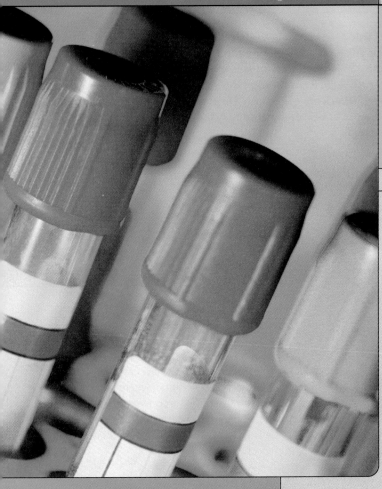

Basic Medical Terminology, the Human Body, and the Cardiovascular System

CHAPTER OBJECTIVES

Upon completion of Chapter 3, the learner should be able to:

1. Define word elements such as roots, prefixes, and suffixes.

2. Combine elements to make words and divide complex words into these elements.

3. Define basic terms used in the laboratory.

4. Describe the basic functions of the cardiovascular system.

5. Distinguish the characteristics of arterial, venous, and capillary blood.

6. Locate the veins most commonly used for phlebotomy.

7. Define *hemostasis*.

KEY TERMS

antecubital

anterior

arteriole

artery

blood cells

capillary

cardiovascular

cerebrospinal fluid

distal

dorsal

hematology

hemostasis

homeostasis

KEY TERMS *(continued)*

immunology	pathology	superficial
lateral	phlebotomy	synovial fluid
medial	pleural fluid	vascular
microbiology	posterior	veins
osteoporosis	proximal	ventral
pathogenesis	steady state	venules

Basic Medical Terminology

To be an effective member of a health care team, you must learn how to pronounce basic medical terms and know what they mean. Medical terminology becomes easier with practice and fundamental tools to understand how words are formed. Medical terms consist of several parts:

- **Word root**—The main part of the word that describes what the word is about; for example, *cardio-* is the word root for heart, so every time a medical term contains cardio-, it means it has something to do with the heart, and *phleb-* is a word root relating to vein.

- **Prefix**—A word element that is added *before* the root, at the *beginning of the word*. It makes the word more specific; for example, *endo-* is the prefix meaning inside.

- **Suffix**—A word element that is added *after* the root, at the *end of the word*. It also adds to the meaning of the root; for example, *-itis* is the suffix for inflammation, and *-tomy* is the suffix for cut or incision.

- **Combining vowel**—Sometimes a vowel (usually i, o, u, or y) is added to make a word easier to pronounce.

Combining the examples above results with the words:

> **endocarditis** (endo/card/itis), which means an inflammation of the inside lining of the heart. In this example, there was no need to add a combining vowel.

> **phlebotomy** (phleb/o/tomy), which means a cut or incision into the vein. In this example, the *o* in the middle helps make the pronunciation easier.

When different prefixes or suffixes are added to the word root, the meaning changes. You can build a huge medical vocabulary by learning the meanings of word parts and how to combine them (Figure 3-1 ■ and Tables 3-1 ■, 3-2 ■, and 3-3 ■).[1]

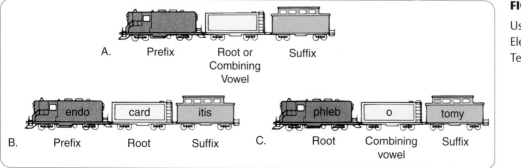

FIGURE ■ 3-1

Using Word Elements in Medical Terminology

TABLE ■ 3-1	**Prefixes That Pertain to Position or Placement**

Primary Word Elements: Prefixes

ab away from	**epi** upon, above	**intra** within
ad toward	**ex** out, away from	**meso** middle
ana up	**extra** outside, beyond	**para** beside
ante before	**hyper** above, excessive	**retro** backward
cata down	**hypo** below, deficient	**sub** below, under
circum, peri around	**infra** below	**supra** above, beyond
endo within	**inter** between	

Prefixes That Pertain to Numbers and Amounts

ambi both	**milli** one-thousandth	**quint** five
bi two, double	**multi** many, much	**semi, hemi** half
centi a hundred	**nulli** none	**tetra** four
deca ten	**poly** many	**tri** three
dipl double	**primi** first	**uni** one
di (s) two	**quadri** four	

Prefixes That Are Descriptive and Are Used in General

a, an without, lack of	**dia** through	**mega** large, great
ante, anti, contra against	**dys** bad, before, difficult	**micro** small
auto self	**eu** good	**oligo** scanty, little
brachy short	**hetero** different	**pan** all
brady slow	**homeo** similar, same	**pseudo** false
cac, mal bad	**hydro** water	**sym, syn** together

Adapted from J. Rice: The Terminology of Health and Medicine, 2nd ed. Upper Saddle River, NJ: Prentice Hall, 2003.

TABLE ■ 3-2	Root	Meaning	Root	Meaning
Primary Word Roots Related to the Cardiovascular System	**ang/i, angi/o, vas/o**	vessel	**lipid**	fat
	angin	to choke	**log**	study
	arter	artery	**man/o**	thin
	arteri/o	artery	**my/o**	muscle
	ather/o	fatty substance, porridge	**phleb**	vein
	capillus	hairlike	**phleb/o**	vein
	card	heart	**pulmonar**	lung
	card/i, cardi/o	heart	**rrhyth**	rhythm
	cubitum	elbow, forearm	**scler**	hardening
	cyte	cell	**sera**	serum
	derm	skin	**sphygm/o**	pulse
	electr/o	electricity	**steth/o**	chest
	embol	to cast, to throw	**tens**	tension

Root	Meaning	Root	Meaning
erg/o	work	**thromb**	clot
erythr/o	red	**ven/i**	vein
hem/o	blood		
infarct	infarct (necrosis of an area)		

Adapted from J. Rice; The Terminology of Health and Medicine, 2nd ed. Upper Saddle River, NJ: Prentice Hall, 2003.

BASIC RULES FOR COMBINING WORD ELEMENTS

Medical terms are different from everyday English language because they sound different, they come primarily from Greek or Latin origins, there can be more than one word element for a particular meaning, and changing a simple prefix can change the entire meaning. Many terms for the body's organs or structures originate from Latin; for example, *vessel* comes from the Latin word *vascillum*, or little vessel; and **capillary** originates from *capillus*, or hairlike. Most of the terms that describe diseases originate from Greek: for example, *lipo-* means fat and *-oma* means tumor, so *lipoma* means a fatty tumor; *hepat-* means liver and *-itis* means inflammation, so hepatitis means inflammation of the liver.[2]

Suffixes That Pertain to Pathologic Conditions			**TABLE ■ 3-3**
-algia, dynia pain	**-oma** tumor	**-ptosis** drooping	Primary Word Elements: Suffixes
-cele hernia, tumor, swelling	**-osis** condition of	**-ptysis** spitting	
-emesis vomiting	**-pathy** disease	**-rrhage** bursting forth	
-itis inflammation	**-penia** deficiency	**-rrhagia** bursting forth	
-lysis destruction, separation	**-phobia** fear	**-rrhea** flow, discharge	
-megaly enlargement, large	**-plegia** paralysis, stroke	**-rrhexis** rupture	
-oid resemble			

Suffixes Used in Diagnostic and Surgical Procedures		
-centesis surgical puncture	**-opsy** to view	**-scopy** to view
-desis binding	**-plasty** surgical repair	**-stasis** control, stopping
-ectomy surgical excision	**-plexy** surgical fixation	**-stomy** new opening
-gram a weight, mark, record	**-rrhaphy** suture	**-tome** instrument to cut
-graph to write, record	**-scope** instrument	**-tomy** incision
-meter measure		

Suffixes That Are Used in General		
-blast immature cell, germ cell	**-philia** attraction	**-therapy** treatment
-cyte cell	**-phraxis** to obstruct	**-trophy** nourishment, development
-ist one who specializes, agent	**-physis** growth	
-logy study of	**-plasia** formation, produce	**-uria** urine
-phagia to eat	**-pnea** breathing	
-phasia to speak	**-poiesis** formation	

Adapted from J. Rice: The Terminology of Health and Medicine, 2nd ed. Upper Saddle River, NJ: Prentice Hall, 2003.

BOX 3-1   The Study of . . .

-logy is a common suffix used in health care. It means "the study of." Here are some examples:

	The Study of:
Cardiology	Diseases of the heart, arteries, veins, and capillaries
Cytology	Cellular structure and functions
Dermatology	Skin
Endocrinology	Diseases of the endocrine (glands and hormones) system
Gastroenterology	Diseases of the intestinal or digestive system
Gynecology	Diseases of the female reproductive system
Hematology	Blood
Histology	Microscopic structures of tissues
Immunology	Diseases of the immune system
Microbiology	Microbes
Nephrology	Diseases of the kidney and urinary system
Neurology	Diseases of the nervous system
Oncology	Tumors
Parasitology	Parasites
Pathology	Pathogens or disease causing agents
Serology	Antibodies in the serum
Urology	Urinary system

A few basic rules make medical terminology easier to learn and use and help us to avoid mistakes. Remember that changing a simple prefix can change the entire meaning of a word, as you can see in Box 3-1.

■ Practice using medical terminology with someone who is familiar with the correct pronunciation. A study partner can give you tips about the sound of the word so that confusion is avoided. It is even recommended that you read this section out loud. Following are some basic tips on pronunciation:

  ◦ *ch* sounds like *k*; for example, chronic (kro-nic)
  ◦ *ps* sounds like *s*; for example, psychology (si-kol-o-ji)
  ◦ *pn* sounds like *n*; for example, pneumonia (nu-mo-ni-a)
  ◦ *c* sounds like an *s* when it comes before e, i, and y; for example, cytoplasm (si-to-plazm), centrifuge (sen-tri-fuj)
  ◦ *g* sounds like *j* when it comes before e, i, and y; for example, generic (jen-er-ik)
  ◦ *i* sounds like *eye* when added to the end of a word to form a plural; for example, bacilli (ba-sil-li), bronchi (bron-ki)

■ The combining vowel is often an *o*. For example, **osteoporosis** (oste/o/por/osis) is a condition in which the bone becomes porous. It is easier to say with the addition of the *o* than to say "osteporosis."

■ When changing a word from the singular to plural, substitute the plural endings as follows:

  ◦ *-ax* as in thorax to *-aces* as in thoraces
  ◦ *-nx* as in phalanx to *-ges* as in phalanges
  ◦ *-en* as in foramen to *-ina* as in foramina
  ◦ *-is* as in crisis to *-es* as in crises

- ○ *-ix* as in appendix to *-ices* as in appendices
- ○ *-on* as in spermatozoon to *-a* as in spermatozoa
- ○ *-um* as in ovum to *-a* as in ova
- ○ *-us* as in nucleus to *-i* as in nuclei
- ○ *-y* as in **artery** to *-i* and add *-es* as in arteries or phlebotomy to phlebotomies

Table 3-1 lists selected prefixes and their meanings that you will use as you build medical terms. Please commit these prefixes to memory.

The word roots listed in Table 3-2 are used to build medical terms that relate to the cardiovascular system. Please commit these terms to memory.

The terms listed in Table 3-3 are selected suffixes and their meanings that you will use as you build medical terms. Please commit these terms to memory.

Anatomical terms provide a description of the body's landmarks. These terms are helpful during an assessment of a patient to make the patient's condition understandable to others. The following terms may be useful when describing or evaluating a venipuncture complication, an interfering surgical wound site, the location of a vein or artery, or a potential venipuncture site (see Figure 3-2 ■ and Box 3-2).

- ■ **Anterior**—In front of (example: I will draw blood from the *anterior* side of the arm.)
- ■ **Posterior**—Toward the back (example: There is a large bandage on the *posterior* side of the arm.)
- ■ **Medial**—Toward the midline (example: The heart is *medial* to the right shoulder.)
- ■ **Lateral**—Toward the sides of the body (example: The hip is *lateral* to the navel.)
- ■ **Dorsal**—Back side (example: The mole was on the *dorsal* side of her shoulder.)
- ■ **Ventral**—Front side (example: The scrape was on the *ventral* side of the knee.)

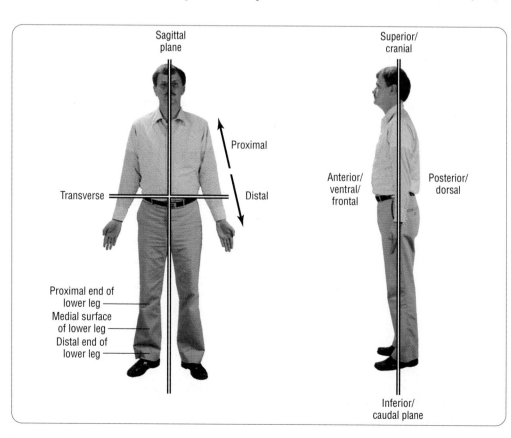

FIGURE ■ 3-2

Terms Related to Body Orientation

Areas of and the direction on the body can be described in terms related to imaginary planes that divide the body

BOX 3-2	**Right and Left Sides: The Patient's or the Health Care Worker's?**

When speaking with patients, health care workers should refer to the *patient's right* and the *patient's left* sides. This comes up when the health care worker asks to see a patient's right or left arm prior to vein selection for venipuncture. Even though the task seems easy, some health care workers confuse right and left arms when they are face to face with a patient. Practice using the terms by directly facing a friend and pointing to the friend's right and left side until it is done correctly each time. Do not confuse your own right and left side with the patient's right or left side. This task becomes important when there are specific instructions to draw blood from only one side of a patient because of a clinical condition.

- **Proximal**—Near the point of attachment (example: The leg broke on the *proximal* side of the knee.)
- **Distal**—Distant or away from the point of attachment (example: The birthmark was *distal* to the wrist.)
- **Superficial**—Near the surface of the body (example: *Superficial* veins show up easily on her skin.)
- **Deep**—Far from the surface of the body (example: Major arteries are in the *deep* tissues.)

Terms that describe body positioning can help you communicate details related to the patient prior to, during, or after a phlebotomy procedure. These include the following:

- Normal anatomic position—Erect, standing position with arms at rest and palms forward (never perform a venipuncture on a patient who is standing because of the risk of fainting or falling)
- Supine position—Lying or reclining face-up on his or her back (the best position for performing phlebotomy on patients who are in bed)
- Prone position—Lying face-down on his or her stomach (not a recommended position for venipuncture because of awkward orientation of the arms)
- Lateral recumbent position—Lying on left or right side (not a recommended position for venipuncture because the patient can easily roll over, increasing the risk of harmful needle insertion)

The Human Body

HOMEOSTASIS

The design of the human body is elaborate and sophisticated. Trillions of cells make up each individual. Similar groups of cells are combined into tissues, such as muscles or nerves, and tissues are combined into organ systems, such as the circulatory or reproductive system. These organ systems work simultaneously to serve the needs of the body for survival. No one system works independently of the others. The body strives for a **steady state**, or **homeostasis**. Literally, homeostasis means "remaining the same." It is a condition in which a healthy body, although constantly changing and functioning, remains in a normal, healthy condition. Homeostasis, or a steady-state condition, allows the normal body to stay in balance by compensating with changes. For example, if the body is taking in too much water, it responds to this imbalance by excreting water from the kidneys (urine), skin (perspiration), intestines (feces), and lungs (water in one's breath). A healthy body maintains constancy of its chemical components and processes in order to survive. Each organ system and body structure plays a part in main-

BOX 3-3	Laboratory Specimens

Laboratory test results provide information about an individual's organ systems. Specimens, such as blood, bone marrow, urine, **cerebrospinal fluid** (CSF, from around the spinal cord), **synovial** or joint fluid, **pleural fluid** (from around the lungs), biopsy tissue, semen, and others, can be microscopically analyzed, assayed, and cultured to determine **pathogenesis** (the origin of the disease). You may have a part In the collection, transportation, processing, or testing of these specimens.

taining homeostasis. Health care workers can assess homeostasis, or normal functioning, by taking "vital signs"; for example, temperature, pulse rate, respiration rate (together known as TPR), and blood pressure. Another way to monitor normal functioning is to perform laboratory analyses on blood specimens (Box 3-3). Refer to Figure 3-3 ■ to learn more about each organ system and the types of laboratory tests that are useful in evaluating each system.

Organ System	Major Functions	Common Disorders*	Common Laboratory Tests*
Integumentary system	Protection, temperature regulator, and sensory receptor.	Infections, cancers	Skin scrapings potassium hydroxide (KoH) preparation Biopsy staining procedures
Skeletal system	*Framework and Movement:* Shape, support, protection, and storage place for minerals. Movement is made possible through joints.	Arthritis, gout, tumors, infections, developmental conditions, eg., dwarfism	Calcium, phosphate, alkaline phosphatase uric acid, Vitamin D, blood cell counts, cultures, cytogenetic analysis
Muscular system	*Framework and Movement:* Muscles produce movement, maintain posture, and produce heat.	Muscular dystrophy, multiple sclerosis tendinitis, infections	Muscle enzymes, eg., creatine phosphokinase (CK), lactate dehydrogenase
Nervous system	*Communication and Control:* Transmits impulses, responds to change, is responsible for communication, and exercises control over all parts of the body.	Infections, eg., meningitis, encephalitis, tumors, epilepsy, Parkinson's disease amyotrophic lateral sclerosis (ALS)	Hormone, protein, and enzyme analysis microbial cultures
Endocrine system	*Communication and Control:* The glands of the endocrine system produce hormones, chemical messengers, that provide for communication and control over various parts of the body.	Addison's disease, Cushing's Syndrome, diabetes, hyper or hypothyroidism, goiter	Hormone analysis, thyroid function tests
Cardiovascular system	*Transportation and Immunity:* Transports oxygen and carbon dioxide, delivers nutrients and hormones, regulates blood clotting and removes waste products.	Tumors, heart disease, hemophilia	Heart enzymes, hemoglobin, hematocrit (H&H), cell counts, platelet function tests, coagulation factors, bone marrow analysis, cytogenetic analysis
Lymphatic system	*Transportation and Immunity:* The lymphatic system stimulates immune response, protects the body, and transports proteins and fluids.	Tumors, eg., lymphoma, Hodgkin's disease, immune disorders, infections	Bone marrow analysis, immune function tests
Respiratory system	*Distribution and Elimination:* Furnishes oxygen for use by individual tissue cells and removes their gaseous waste products, carbon dioxide.	Infections, eg., pneumonia, tuberculosis, sore throats, laryngitis, coughs, colds, influenza	Blood gases, eg., CO_2, & O_2, blood pH, electrolytes (sodium, chloride, potassium), bicarbonate, microbial cultures
Digestive system	*Distribution and Elimination:* Digestion, absorption, and elimination.	Peridontal disease, stomach disorders, eg., ulcers, acid reflux, hernias, intestinal disorders, eg., appendicitis	Occult blood test, microbial cultures, and parasitic analysis
Urinary system	*Distribution and Elimination:* Produces urine, transports urine, and eliminates urine. The kidneys help maintain electrolyte, water, and acid—base balance of the body.	Acidosis and alkalosis	Protein, glucose, ammonia, creatinine, blood urea nitrogen, electrolytes
Reproductive system	*Cycle of Life:* Responsible for sexual characteristics of the male and/or female. Proper functioning ensures survival of the human race.	Tumors, infertility, cysts, cancer, sexually transmitted diseases (STD)	Cytogenetic analysis, semen analysis, biopsies, hormone analysis, prostatic specific antigen (PSA)

* Disorders and laboratory tests listed are only a few examples. The lists are not comprehensive.

FIGURE ■ **3-3** Organ Systems of the Human Body

CARDIOVASCULAR SYSTEM

All body systems are linked by the **cardiovascular** system, a transport network that affects every part of the body within seconds (see Table 3-4 ■). To maintain homeostasis, the cardiovascular system must provide rapid transport of water, nutrients, electrolytes, hormones, enzymes, antibodies, cells, and gases (oxygen and carbon dioxide) to all cells. In addition, the cardiovascular system helps bodily defenses, controls the blood coagulation process, and controls body temperature. The term *cardiovascular* refers to the cardiac muscle (e.g., the heart), the **vascular** system (e.g., a network of blood vessels that includes **veins**, arteries, and capillaries), and the circulating blood (refer to Box 3-4).

TABLE ■ 3-4	Organ/Structure	Primary Functions
The Cardiovascular System	Heart	• Muscular organ about the size of an adult's closed fist • Contractions push blood throughout the body • Average heart beats 60 to 80 times per minute
	Arteries	• Transport blood from the right and left chambers of the heart to the entire body • Large arteries branch into **arterioles** the farther they are from the heart • Carry oxygenated blood that is bright red in color • Have thicker elastic walls than veins do • Have a pulse • Are located deep in muscles/tissues
	Veins	• Transport blood from peripheral tissues back to the heart and lungs • Large veins branch into **venules** in the peripheral tissues • Carry deoxygenated blood back to the lungs to release carbon dioxide • Carry blood that is normally dark red in color • Have thinner walls than arteries that appear bluish • Have valves to prevent backflow of blood • Are located both deep and superficially (close to the surface of the skin)
	Capillaries	• Connect arterioles with venules via microscopic vessels • Exchange oxygen and carbon dioxide, nutrients, and fluids in tissue capillaries • Pass waste products from tissue cells into capillary blood, then onto removal from the body • Carry blood that is a mixture of arterial blood and venous blood
	Circulating Blood	• Transports oxygen and carbon dioxide, nutrients, and fluids • Removes waste products • Disburses nutrients • Regulates body temperature and electrolytes • Regulates the blood clotting system

BOX 3-4 Study Your Veins

Take a look at the superficial veins in one of your hands or in the hands of a friend. Try to find veins that are prominent and easy to see. (Remember that arteries are located deeper in the tissues and are not visible.) Study the characteristics:

Bluish color—Caused by the low oxygen/high carbon dioxide content

Direction of blood flow—Venous blood flow is from the tips of fingers toward the heart, because veins are taking blood back to the heart and lungs to get more oxygen. This can be visible by hanging your hand down low for a minute so that venous blood pools in the veins. Take note of how they become more prominent. Next, raise your hand up: the venous blood empties and veins become less visible.

Firmness—Some veins feel rather soft, whereas others are slightly firm. Try to compare the feeling of veins from different people of different ages. The more practice you have feeling (not seeing) veins, the better your venipuncture outcomes will be (Figure 3-4 ■).

Become familiar with the principal veins of the arms and legs (Figures 3-5 ■, 3-6 ■, 3-7 ■, and 3-8 ■). Although every individual has a slightly different venous pattern, always rely on feeling the "best" vein for a venipuncture. Also note the figure on the inside front cover that shows the positions of nerves of the arm. Keep in mind that "nerve damage" can occur if appropriate venipuncture procedures are not followed.

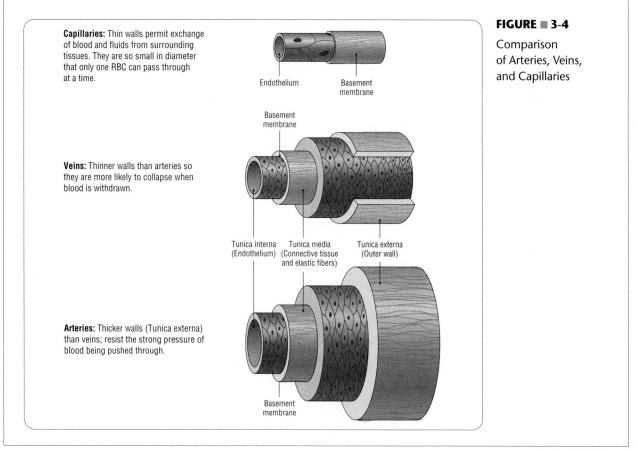

Capillaries: Thin walls permit exchange of blood and fluids from surrounding tissues. They are so small in diameter that only one RBC can pass through at a time.

Endothelium   Basement membrane

Basement membrane

Veins: Thinner walls than arteries so they are more likely to collapse when blood is withdrawn.

Tunica interna (Endothelium)   Tunica media (Connective tissue and elastic fibers)   Tunica externa (Outer wall)

Arteries: Thicker walls (Tunica externa) than veins; resist the strong pressure of blood being pushed through.

Basement membrane

FIGURE ■ 3-4

Comparison of Arteries, Veins, and Capillaries

(continued)

BOX 3-4 **Study Your Veins** (continued)

FIGURE ■ 3-5

Venous System of the Upper Torso and Arm

The antecubital area of the forearm (around the crease of the elbow) is most commonly used for venipuncture. The median cubital vein is best for venipuncture because it is generally the largest and best anchored vein. Others in the antecubital area that are acceptable are the basilic vein and the cephalic vein

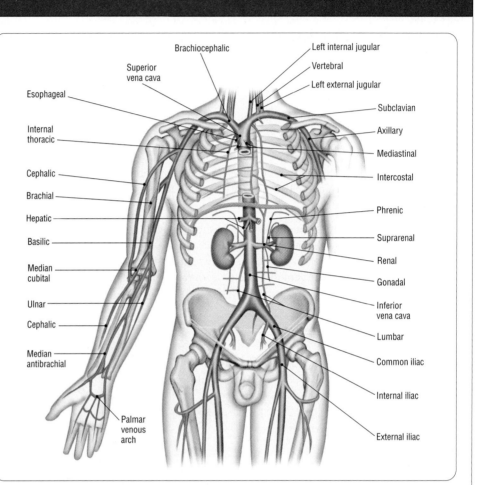

FIGURE ■ 3-6

Major Arm Veins

Note that the *cephalic vein* extends almost the entire length of the arm. The superficial *median cubital vein* serves as a connection between the cephalic and basilic veins. The subclavian, brachial, and axillary veins are deeper veins

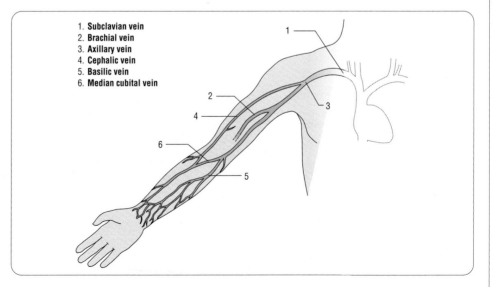

1. **Subclavian vein**
2. **Brachial vein**
3. **Axillary vein**
4. **Cephalic vein**
5. **Basilic vein**
6. **Median cubital vein**

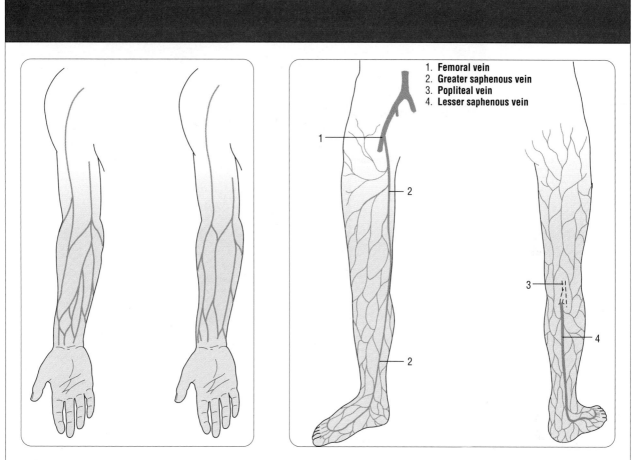

1. Femoral vein
2. Greater saphenous vein
3. Popliteal vein
4. Lesser saphenous vein

FIGURE ■ 3-7 Variations in Venous Patterns

Because all individuals are unique, the exact location of veins may vary from one to another. This figure depicts variations in venous patterns in the arms of two individuals

FIGURE ■ 3-8 Major Veins of the Leg

The *femoral vein* (1) is a deep vein. Note that the *greater saphenous vein* (2) is the longest vein in the body. It ascends up the medial side of the leg and the medial thigh and empties into the femoral vein in the groin area. The *lesser saphenous vein* (4) comes up the lateral side of the ankle and enters the deeper *popliteal vein* (3) behind the knee

Clinical Alert ❗

Nerve damage can occur as a result of accidental injury during phlebotomy procedures. Injury may be the result of excessive probing with the needle, sticking the needle in a poor site for venipuncture, deep needle penetration all the way into the nerve, and/or if the patient suddenly jerks his or her arm during the venipuncture procedure, causing the needle to puncture a nerve.

Choose sites that are least likely to cause nerve damage, and take precautions to have the patient's movements stabilized as much as possible. Even though the **antecubital** area (anterior side) of the arm is preferred for venipuncture, in some circumstances, the puncture site must be on the back or posterior side of the hand (Figure 3-9 ■). *Never use the anterior or palm side of the wrist or hand* to collect a blood specimen because the risk of hitting a nerve is very high because of nerve locations close to the skin's surface.

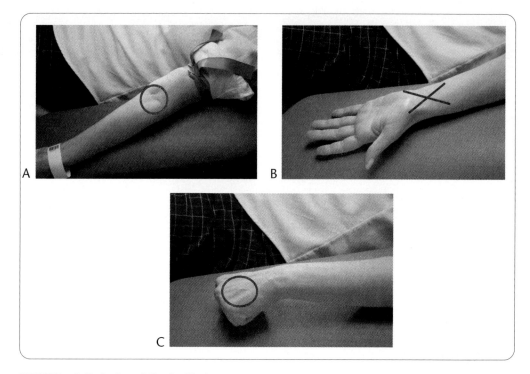

FIGURE ■ 3-9 Preferred Site for Venipuncture
A. The preferred site for venipuncture is the antecubital area of the arm. B. Avoid using the wrist area for venipuncture. C. If other preferred sites are not available, use the back (posterior) side of the hand

Blood

Circulating blood is essential to homeostasis and to sustaining life. Any region of the body that is deprived of blood may die within minutes. Humans contain approximately 5 quarts (4.73 liters) of whole blood that is composed of water, solutes (dissolved substances), and cells. The volume of blood in an individual varies according to body weight; for example, men have 5 to 6 liters of whole blood, whereas adult women usually have 4 to 5 liters.

Blood is made up of the liquid portion (plasma) and the cells. There are three main types of circulating **blood cells**. See Table 3-5 ■ and Figure 3-10 ■.

PLASMA

The liquid portion of blood is called plasma. It is about 90% water and 10% dissolved substances and cells. Normally, blood cells, gases (oxygen or carbon dioxide), proteins, glucose, and other chemical substances are suspended in plasma. It is the medium for transporting constituents in the bloodstream. If a chemical agent called an anticoagulant is added to the blood specimen to prevent it from coagulating or clotting, the specimen can be centrifuged and will result in a layer of cells and the liquid plasma. The cellular portion of the specimen contains white blood cells (WBCs), red blood cells (RBCs), and platelets. If the specimen is centrifuged or allowed to settle, the WBCs and platelets settle in a layer above the RBCs, called the buffy coat. The fluid portion is straw-colored and remains on

Cells	Number/Size	Function	Formation	Destruction
Erythrocytes (RBCs)	4–6 million/μl(mm³); size 6–7 μm	Transport O_2 and CO_2	Bone marrow	Fragmentation and removal in spleen, liver, and bone marrow; life span: 120 days
Leukocytes (WBCs)	5000–9000/μl(mm³); size 9–16 μm	Defense	Granulocytes in bone marrow; nongranular WBCs in all lymphatic tissue	Removed in spleen, liver, bone marrow; life span: 1 day to 1 year
Thrombocytes (platelets)	250,000–450,000/μl(mm³); size 1–4 μm	Clotting	Bone marrow	Removed in spleen; life span: 9–12 days

TABLE ■ 3-5

Blood Cells

RBCs, red blood cells; WBCs, white blood cells.

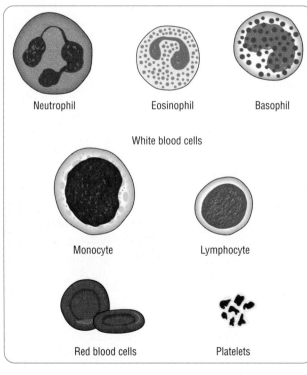

Neutrophil   Eosinophil   Basophil

White blood cells

Monocyte   Lymphocyte

Red blood cells   Platelets

FIGURE ■ 3-10 Human Blood Cells

the top of the cells. It contains fibrinogen, a clotting factor, and other chemical substances. However, if the sample is mixed, the cells will again become suspended in the plasma and it will again look like normal blood.

FIGURE ■ 3-11

Centrifuged Blood
Specimens With
and Without
Anticoagulant

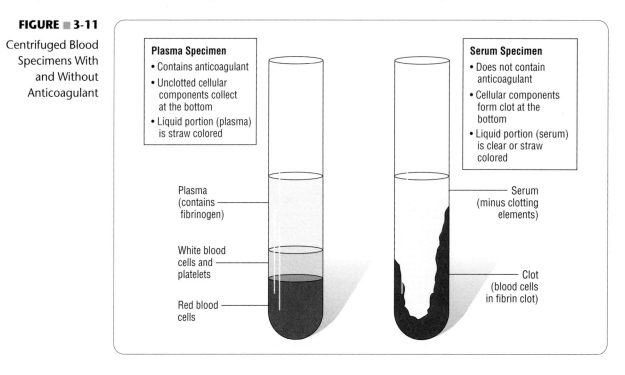

FIGURE ■ 3-11

Centrifuged Blood Specimens With and Without Anticoagulant

Plasma Specimen
• Contains anticoagulant
• Unclotted cellular components collect at the bottom
• Liquid portion (plasma) is straw colored

Serum Specimen
• Does not contain anticoagulant
• Cellular components form clot at the bottom
• Liquid portion (serum) is clear or straw colored

Plasma (contains fibrinogen)

White blood cells and platelets

Red blood cells

Serum (minus clotting elements)

Clot (blood cells in fibrin clot)

SERUM

If the blood specimen is allowed to clot, the resulting liquid portion changes from plasma to serum (also straw-colored) plus blood cells meshed in a fibrin clot. Serum contains essentially the same chemical constituents as plasma, except that the clotting factors (fibrinogen) and the blood cells are contained within the fibrin clot (Figure 3-11 ■).

Hemostasis and Coagulation

Hemostasis (*hemo* = blood, *stasis* = standing still), not to be confused with the term homeostasis, is the maintenance of circulating blood in the liquid state so that it does not clot spontaneously. Hemostasis is the body's mechanism to prevent blood loss. When a blood vessel is injured by an incision or puncture, the hemostatic process (blood clotting response) repairs the break and stops the hemorrhage by forming a blood clot (Figure 3-12 ■). Essentially, the blood clot bridges the torn or punctured edges together. This entire coagulation process is the result of numerous factors and steps taking place.

Normally, slight pressure over a puncture site will stop bleeding. However, there are some drugs, such as aspirin, heparin, and coumadin (warfarin), that may cause a patient to bleed excessively and would require extra pressure or assistance (Figure 3-13 ■). Make sure bleeding has stopped before leaving a patient.

Health care workers regularly deal with patients who are bleeding. External bleeding is described according to the type of blood vessel injured and the color of the blood:

Arterial bleeding

■ Bright red in color (because of the high oxygen content)
■ Bleeding is quicker, more abundant (because of higher pressure), and in spurts (with each heartbeat)

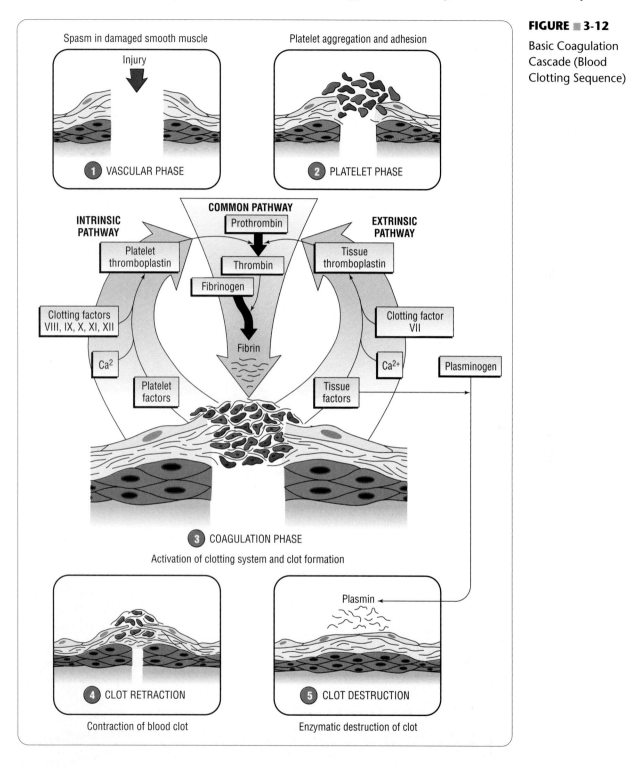

Basic Coagulation Cascade (Blood Clotting Sequence)

■ Harder to control and requires special attention from a nurse and/or doctor

■ If an artery is accidentally punctured, take immediate steps to terminate the procedure, apply pressure to the site for at least 5 minutes, and seek assistance

■ Report accidental arterial punctures immediately to a supervisor

Medications That Increase Bleeding

Some medications, such as aspirin, may increase bleeding. Make sure the bleeding has stopped after the venipuncture

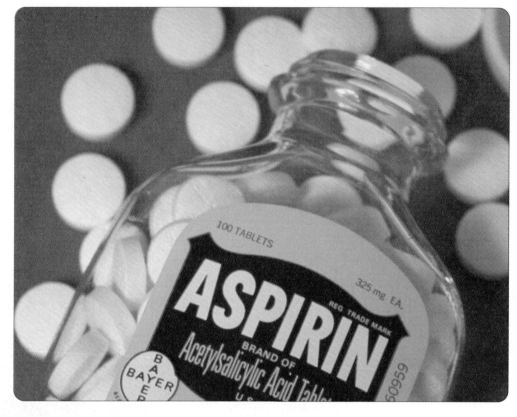

Clinical Alert ❗

Bleeding should be anticipated during or after a venipuncture. Therefore, always use precautions, including gloves, to avoid direct exposure. A mask, protective eyewear, a face shield, or a gown should be worn if there is a chance of blood splatters or if the patient is coughing up blood. And always ensure that bleeding has stopped before leaving the patient.

Venous bleeding

- Blood is dark red in color (because it lacks oxygen)
- Occurs in a steady flow
- Normal bleeding is easily stopped by applying pressure (because venous pressure is lower than arterial pressure)

Capillary bleeding

- Occurs slowly and evenly because of smaller size of vessels and lower pressure
- Easily controlled with slight pressure; sometimes stops without intervention
- Blood is a color between the bright red of arterial blood and dark red of venous blood

Self Study

Study Questions

For the following questions, select the one best answer

1. Homeostasis refers to which of the following?

   a. chemical imbalance
   b. steady-state condition
   c. balanced chemistry
   d. thousands of genes

2. The term *superficial vein* means which of the following?

   a. deep vein
   b. vein that has a blockage
   c. vein that is close to the skin surface
   d. vein that is cut open and bleeding

3. What is the best position for a patient to be in when the health care worker performs a phlebotomy procedure?

   a. prone position
   b. standing position
   c. supine position
   d. ventral position

4. Arteries differ from veins in which way(s)?

   a. arteries have thin walls
   b. arteries do not have a pulse
   c. blood from arteries appears dark red
   d. blood from arteries appears bright red

5. Capillary blood contains the following?

   a. cells, plasma, arterial blood, venous blood
   b. plasma and cells
   c. only arterialized blood
   d. only venous blood

6. A patient has a severe burn on his left wrist. Select the best description of its location relative to his fingers. The burn is:

   a. proximal to his fingers
   b. distal to his fingers
   c. lateral to his elbow
   d. posterior to his elbow

7. Venous blood is:

   a. blue
   b. dark red
   c. bright red
   d. straw-colored

8. What volume of blood (in liters) does a normal adult have?

   a. 0.5–1.0
   b. 2–3
   c. 4–5
   d. 6–7

9. A patient is taking aspirin. How might this affect a venipuncture?

   a. blood will appear thicker
   b. blood will appear darker than usual
   c. bleeding may be excessive or prolonged
   d. aspirin does not affect the venipuncture at all

10. Hemostasis refers to:

    a. steady state condition
    b. anticoagulant therapy
    c. blood leakage into tissues
    d. control of blood clotting

Case Study

A young man who was from China was scheduled to have laboratory work done in the University Health Clinic. The health care worker was visiting with him prior to the procedure. He asked "Why do my veins look blue? Please explain this to me before you stick a needle in me."

Question

What should the health care worker say to the patient?

Self Assessment

Check Yourself

Basic Medical Terminology.

1. In the space provided, write the definition of these prefixes, roots, and suffixes. Do not refer back to the chapter, and leave the space blank for the words that you do not know.

2. After answering as many as you can, go back to the list to check your work. Note the ones that you missed.

Competency Checklist: Prefixes

Write the definitions of the following prefixes:

1. a _____
2. ab _____
3. ad _____
4. ambi _____
5. an _____
6. ana _____
7. ante _____
8. anti _____
9. auto _____
10. bi _____
11. brachy _____
12. brady _____
13. cac _____
14. cata _____
15. centi _____
16. circum _____
17. contra _____
18. deca _____
19. dia _____
20. dipl _____
21. dl(s) _____
22. dys _____
23. endo _____
24. epi _____
25. eu _____
26. ex _____

27. extra _____
28. hemi _____
29. hetero _____
30. homeo _____
31. hydro _____
32. hyper _____
33. hypo _____
34. infra _____
35. inter _____
36. intra _____
37. mal _____
38. mega _____
39. meso _____
40. micro _____
41. milli _____
42. multi _____
43. nulli _____
44. oligo _____
45. pan _____
46. para _____
47. peri _____
48. poly _____
49. primi _____
50. pseudo _____
51. quadri _____
52. quint _____

53. retro _____

54. semi _____

55. sub _____

56. supra _____

57. sym _____

58. syn _____

59. tetra _____

60. tri _____

61. uni _____

Competency Checklist: Root Words

Write the definitions of the following roots:

1. angio _____

2. angin _____

3. arter _____

4. arterio _____

5. athero _____

6. capillus _____

7. card _____

8. cardi _____

9. cardio _____

10. cubitum _____

11. cyte _____

12. derm _____

13. electro _____

14. embol _____

15. ergo _____

16. erythro _____

17. hemo _____

18. infarct _____

19. lipid _____

20. log _____

21. mano _____

22. myo _____

23. phleb _____

24. phlebo _____

25. pulmonar _____

26. rrhyth _____

27. scler _____

28. sera _____

29. sphygmo _____

30. stetho _____

31. tens _____

32. thromb _____

33. vaso _____

34. veni _____

Competency Checklist: Suffixes

Write the definitions of the following suffixes:

1. algia _____

2. blast _____

3. cele _____

4. centesis _____

5. cyte _____

6. desis _____

7. dynia _____

8. ectomy _____

9. emesis _____

10. gram _____

11. graph _____

12. ist _____

13. itis _____

14. logy _____

15. lysis _____

16. megaly _____

17. meter _____

18. oid _____

19. oma _____

20. opsy _____

21. osis _____

22. pathy _____

23. penia _____

24. pexy _____

25. phagia _____

26. phasia _____

27. philia _____

28. phobia _____

29. phraxis _____

30. physis _____

31. plasia _____

32. plasty _____

33. plegia _____

34. pnea _____

35. poiesis _____

36. ptosis _____

37. ptysis _____

38. rrhage _____

39. rrhagia _____

40. rrhaphy _____

41. rrhea _____

42. rrhexis _____

43. scope _____

44. scopy _____

45. stasis _____

46. stomy _____

47. therapy _____

48. tome _____

49. tomy _____

50. trophy _____

51. uria _____

Competency Checklist: Identifying Medical Terms

Write the medical terms for the following definitions:

1. _____ Process of forming a blood clot

2. _____ Substance that prevents blood clotting

3. _____ The study of diseases of the blood

4. _____ Excess sugar in the blood

5. _____ White blood cell

6. _____ Red blood cell

7. _____ Study of diseases

8. _____ Front area of the elbow

9. _____ Decrease in white blood cells

10. _____ Hardening of the arteries

Competency Checklist: Spelling

In the spaces provided, write the correct spelling of these misspelled terms:

1. imumology _____

2. phlebtomy _____

3. hemmorage _____

4. hemacrit _____

5. leukema _____

6. erthocyte _____

7. homatology _____

8. embollis _____

9. thrombes _____

10. millemeter _____

Competency Checklist: Cardiovascular System

Match the appropriate lettered meaning to the numbered word:

1. Erythrocyte	A. steady state condition of the body
2. Leukocyte	B. heart
3. Arteries	C. carbon dioxide
4. Venules	D. blood clotting mechanism in the body
5. Capillary	E. a blood clotting factor
6. Veins	F. deep vessel in the leg
7. Plasma	G. thrombocytes
8. Serum	H. RBC
9. Antecubital	I. WBC
10. Median cubital vein	J. near the bend of the elbow
11. Basilic vein	K. thick-walled vessels
12. Saphenous vein	L. thin-walled vessels
13. Fibrinogen	M. branching vessels that flow back to the heart
14. Femoral artery	N. contains a mixture of arterial and venous blood
15. Platelets	O. blood specimen that does not contain anticoagulant
16. CO_2	P. blood specimen that does contain an anticoagulant
17. Hemostasis	Q. best vein to use for venipuncture
18. Homeostasis	R. alternate vein to use for venipuncture
19. Deoxygenated blood	S. blood that is carried in the veins
20. Cardiac muscle	T. the longest vessel in the body

References

1. Badasch SA, Chesebro DS: *Introduction to Health Occupations: Today's Health Care Worker,* 5th ed. Upper Saddle River, NJ: Prentice Hall Health, 2000.

2. Rice J: *The Terminology of Health and Medicine,* 2nd ed. Upper Saddle River, NJ: Prentice Hall Health, 2003.

Additional Resources

www.medterms.com provides easy-to-understand descriptions of medical terms.

www.familydoctor.org provides a dictionary of common medical terms.

www.medilexicon.com provides medical terminology definitions.

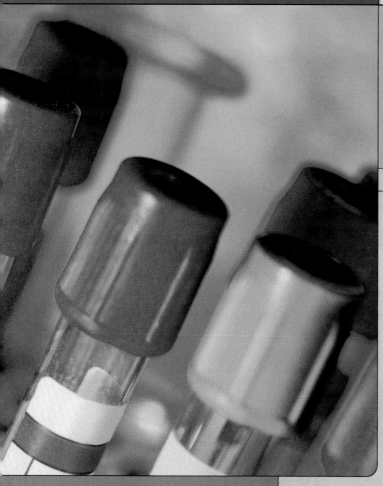

Chapter 4

Safety and Infection Control

CHAPTER OBJECTIVES

Upon completion of Chapter 4, the learner should be able to do the following:

1. Explain the safety policies and procedures that must be followed in specimen collection and transportation.

2. Define the term *health care–acquired (nosocomial) infection.*

3. Identify the basic programs for safety, infection control, and isolation procedures.

4. Explain the proper techniques for handwashing, gowning, gloving, masking, double bagging, and entering and exiting the various isolation areas.

5. Identify steps to avoid transmission of bloodborne pathogens.

6. Explain the measures that should be taken for fire, electrical, radiation, and chemical safety in a health care facility.

7. Describe the essential elements of a disaster emergency plan for a health care facility.

8. List three precautions that can reduce the risk of injury to patients.

KEY TERMS

antiseptics

aseptic

bloodborne pathogens (BBP)

Centers for Disease Control and Prevention (CDC)

chain of infection

disinfectants

double-bagging

Environmental Protection Agency (EPA)

fomites

The goal of safety for health care facilities is to get rid of hazards for patients and employees and provide safety education for health care workers. Safe working guidelines for health care facilities and employees have been developed by the federal **Occupational Safety and Health Administration (OSHA)** and the **Centers for Disease Control and Prevention (CDC)**. Providing protection from hazardous events in the health care environment for the patient is an important part of the health care worker's everyday responsibilities.

Personal Safety from Infection During Specimen Handling

Patients' specimens should be handled with caution to prevent the possibility of acquiring **bloodborne pathogens (BBP)**, which are infectious organisms found in blood and other body fluids (i.e., hepatitis B and C viruses and human immunodeficiency virus [HIV]). This preventive approach is called **universal precautions**.[1] OSHA requires health care facilities to protect workers exposed to biological hazards. Health care workers who are routinely exposed to blood and body fluids must wear gloves and other **personal protective equipment (PPE)** (facial shields, gowns, etc.) to protect themselves from infection as well. These requirements have occurred because of the 1991 OSHA standards for occupational exposure to bloodborne pathogens (29 CFR 1930.1030) and the Needlestick Safety and Prevention Act (2001).[2] These federal regulations require that, in most cases, warning labels be placed on containers (refrigerators, freezers, infectious waste, etc.) that contain blood or other potentially infectious materials. The labels required are fluorescent orange or orange-red and feature the biohazard alerts shown in Figure 4-1 ■ and Figure 4-2 ■.

EXPOSURE CONTROL

If an accident occurs, such as a needlestick, the injured health care worker should immediately cleanse the area with isopropyl alcohol and apply an adhesive bandage. Any incident of exposure to potentially harmful bloodborne pathogens or other infectious body fluids should be reported immediately to the supervisor.[3] Each health care worker should know whom to contact, where to go, and what to do if exposed to harmful pathogens. The report must include the blood collection device that did not work effectively to protect the health care worker during blood collection. If exposures are not reported, it is difficult to prove retrospectively that an exposure to an infection was caused by working conditions.

HEALTH CARE–ACQUIRED (NOSOCOMIAL) INFECTIONS

Health care–acquired (nosocomial) infections are those that are acquired by a patient after admission to a health care facility, such as a hospital, clinic, or nursing home. In an

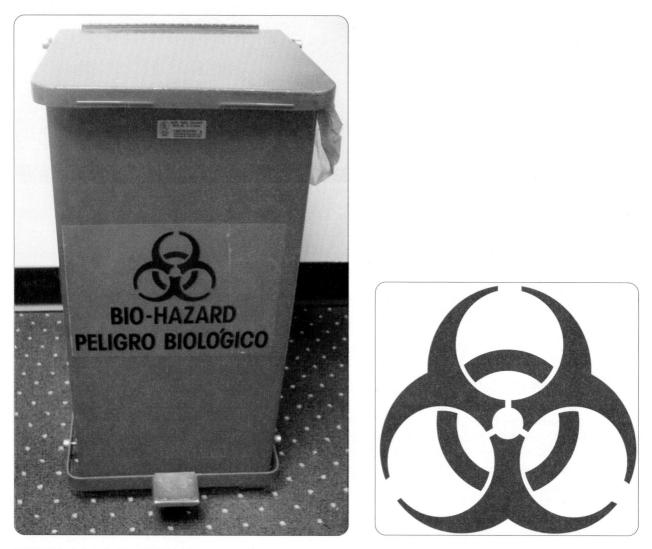

FIGURE ■ 4-1 Label for Biohazard   **FIGURE ■ 4-2** Label for Biohazard

attempt to control them, **infection control programs** have been developed. Using guidelines established by the CDC, The Joint Commission, and state regulatory agencies, managers of health care institutions address the issues of proper **aseptic** technique (i.e., to prevent growth of microorganisms), **isolation procedures**, education, and management of health care–acquired infections. The CDC provides infection control and safety guidelines to protect health care workers and patients from infection. The cornerstones of infection protection of patients and health care workers are aseptic techniques, which include the following:

- Frequent handwashing
- Use of barrier garments and personal protective equipment (PPE)
- Waste management of contaminated materials
- Use of proper cleaning solutions
- Following standard precautions
- Using sterile procedures when necessary

These protective procedures must become part of a health care worker's routine procedures and standards for practice. Because each health care facility has its own infection control program and policy manual, the health care worker should read and be familiar with both.

Chain of Infection

Nosocomial (health care–acquired) infections result when the **chain of infection** is complete (Table 4-1 ■).

The three components that make up the chain are the (1) **source**, (2) **mode of transmission**, and (3) **susceptible host**. Infection control programs aim at breaking the infection chain at one or more links, as shown in Figure 4-3 ■. Handwashing procedures for sterile technique, proper waste disposal, appropriate laundry services, and housekeeping are ways of controlling the sources. Isolation techniques, control of insects and rodents, and the use of disposable equipment and supplies help interrupt the modes of transmission. Host susceptibility is controlled by speeding the patient's recovery. Immunizations, transfusions, proper nutrition, medication, and adequate exercise all help the patient to become healthy.

TABLE ■ 4-1

Chain of Infection

A pathogen must be present

A source of disease, including patients who have a disease and human carriers of disease (i.e., health care provider and patient's family members) who are unaware they have the disease but can still transmit it to another

A mode of transmission for the pathogen to pass directly from the source to the new host (i.e., touching infected individuals, individuals spreading infection through coughing or sneezing, inadequate ventilation, and invasive medical instruments)

A susceptible host (i.e., hospital patient) that cannot fight off the pathogen (i.e., elderly persons and patients with cancer)

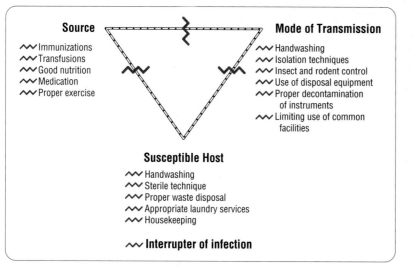

FIGURE ■ 4-3 The Chain of Infection
Health care–acquired infection can be interrupted by infection control procedures

Standard Precautions

Standard precautions (Figure 4-4 ▣) have been designed through the CDC to decrease the risk of transmission of microorganisms from both recognized and unrecognized sources of infection in hospitals. Standard precautions include *universal precautions* that are designed to prevent transmission of all infectious agents in the health care setting.

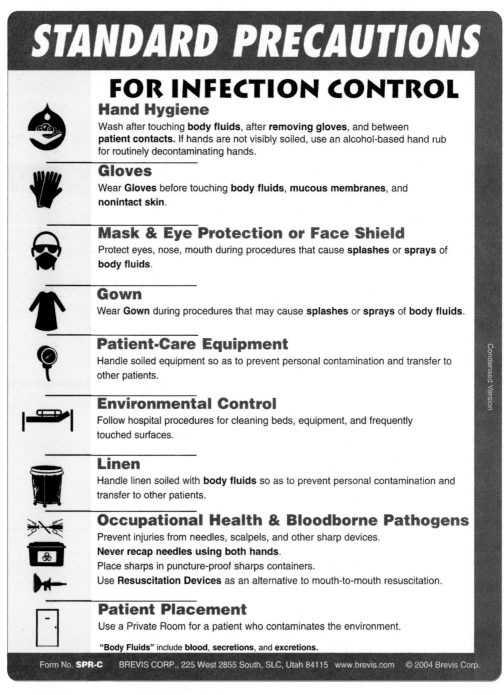

FIGURE ▣ **4-4** Infection Control
Courtesy of BREVIS Corp.

They provide protection from contact with blood, all body fluids, mucous membranes, and nonintact skin. **Transmission-based precautions** are used in addition to standard precautions for patients with known or suspected infections that are spread in one of three ways, by (1) airborne transmission; (2) droplet transmission; or (3) contact transmission (Figures 4-5 ■ and 4-6 ■).[4,5,6]

- **Airborne precautions** decrease the spread of airborne droplet transmission of infectious diseases such as rubeola, varicella, and tuberculosis.[7]

- **Droplet precautions** are used to decrease the transmission of diseases such as pertussis (whooping cough) and pneumonia. These diseases can be transmitted through contact with eye, mouth, or nose secretions from sneezing, coughing, or talking.

- **Contact precautions** decrease the risk of infection to other patients and health care workers from diseases such as herpes simplex that can occur through direct or indirect contact.

All three types of precautions may be used at one time when multiple infectious microorganisms are suspected in a patient. These precautions are *always* used with standard precautions.

USE OF STANDARD PRECAUTIONS

Health care workers should follow these guidelines when collecting blood from a patient in order to reduce the possibility of obtaining an infection from a patient.

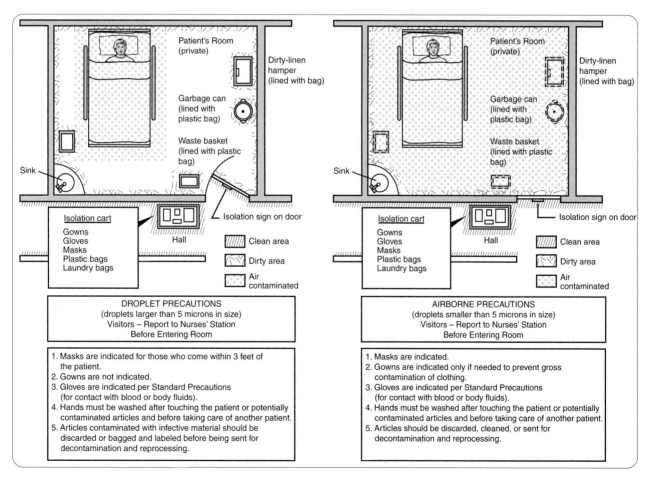

FIGURE ■ 4-5 Transmission-Based Precautions

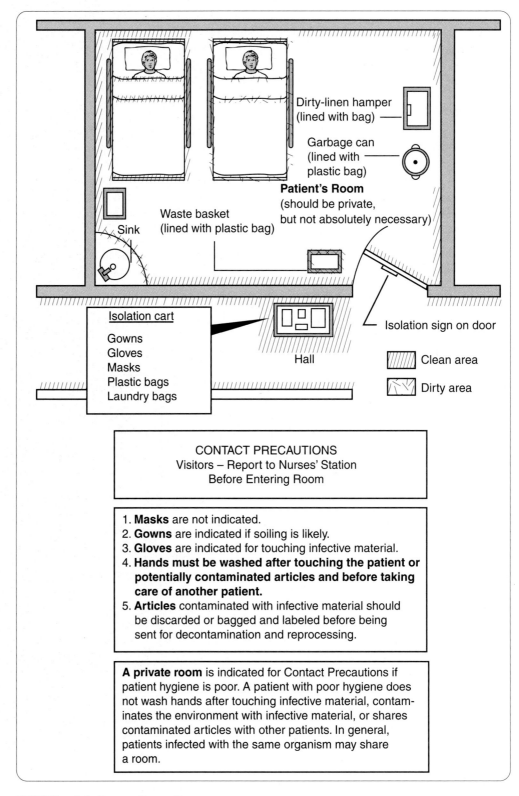

FIGURE ■ 4-6 Contact Precautions

1. Use personal protective equipment (i.e., gloves, facial masks, gowns, and respirators) to prevent skin and mucous membrane exposure when contact with blood or other body fluids of any patient is anticipated. This will prevent transmission by **fomites** (objects that transmit infection, such as door knobs, telephones, countertops, etc.).

   a. Gloves should be worn for

      i. Handling objects or surfaces soiled with blood or body fluids; and
      ii. Performing venipunctures, skin punctures, and intravenous (IV) line collections.

   b. Gloves should be changed after contact with each patient and wash the hands or use alcohol hand sanitizers after glove removal and before donning new gloves.

   c. Masks and protective eyewear or face shields should be worn to prevent exposure of mucous membranes of the mouth, nose, and eyes during procedures that are likely to cause droplets or splashes of blood or other body fluids.

   d. A personal respirator should be used if the risk of tuberculosis is present.

   e. Footwear (i.e., covers the entire foot) should be worn that protects against broken glass possibly contaminated with blood or other body fluids (i.e., flip flops, sandals, and clogs are **not** recommended).

2. Hands and other skin surfaces should be washed immediately and thoroughly if contaminated with blood or other body fluids. Hands should be washed immediately after gloves are removed! If hands are not visibly soiled, either an alcohol-based rub or soap and water may be used.[8] Proper handwashing technique is shown in Procedure 4-1.

Clinical Alert !

- Do not wear artificial fingernails or extenders because of the possible spread of pathogenic infections and fungus to patients.
- Remove gloves after collecting blood from a patient. DO NOT wear the same pair of gloves for the blood collection of more than one patient.
- Wash or decontaminate hands with alcohol-based rub before placing new gloves on hands.

---

3. Take precautions to prevent injuries caused by needles and other sharp instruments or devices

   a. During blood collection procedures,
   b. During the disposal of used needles, lancets, etc., and
   c. When handling any sharp instruments after procedures.

4. To prevent infections from BBPs as a result of needlestick injuries, health care workers should

   a. Only use safety engineered needle and sharps devices.
   b. NOT recap needles, purposely bend or break them by hand, remove them from disposable syringes or holders, or handle them for any reason.
   c. Immediately dispose of the blood tube holder and safety needle as a single unit after blood collection.
   d. Place disposable syringes and needles, lancets, and other sharp items, after they are used, in puncture-resistant containers for transport to the biohazardous waste center.

Handwashing Technique

RATIONALE

To perform proper handwashing technique.

PROCEDURE

---

(1) Remove jewelry (including rings, with the exception of watches, wedding bands, and bracelets) and stand at the sink without allowing clothing to touch the sink. Wet hands with water. Foot pedals are preferable for controlling the flow of water but they are not available in all health care facilities (Figure 4-7 ■).

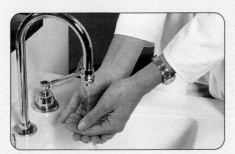

FIGURE ■ 4-7

(2) Dispense a small amount of soap to the hands (1–2 teaspoonfuls or the amount recommended by the manufacturer) (Figure 4-8 ■). If using bar soap, keep the bar in hands and use enough soap to form a lather by moving your hands over each other and between the fingers of each hand.

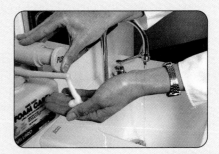

FIGURE ■ 4-8

Clinical Alert ❗

- Standard precautions have been designed to be used for patients, health care providers, and visitors in health care facilities.
- Standard precautions reduce the risk of infections being transmitted from health care workers to patients, patients to patients, patients to health care workers, and health care workers to other health care workers or visitors.
- These precautions apply in the following situations:
  ◦ Contact with blood
  ◦ Contact with body fluids
  ◦ Contact with mucous membranes and wounds

ISOLATION FOR HOSPITAL OUTBREAKS

Occasionally, outbreaks of particular infections occur in one or more hospital areas. To control the outbreak, the need for special precautions and isolation procedures might

3 Rub hands together vigorously for at least 15 seconds, covering all surfaces of the hands and fingers (Figure 4-9).

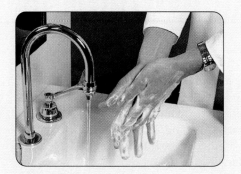

FIGURE ■ 4-9

4 Rinse hands in a downward motion with water (Figure 4-10) and dry thoroughly with a clean disposable towel. Multiple-use cloth towels of the hanging or roll type are not acceptable for use in health care settings, because they can transmit microorganisms.

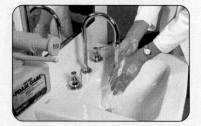

FIGURE ■ 4-10

5 Turn off the faucet with a dry disposable towel if not using a foot pedal (Figure 4-11 ■).

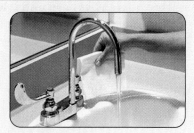

FIGURE ■ 4-11

occur. Any health care worker entering or exiting these areas should be made aware of the special circumstances.

PROTECTIVE, OR REVERSE, ISOLATION

A few hospitals in the United States have large **protective isolation** facilities for patients with immunodeficiencies (suppression of their immune system) who must live in an environment that is completely sterile. All food and articles are sterilized before they are taken into the patient's room. Some patients must live in these protected environments when they are recovering from, for example, cancer treatments.

INFECTION CONTROL IN SPECIAL HOSPITAL UNITS

Infection Control in a Nursery Unit

Newborns are easy targets for infections of all sorts, because their immune systems are not fully developed at birth. Neonates may pick up pathogens from their mothers, other babies, or hospital personnel. The best way to minimize infection is to use gloves and an **antiseptic** for handwashing. Special clothing may be worn by nursery personnel, changed daily, and limited to the unit. Bibs should be used and discarded after contact with only one baby. Often, a baby is assigned a single nurse, to limit the possible sources of infection transmission. Babies whose mothers have genital herpes must be isolated from other infants. Mothers with genital herpes must also be isolated. All individuals having contact with either the mothers or the children must be gowned and gloved, and **double-bagging** (as described later in this chapter) procedures must be used for the disposal of contaminated articles in the patient's room.

Infection Control in a Burn Unit

Patients with burns are also highly susceptible to infection. Each bed is surrounded by a plastic curtain with sleeves. Hospital personnel use these sleeves to have contact with the patient. All supplies and equipment are kept outside the curtain. In hospitals lacking these facilities, burn patients are housed in private rooms. Gowning, gloving, **double-bagging**, and strict handwashing procedures should be used. All articles in the room, as well as the room itself, should be disinfected or sterilized frequently.

Infection Control in an ICU or Postoperative Care Unit

Patients in **intensive care units (ICUs)** are more critically ill and, by nature, are more susceptible to infections. In most hospitals, ICUs are open areas, with numerous patients in one large room. Patients with known infections are isolated according to the types of infections they have, and strict handwashing and gloving policies are necessary in all ICUs.

Specific Isolation Techniques and Procedural Steps

In most hospitals, all supplies required for isolation procedures (see Procedures 4-2, 4-3, and 4-4) are located in an area or on a cart just outside the patient's room (Figure 4-12 ▒). These include:

- Disposable gloves
- Gown
- Mask
- Protective eyewear

The type of PPE used will vary on the basis of the level of precautions required (i.e., standard and contact, droplet, or airborne infection isolation).

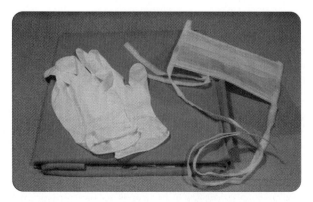

FIGURE ▒ **4-12** Supplies for Isolation Procedures

Gowning, Masking, and Gloving

RATIONALE

To prevent the transmission of microorganisms from health care workers to patients, or from patients to health care workers.

EQUIPMENT

- Alcohol-based rub or soap and water
- Gown
- Mask

- Face shield or goggles
- Chemically clean disposable gloves or sterile disposable gloves

PROCEDURE

Follow these isolation procedural steps:

① Decontaminate hands using an alcohol-based hand rub or soap and water as described in Procedure 4-1 (Figure 4-13 ■).

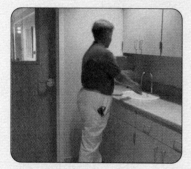

FIGURE ■ 4-13

② Use gowns large enough to cover all clothing (Figure 4-14 ■).

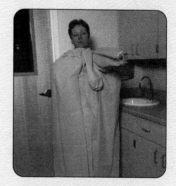

FIGURE ■ 4-14

③ Touching only its inside surface, place one arm at a time through the gown's sleeves and wrap the gown completely around the body. Gowns are generally made of cloth and paper (Figure 4-15 ■).

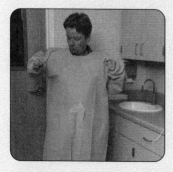

FIGURE ■ 4-15

④ Pull down the sleeves, then bring the waist ties from the back to the front of gown and tie them in back (Figure 4-16 ■).

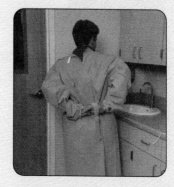

FIGURE ■ 4-16

(continued)

5 Tie or use the Velcro strap to close the gown around the neck (Figure 4-17 ■).

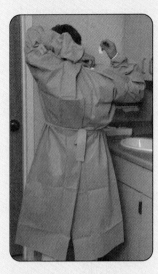

FIGURE ■ 4-17

6 Don mask (Figure 4-18 ■). Masks protect the health care worker from small-particle droplets that may carry pathogens. Often, a small metal band on the mask can be shaped to fit the nose. Two ties are usually made, the first around the upper portion of the head and the second around the upper portion of the neck. Most masks become ineffective after prolonged use (20 minutes) or if they become wet.[5]

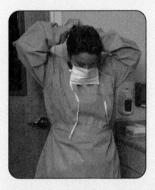

FIGURE ■ 4-18

7 Wear a face shield or goggles during procedures that may possibly generate blood or body fluid droplets (i.e., splashes or sprays), such as from severe patient coughing (Figure 4-19 ■).

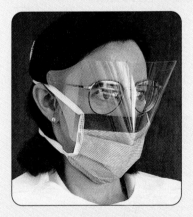

FIGURE ■ 4-19

8 Pull gloves over the ends of gown sleeves (Figure 4-20 ■). Chemically clean disposable gloves may be used for most isolation procedures. For isolation procedures in which the patient must be protected from any microorganisms, use sterile disposable gloves. Do not wear rings and other pieces of jewelry, because they may puncture a glove during patient contact.

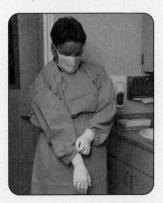

FIGURE ■ 4-20

Removal of Isolation Gown, Mask, and Gloves

RATIONALE

To prevent the transmission of microorganisms, remove the PPE at the doorway or in the interior room (anteroom), except for the respirator. Remove the respirator after leaving the patient's room and closing the door.

EQUIPMENT

- Large red isolation bag
- Linen hamper
- Special container for disposing masks

PROCEDURE

After the completion of blood collection in an isolation room, follow these steps for removing the isolation gown, mask, and gloves:

1. Remove the gloves as shown in (Figure 4-21 ■). Pull off the first glove in such a manner to turn it inside out. Place the rolled-up glove into the palm of the hand that is still gloved. Remove the second glove by slipping the index finger of the ungloved hand between the glove and the hand. Then pull the glove down and off as it turns inside out. Dispose of both gloves in a red garbage bag in the isolation room.

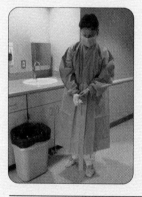

FIGURE ■ 4-21

After the removal of gloves, remove the goggles or face shield by touching the head band or ear pieces. (DO NOT TOUCH THE OUTSIDE OF GOGGLES OR FACE SHIELD BECAUSE OF CONTAMINATION.)

2. Unfasten the gown's ties. Take off the gown by pulling down from the neck and shoulders first and then pull the arms out of the gown (Figure 4-22 ■). Remove the gown and fold it with the contaminated side turned inside and with care taken not to touch the uniform.

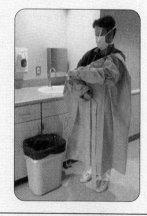

FIGURE ■ 4-22

3. Only use gowns once to prevent contamination. Dispose of the gown in the linen hamper or, if disposable, in a garbage bag in the isolation room (Figure 4-23 ■).

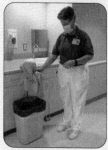

FIGURE ■ 4-23

(continued)

④ Remove the mask by carefully untying the lower tie first, then the upper one (Figure 4-24 ■). Only hold the ends of the ties. Properly dispose of the mask inside the room. In some cases, a special container for masks is placed just outside the room to prevent exposure of hospital personnel to airborne pathogens while inside the isolation room.

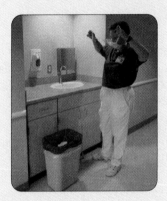

FIGURE ■ 4-24

⑤ Wash hands in the room and again at the nearest sink after exiting the room (Figure 4-25 ■). Use a clean paper towel to open the door. Hold the door open with one foot and discard the used paper towels in the wastebasket directly inside the patient's room.

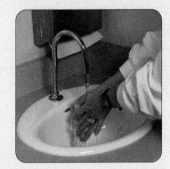

FIGURE ■ 4-25

ISOLATION ITEM DISPOSAL

The supplies needed for isolation item disposal include:

- Garbage bag
- Linen hamper
- Large red isolation bag
- Specimen container
- Plastic bag with biohazard label
- Laundry bag
- Puncture-resistant disposal container for needle and sharps
- Gloves
- Antiseptic agent or antimicrobial agent

Isolation bags for transporting specimens should be turned halfway inside out and left near the door outside the room; someone may be available to hold the bag outside the door. Only the needed supplies should be taken into the room. Phlebotomy requisitions may be left outside the room on the isolation cart. If collecting a blood specimen, the health care provider may use a tourniquet in the room or leave the one brought in. The specimen should be labeled at the bedside and the pen left in the room. Used needles, swabs, and so forth should be put in appropriate containers inside the room. Any blood on the outside of the specimen container should be removed with a paper towel. While standing in the doorway and touching only the inside of the isolation bag, the health care worker should place the specimen inside the bag. Gloved hands should be washed in the room. The faucet may be turned off with a paper towel.

Disposing of Contaminated Items

RATIONALE

To properly dispose of contaminated items and prevent the transmission of microorganisms.
Trash, linens, and other articles in an isolation room may be removed by using one sturdy biohazard bag or the double-bagging procedure.

EQUIPMENT

- Two large red isolation bags

PROCEDURE

(1) Put contaminated material in one bag and seal the bag inside the room as shown in Figure 4-26 ■.

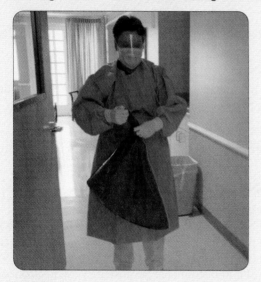

FIGURE ■ 4-26

(2) Have another person stand outside the room with another opened, clean, impermeable bag (Figure 4-27 ■). The person standing outside the room should have the ends of the bag folded over their hands to shield from possible contamination. Place the sealed bag from the room in the clean bag. The person outside the room can then fold over the edges, expel the air, and seal the outer bag. Label the bag with biohazard warnings.

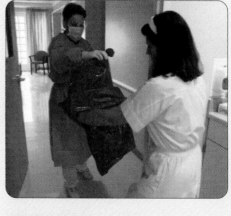

FIGURE ■ 4-27

INFECTION CONTROL AND SAFETY IN THE CLINICAL LABORATORY

The laboratory receives numerous patients' specimens for diagnostic procedures to be performed to determine causes of diseases and disorders. Health care workers in the laboratory must be extremely cautious, because they often handle specimens with infectious agents. The following essentials of standard precautions and safe laboratory work practices should be adhered to when in the laboratory:

- Frequent handwashing
- Assuming all patients are infectious for HIV and other bloodborne pathogens
- Using personal protection equipment

- Using appropriate waste-disposal practices
- Maintaining good personal hygiene, including wearing clean clothes, keeping hair clean and tied back if necessary, keeping fingernails clean, and washing hands frequently
- Not eating, drinking, smoking, or applying cosmetics (including lip balm)
- Not inserting or removing contact lenses
- Avoiding biting nails or chewing on pens
- Carefully disposing of safety needles, lancets, and other blood-collection supplies in appropriate biohazardous labeled containers
- Maintaining good health by eating balanced meals, getting enough sleep, and getting enough exercise
- Reporting personal illnesses to supervisors
- Becoming familiar with and observing *all* isolation policies
- Learning about the job-related aspects of infection control, and sharing this information with others
- Cautioning all personnel working with known hazardous material (this can be done with proper warning labels)
- Reporting violations of the policies
- Covering patients' specimens at all times during transportation and centrifugation
- Centrifuging specimens within a biohazard safety hood
- Cleaning phlebotomy trays at least once a week with a 1:10 bleach solution
- Cleaning the specimen collection area with a decontaminating 1:10 bleach solution

DISINFECTANTS AND ANTISEPTICS

Disinfectants are chemical compounds used to remove or kill pathogenic microorganisms. Chemical disinfectants are regulated by the Environmental Protection Agency (EPA). Antiseptics are chemicals used to inhibit the growth and development of microorganisms, but they do not necessarily kill them. Antiseptics may be used on human skin, whereas disinfectants are generally used on surfaces and instruments because they are too corrosive for direct use on skin. A disinfectant with a product label claiming that the disinfectant is HIV-cidal or tuberculocidal, or a disinfectant having a chlorine bleach dilution of 1:10, should be used to disinfect items contaminated with blood or other body fluids. A more dilute solution of chlorine bleach (1:100) can be used for routine cleaning of surfaces. Gloves and gowns should be worn when performing decontamination procedures. The minimal contact time for disinfectants to be effective is 10 minutes. Table 4-2 ■ lists some of the more common hospital disinfectants and antiseptics.

Fire Safety

Fire safety is the responsibility of all employees in the health care institution. Fire or explosive hazards may occur in the laboratory or other areas of the health care facility. Health care workers should be familiar with not only the use and location of the fire extinguishers but also the procedures to follow during a fire. They should also be knowledgeable of the exact locations of fire extinguishers and fire blankets. The blankets should be available to smother burning clothes or to use as a fire shield if fire is blocking the exit. Health care institutions usually conduct periodic safety education programs in which the health care worker can participate to become skillful in and knowledgeable about the use of fire safety equipment (Figure 4-28 ■).

Compound	Uses and Restrictions
Alcohols	
Ethyl (70%)	Antiseptic for skin
Isopropyl (70%)	Antiseptic for skin
Chlorine	
Chloramine	Disinfectant for wounds
Hypochlorite solutions	Disinfectant
Ethylene oxide	Disinfectant (toxic)
Formaldehyde	Disinfectant (noxious fumes)
Glutaraldehyde	Disinfectant (toxic)
Hydrogen peroxide	Antiseptic for skin
Iodine	
Tincture	Antiseptic for skin (can be irritating)
Iodophors	Antiseptic for skin (less stable)
Phenolic compounds	
1%–2% phenols	Disinfectant
Chlorophenol	Disinfectant (toxic)
Chlorhexidine	Antiseptic for skin
Hexylresorcinol	Antiseptic for skin
Quaternary ammonium compounds	Antiseptic for skin (ingredient in many soaps)

TABLE ■ 4-2

Common Antiseptics and Disinfectants for the Health Care Setting

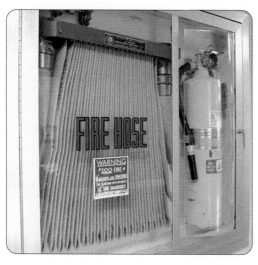

FIGURE ■ 4-28 Fire Extinguisher and Fire Hose

Health care workers need to learn how to use fire extinguishers.[9] As shown in Figure 4-29 ■, Class A fires require an ABC extinguisher or pressurized water extinguisher for wood, paper, clothing, and trash. The Class B fires need an ABC extinguisher or carbon dioxide (CO_2) extinguisher for liquids, grease, and chemical fires. Class C fires are electrical fires and a CO_2, halon, or ABC extinguisher can be used. The ABC extinguisher is found in most health care facilities, so health care workers need not worry about which extinguisher to use in case of a fire.

FIGURE ■ 4-29

Proper Use of Fire
Extinguishers

*Source: Courtesy of Health
and Environmental Safety,
The University of Texas Health
Science Center at Houston.*

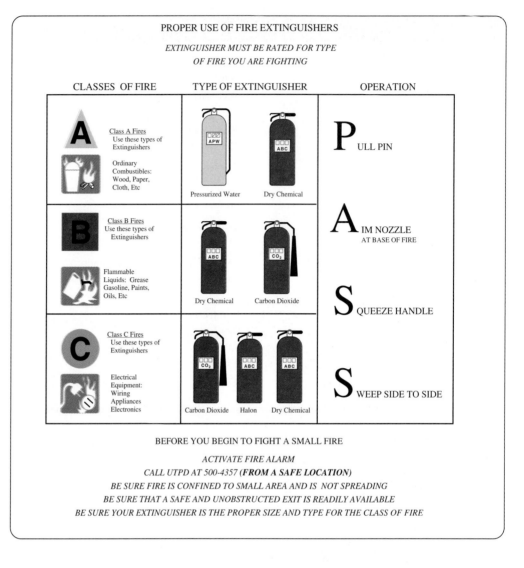

EMERGENCY RESPONSE TO POSSIBLE FIRE

If a fire or explosion occurs in the workplace, the health care worker should ***not*** do the following:

- Block entrances
- Reenter the building
- Panic
- Run

Instead the health care worker should **RACE**: ***Rescue Alarm Contain Exit. RACE*** by doing the following:

- Pull the nearest fire alarm.
- Call 911 or the hospital's fire emergency number, which should be posted on or near the phone.

- Remove patients from danger if on patient floor.
- Close windows and doors to prevent spreading of the fire.
- If the fire is small and isolated from other possible fuel sources, use an ABC extinguisher to fight it:

  1. Pull the plastic lock off of the extinguisher.
  2. Aim the extinguisher at the base of the fire and squeeze the handle.
  3. Spray the solution toward the base of the fire but do not point it directly at an individual.

- If the fire threatens to block exits or is not small, leave the area immediately. Take the stairs, not the elevator.
- If clothing is on fire, drop to the ground and roll, preferably in a fire blanket.
- If caught in a fire, crawl to the exit. Because smoke rises, breathing is easier at floor level. Breathing through a wet towel is also helpful.

Electrical Safety

A major hazard in any area of a health care institution is the possibility of electrical current passing through a person. The important safety points to remember are:

- Do not use power cords that are frayed.
- Avoid using extension cords.
- While collecting blood, avoid contact with any electrical equipment, because the electricity may pass through you and the needle and shock the patient.
- Use three-prong electrical plugs for all equipment (Figure 4-30 ■).

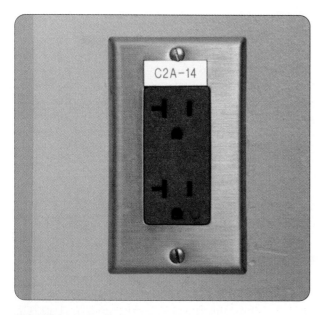

FIGURE ■ **4-30** Three-Prong Electrical Outlet

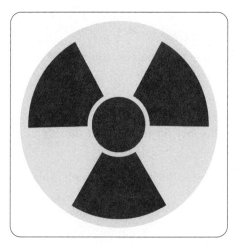

FIGURE ■ 4-31 Radiation Hazard Sign

Radiation Safety

The three cardinal principles of self-protection from radiation exposure are time, shielding, and distance. Radiation exposure is cumulative; thus, limiting the length of exposure at any one time is a major factor in minimizing the hazard.

Areas where radioactive materials are in use and stored must have warning signs (Figure 4-31 ■) posted on the entrance doors. The health care worker will probably encounter potential hazards from radiation exposure only if he or she must collect specimens from patients in the nuclear medicine or x-ray department or must take specimens to the radioimmunoassay section of a research or a clinical chemistry laboratory. Thus, the health care worker should be cautious when entering an area posted with the radiation hazard sign and should be knowledgeable about the institution's procedures pertaining to radiation safety.

Chemical Safety

Because a health care worker must sometimes pour preservatives, such as hydrochloric acid (HCl), into containers for 24-hour urine collections and transport these specimens to the patients' floor, he or she should be knowledgeable about chemical safety (Figure 4-32 ■). Labeling may be the single most important step in the proper handling of chemicals. Laboratorians should be able to ascertain from appropriate labels not only the contents of the container but also the nature and extent of hazards posed by the chemicals. Carefully read the label before using any reagents.

> **Clinical Alert** !
>
> When mixing acids with water, ALWAYS add acid to water. NEVER add water to acid because it can explode.

The **National Fire Protection Association (NFPA)** developed a labeling system for hazardous chemicals that is frequently used in health care facilities (Figure 4-33 ■). The system uses a diamond-shaped symbol, four colored quadrants, and a hazard rating scale of 0 to 4. The health hazard is shown in the blue quadrant; the flammability hazard is

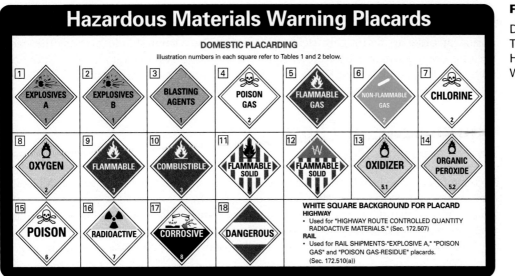

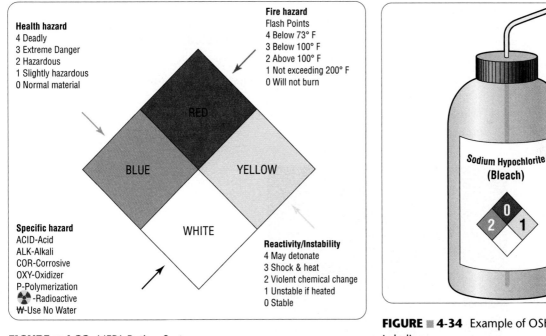

FIGURE ▦ 4-33 NFPA Rating System

FIGURE ▦ 4-34 Example of OSHA-Mandated Labeling

shown in the red quadrant; the instability hazard is indicated in the yellow quadrant; and the specific hazard is shown in the white quadrant. Common laboratory chemicals such as isopropyl alcohol or diluted bleach (sodium hypochlorite) in squirt bottles require regulatory labels (Figure 4-34 ▦).

SAFETY SHOWERS AND THE EYEWASH STATION

Safety showers should be nearby for use if an accidental chemical spill occurs. Because permanent damage to the skin can result from chemical burns, the victim of a chemical accident must immediately rinse for at least 15 minutes after removing contaminated clothing.

In case of a chemical spill in the eye, the victim should rinse his or her eyes at the eyewash station for a minimum of 15 minutes. Contact lenses must be removed before the rinsing in order to thoroughly cleanse the eyes. The victim should not rub the eyes, because doing so may cause further injury. If someone is hurt in a chemical spill, it is preferable to take the victim to the emergency department for treatment after his or her eyes have been rinsed for 15 minutes.

Equipment and Safety in Patients' Rooms

Each member of the health care team is responsible for the safety of the patient. All health care professionals are responsible for patient safety from the time the patient enters the health care setting until his or her departure. First, when collecting blood from a hospitalized patient, provide privacy for the patient during the procedure (Figure 4-35 ■).

As a matter of general patient safety, do the following when in the patient's room:

1. Make certain that all specimen collection supplies, needles, and equipment are either properly disposed of or returned to the specimen collection tray after blood collection.

2. Check to see whether the bed rails are up or down. Always place bed rails up before leaving the patient if they were up when you entered the room.

3. Check for food or liquid spilled on the floor, urine spills, or IV line leakage.

4. If the patient's alarm for the IV drip is sounding, report this problem to the nursing station immediately.

5. If the patient is in unusual pain or is unresponsive, notify the nursing station immediately.

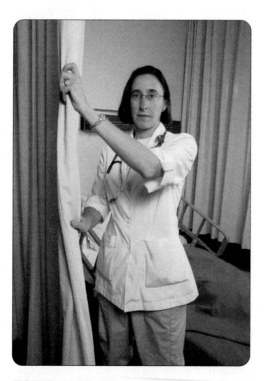

FIGURE ■ 4-35 Patient Privacy

Patient Safety Related to Latex Products

Patients, as well as health care workers, may be allergic to latex products (Figure 4-36 ■).

The signs and symptoms of an allergic reaction to latex may include a skin rash, hives, nasal, eye, or sinus irritation, and sometimes, shock. Table 4-3 ■ provides examples of items frequently used in the health care environment that contain latex. Figure 4-37 ■ shows an example of a Latex-Safe Environment sign.

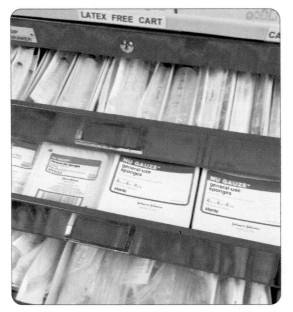

FIGURE ■ **4-36** Latex-Free Cart

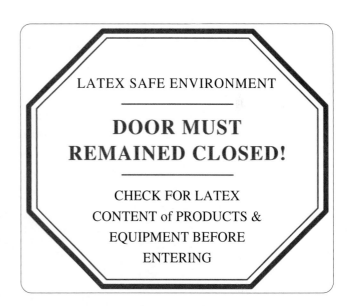

FIGURE ■ **4-37** Latex-Safe Environment Sign

Medical Equipment	Personal Protective Equipment	Office Supplies	Medical Supplies
Tourniquets	Gloves	Adhesive tape	Condom-style urinary collection device
Syringes	Goggles	Erasers	Enema tubing tips
Stethoscopes	Rubber aprons	Rubber bands	Injection ports
Oral and nasal airways	Surgical masks		Rubber tops of stoppers on multidose vials
IV tubing			
Disposable gloves			Urinary catheter
Breathing circuits			Wound drains
Blood pressure cuffs			

TABLE ■ **4-3**

Products Containing Latex

Source: Reprinted from Preventing Allergic Reactions to Natural Rubber Latex in the Workplace. *National Institute for Occupational Safety and Health Alert, June 1997. Atlanta, GA: The Centers for Disease Control and Prevention.*

Disaster Emergency Plan

Many health care institutions have developed procedures to be followed in case of a hurricane, flooding, earthquake, bomb threat, and other disasters. The health care worker should become familiar with these procedures, because he or she must be prepared to take immediate action whenever conditions warrant such action (Figure 4-38 ■).

Clinical Alert !

If someone telephones and threatens to bomb the health care facility:

- Listen to the person and keep him or her talking.
- Listen for background noises to identify the caller's location.
- Listen for the caller's accent, language, and voice characteristics.
- Ask the caller where the bomb is located and what time it will go off.
- Write down everything the caller states.
- Notify the health care facility's security officer.

If a bomb threat procedure is in place, it must be used by all health care workers.

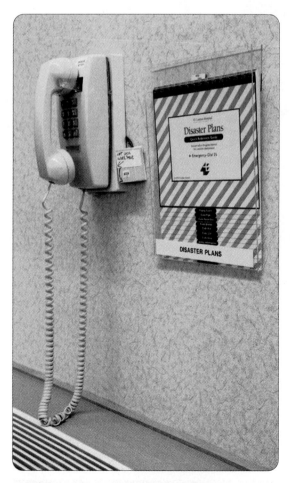

FIGURE ■ 4-38 Disaster Plans and Phone

Self Study

Study Questions

For the following questions, select the one best answer.

1. If a health care worker is caught in a fire in the health care facility, she or he should **not**:

   a. close all the doors and windows before leaving the area
   b. call the assigned fire number
   c. run
   d. attempt to extinguish the fire if it is small

2. What are the major principles of self-protection from radiation exposure?

   a. time, distance, and shielding
   b. distance, shielding, and combustibility
   c. combustibility, anticorrosiveness, and time
   d. shielding, distance, and anticorrosiveness

3. The health care worker was asked to bring a chemical into the chemistry laboratory. The health care worker noticed that a yellow quadrant of a diamond on the chemical's label showed 1. This yellow quadrant of the diamond, according to NFPA, indicates a:

   a. flammability hazard
   b. health hazard
   c. instability hazard
   d. specific hazard

4. If an accident occurs, such as a needlestick, the injured health care worker should first and immediately:

   a. call his or her immediate supervisor from the location of the needlestick accident
   b. cleanse the area with isopropyl alcohol and apply an adhesive bandage
   c. fill out the incident report form
   d. take the needle back to the clinical laboratory for verification of the accident

5. Safe working conditions must be ensured by the employer and have been mandated by law under the:

   a. Occupational Safety and Facility Act
   b. Occupational Safety and Health Administration Act
   c. Health Care Facility and Occupational Safety Act
   d. Health Care Institutional Safety and Health Act

6. Antiseptics for skin include:

   a. formaldehyde
   b. iodine
   c. ethylene oxide
   d. hypochlorite solution

7. In a health care facility, which is a typical fomite?

   a. 95% isopropyl alcohol
   b. iodine
   c. telephone
   d. facial shield

8. Which of the following isolation techniques is used to decrease the spread of whooping cough?

   a. droplet precautions
   b. contact precautions
   c. airborne precautions
   d. enteric precautions

9. Reverse isolation is the same as:

   a. protective isolation
   b. enteric isolation
   c. airborne precautions
   d. contact precautions

10. What is the proper order for removal of isolation PPE?

    a. gloves, gown, and then goggles
    b. goggles, gloves, and then gown
    c. gloves, goggles, and then gown
    d. gown, gloves, and then goggles

Case Study

Clara is a Certified Nursing Assistant who has also been training to be a phlebotomist in a rural health clinic. Her supervisor has asked her to start home health care visits so that she can take history and physical assessments and perform any needed blood collection procedures. On her first assignment, she is sent to four patients' homes that are approximately 65 miles from the clinic to collect *fasting* (has not eaten for 8 to 12 hours) blood samples for glucose testing needed to regulate their insulin injections. When she arrives at the first home, she gathers all of her blood collection equipment and enters the home for the collection. As soon as she opens the blood collection container, she realizes that she does not have gloves for the blood collection. However, because of time commitments, she collects the blood from this patient and the other patients in their homes. She figures that if she washes her hands after collecting the blood from each patient, she will be okay. But upon the last patient's collection, she realizes that she has an open abrasion on her ring finger.

Questions

1. What should she do immediately?

2. What should Clara do when she goes back to the clinic?

Self Assessment

Check Yourself

Infection Control Procedures and Safety

1. When you have completed a phlebotomy procedure, what should you always think of doing before going on to the next patient?

2. If you obtain a skin rash on your hands after working as a phlebotomist over a 3-month period, what could possibly be a cause of the rash?

3. Describe what should occur if a small amount of blood is accidently spilled in the clinical laboratory specimen collection area.

Competency Checklist: Infection Control and Safety

This checklist can be completed in a classroom setting using a make believe health care facility or in the clinical setting.

(1) Completed (2) Needs to improve

_____ 1. Looking at the type ABC extinguisher in the health care facility, what type of fire is this extinguisher used for in emergencies?

_____ 2. If you are performing maintenance checks on the centrifuge used to spin down the blood samples, what is the first thing you should do in the maintenance check?

_____ 3. Describe or show the class three pieces of PPE.

_____ 4. Look at the following chemicals in the classroom and identify whether they are an antiseptic or disinfectant.

isopropyl alcohol

iodine

chloramine

References

1. US Department of Labor and Occupational Safety and Health Administration (OSHA): Occupational exposure to bloodborne pathogens; final rule (29 CFR 1910.1030). *Fed. Register* December 6, 1991, 64004–64182.

2. OSHA Revised Bloodborne Pathogens Standard 1910.1030. Needlestick Safety and Prevention Bill Act; April 18, 2001.

3. Updated US public health service guidelines for the management of occupational exposures to HBV, HCV, and HIV: Recommendations for postexposure prophylaxis. *MMWR Morb Mortal Wkly Rep* June 29, 2001;50(RR11).

4. Centers for Disease Control and Prevention: Guidelines for isolation precautions in hospitals, part I: Evolution of isolation practices. *Am J Infect Control* 1996;24(1):24–31.

5. Garner JS: Guideline for isolation precautions in hospitals. The Hospital Infection Control Practices Advisory Committee. *Infect Control Hosp Epidemiol* 1996;17:53–80.

6. Molinari JA: Infection control: its evolution to the current standard precautions. *J Am Dent Assoc* 2003;134:569–574.

7. Centers for Disease Control and Prevention: Guidelines for preventing the transmission of tuberculosis in health care facilities. *Fed. Register* 1994;59:208.

8. Clinical and Laboratory Standards Institute (CLSI): *Protection of Laboratory Workers from Occupationally Acquired Infections, Approved Guideline,* 3rd ed. CLSI document M29-A3, ISO/TC 212 Standards and 76 Standards. Wayne, PA: CLSI, 2005;34–35.

9. National Fire Protection Association (NFPA): *National Fire Codes.* Available at: http://www.NFPA.org.

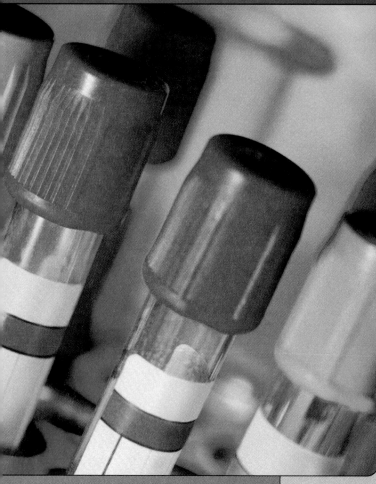

Chapter 5

Documentation, Specimen Handling, and Transportation

CHAPTER OBJECTIVES

Upon completion of Chapter 5, the learner should be able to do the following:

1. Describe the uses of a medical record.

2. List the basic specimen-handling guidelines for maintaining specimen integrity.

3. List examples of policies and procedures important to phlebotomy.

4. Describe the essential elements of requisition and report forms.

5. Name three methods commonly used to transport specimens.

6. Describe which blood constituents are photosensitive or thermolabile.

7. List reasons for specimen rejection.

KEY TERMS

aliquot

bar codes

beta-carotene

bilirubin

centrifugation

clinical (or medical) record

confidentiality

constituents

critical value

date of birth (DOB)

diagnostic test results

electronic medical record (EMR)

KEY TERMS *(continued)*

lipemic

percutaneous

photosensitive

plasma

pneumatic tube systems

porphyrins

radio frequency
identification (RFID)

requisition form

serum

specimen collection
manual

specimen integrity

thermolabile

Documentation Basics

All health care organizations provide a **clinical (or medical) record** or **electronic medical record (EMR)**, the computerized form (see Box 5-1) for each patient that describes the patient's visit, tests and procedures (including laboratory results), and clinical progress. Documentation of all clinical events in the medical record is important for the following reasons (see Box 5-2):[1]

- Monitoring the quality of care, what has been done, how the patient responds.
- Coordination of care among all health care providers involved with the patient.
- Accrediting, licensing, and clinical research.
- Legal protection. (If something is not documented, it is assumed that it was not done!)

BOX 5-1 **Common Components of a Medical Record**

All information should be kept confidential to protect the patient's privacy.

Personal information: Patient's name, **date of birth (DOB)**, social security number (SSN) or other unique identification number, address, marital status, closest relative, known allergies, and physician's name and diagnosis.

Personal and family medical history: Initial assessment completed by the physician (MD or DO), physician assistant (PA), nurse practitioner (NP), and/or nurse (RN).

Ordering documentation: Includes MDs and/or other qualified provider's (nurse practitioner's [NP], clinical nurse specialist's [CNS], physician assistant's [PA]) orders for laboratory, radiology, pharmacy, and so on.

Informed consent and/or release forms: Treatment consent forms, authorization forms for release of medical information, and similar documents.

Patient's plan of care: MD and nursing care diagnoses, interventions, and patient outcomes.

Diagnostic test results: Results from *all* tests performed on the patient.

Medication administration record: Known allergies, medication dosage and timing, route of administration, site, and date.

Progress notes and consultations: Patient's progress, interventions used, and treatment effectiveness.

Discharge plan/summary: Plans for special diets, medications, therapy, home health visits, and follow-up appointments.

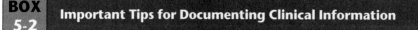

BOX 5-2 Important Tips for Documenting Clinical Information

Health care workers involved in blood collection can provide useful information by making extra notations of circumstances related to the venipuncture site, timing, fasting status, or STAT (priority) status. Some institutions have special procedures for situations that need to be documented and for determining who is authorized to make the notations or electronic entries. If an error is detected:

- **Report it immediately** to a supervisor and document it.

- **Include all relevant information in a timely manner.** For example, if a phlebotomist is unable to identify a patient because of a missing armband, the notation should include the *time*, *date*, and *name* of the nurse who positively identified the patient, and *phlebotomist's name*.

- **Document it** according to institutional policies. If it is a paper copy, note the error by marking a single line through it and writing the word "error" next to it with your signature (first initial and last name, e.g., J. Doe, is sufficient). Do not leave extra space between your notations and your signature. Legally, this "space" on the record becomes your responsibility, so do not leave room for someone else to add information to your notation. If it is an EMR, follow institutional guidelines for making corrections or changes in the computer.

- **Be accurate and legible.** Record facts, not opinions, in short phrases, using ink. Print clearly. Do not erase or use correction fluid.

- **Correcting errors.** Records should never be changed or falsified to cover a mistake. On a paper document, an error should be noted by marking a single line through it, writing the word "error," and signing your initials next to it.

- **Do not assign blame.**

All health care facilities have manuals that detail operating procedures to be followed (Table 5-1 ■). Depending on the facility, there may be several manuals—safety manual, administrative manual, **specimen collection manual**—or just one manual separated by sections. These may also be accessible via computer. Table 5-1 lists the topics generally covered in procedure manuals; these topics are particularly important to health care workers involved in blood collection. Health care workers may be involved in developing, writing, and practicing these procedures.

Clinical Alert !

Remember that it is very tempting to discuss interesting patient situations with peers, friends, or family members. Although patient situations are learning experiences and they may occasionally be discussed with authorized laboratory personnel, this type of information must *not* be shared with anyone else without the prior consent of the patient or prior authorization. This mandate assures compliance with the Health Insurance Portability and Accountability Act (HIPAA) of 1996 (Public Law 104-191), which details specific rights for patients regarding protection of their health information. HIPAA prohibits the disclosure of any health information unless written consent has been obtained from a patient.

TABLE ■ 5-1

Manuals and Procedures Important to Health Care Workers Involved in Blood Collection

Type of Manual	Procedures Included
Specimen collection	Patient preparation Type of collection container and amount of specimen required; type and amount of preservative or anticoagulant needed Timing policies (e.g., creatinine clearance, therapeutic drug monitoring, etc.) Special handling or transportation needs (e.g., refrigeration) Proper labeling requirements Priority status (STAT/emergency specimens) Need for additional data when indicated (e.g., fasting vs. nonfasting, etc.) Reporting of **critical values** (abnormally high or low test results) Handling specimens going to or coming from outside organizations
Administrative procedures	Performance evaluation procedures and job descriptions Disciplinary policies and **confidentiality**/nondisclosure policies Compensatory time, attendance, annual leave, and overtime policies Other human resources procedures (nondiscrimination, benefits, etc)
Safety	Fire and radiation safety Internal and external disaster plan Exposure control plan Hazard communication manual
Infection control (IC)	Precautions/isolation procedures Disposal policies Decontamination procedures Hand-hygiene procedures Accidental **percutaneous** (through the skin) needle sticks Postexposure procedures
Quality control (QC) and preventive maintenance (PM)	Maintaining appropriate supplies; proper use, storage, and handling of supplies; supplies and equipment maintenance and inventory procedures Monitoring reagents and equipment Stability of reagents and expiration dates (when the item should no longer be used) Measuring precision and accuracy; acceptable symbols, abbreviations, and units of measure Maintaining confidentiality

Laboratory Test Requisition Forms

TRANSMITTAL OF THE TEST REQUEST TO THE LABORATORY

A test request initiates the cyclic procedure of the laboratory communication network. Two systems are commonly used for this activity:

■ an online interactive computer system; or

■ a manual request system (paper-based, color-coded, sometimes also used for final test results)

FIGURE ▓ 5-1

Example of a Multipart
Laboratory Test
Requisition Form

Use of multiple-part
requisition forms is
helpful in a manual
system or as a
temporary request
until the formal
request can be
entered into a
computer system

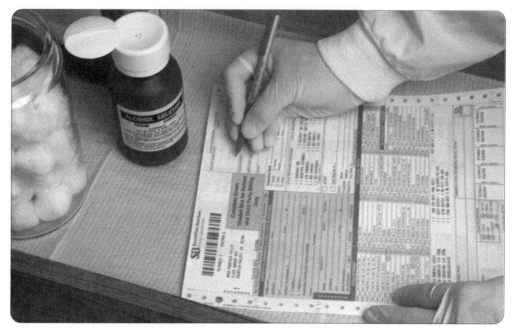

In a manual system, the multipart request forms are more subject to human error, such as transcription mistakes, lost requisitions, and duplicate orders (see Figure 5-1 ▓). Regardless of the method used for submitting a laboratory test request, the information submitted must include the following:[2]

■   patient identification (name, registration or identification number and location, or unique confidential specimen code that has an audit trail to the patient);

■   patient's gender, date of birth, or age;

■   name of physician or legally authorized person ordering the test (the physician's address is needed if it is different than the receiving laboratory);

■   tests requested;

■   time and date of specimen collection;

■   source of specimen, when appropriate; and

■   other pertinent clinical information when appropriate.

In cases of emergency, the test request is called a *STAT request* and should be documented.

BAR CODES

Bar-coded labels are often used for identifying patients and their specimens and have the following characteristics (Figure 5-2 ▓):

■   **Bar codes** consist of a series of light and dark bands that relate to specific alpha-numeric symbols (i.e., numbers and letters).

■   When bands are placed together in a series, they can correspond to a name (of a patient, health care worker, or test) or a number (identification or test code).

■   A reading device is used to scan the actual bar code.

■   Bar codes are very accurate and fast because of the elimination of typing, which reduces transcription errors.

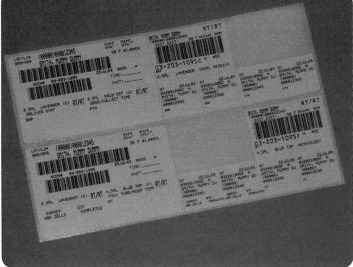

A

B

FIGURE ■ 5-2 Bar Code Labels and Identification Armbands

A. Note that various sizes of labels are printed on one sheet and can be peeled off as needed for each collection tube or microscopic slide. B. There are many styles of identification armbands available

RADIO FREQUENCY IDENTIFICATION

Radio frequency identification (RFID) is a newer form of identification for specimens with the following characteristics:

- RFID tags are tiny silicon chips that transmit data to a wireless receiver.
- In contrast to a bar code, RFID does not require line-of-sight reading with a scanner. The tag can be detected at various distances.
- It is possible to identify and/or track many items simultaneously.
- RFID can also be used in combination with a bar code for multiple purposes.

Specimen Labels and Blood Collection Lists

Accurate specimen identification is essential and must continue from the time of collection through disposal of the specimen. Identification methods vary from manually copying all patient identification information onto the container to using prenumbered, bar-coded labels. Manually labeling specimens can be time-consuming and prone to transcription errors, so these problems can be minimized by using preprinted, commercially available labels. Labeling systems include those that can imprint a patient identification card or electronically print patient identification information onto the specimen label. The computer can generate the correct number of labels containing the following information:

- patient identification information for each tube required to be drawn;
- specific tests requested;
- types of specimen collection tubes required for the requested tests;
- unique accession numbers or sample numbers to be used for that particular collection time;
- smaller transfer labels may be used to label **aliquot** tubes, collection tubes, cuvettes, and microscope slides; and
- blood drawing lists by floor or unit.

Specimen Handling and Transport

Specimen integrity can be affected by the method of transport, timing delays, temperature, agitation, exposure to light, and **centrifugation** methods. Some, but not all, specimens need to be centrifuged before analysis. The Clinical and Laboratory Standards Institute (CLSI) defines standards for the handling and processing of blood samples after consideration of numerous variables that might affect laboratory testing during precentrifugation (after the specimen is collected but before centrifugation), centrifugation (while the specimen is in the centrifuge), and postcentrifugation (after centrifugation of the specimen but before removal of an aliquot of **serum** or **plasma** for testing). There are at present hundreds of laboratory assays, chemical reagents, and manufacturers' instructions for testing specimens. With all of these data, it is not surprising that some evidence on specimen variables may be conflicting. Table 5-2 ■ summarizes basic CLSI recommendations for the handling and processing of blood specimens. It provides an overview of essential recommendations adapted from the CLSI approved guideline entitled *Procedures for Handling and Processing of Blood Specimens*.[3] The guideline is much more detailed and provides numerous references and resources for further information. Every laboratory is under pressure to balance transportation, time, test accuracy, and specimen rejection issues, so each laboratory has its own guidelines, and health care workers must follow their own institution's policies.

Basic Rules of Thumb	**TABLE ■ 5-2**

Tubes with additives should be gently inverted 5–10 times to mix the specimen with the additive as soon as the specimen is withdrawn. Excessive agitation causes hemolysis.

Serum or plasma should be removed from cells as soon as possible, no more than 2 hours after the time of collection.

Not all specimens require centrifugation.

Precentrifugation refers to specimen handling and processing after collection and before centrifugation.

Specimens without anticoagulant additives (serum specimens) should be clotted before centrifugation, which usually takes 30 to 60 minutes at room temperature (22°C–25°C).

- Clotting time is affected (often delayed) by anticoagulant therapy/medications that the patient may be taking.
- Chilling the specimen will delay clotting.
- Clotting may be accelerated by 15–30 minutes with the use of activators.

Anticoagulated specimens (plasma specimens) can be centrifuged immediately after collection. Some **constituents** are **thermolabile**—that is, they degrade if exposed to warm temperatures, so they need to be chilled immediately.

- Chilling a specimen stabilizes most constituents.
- If potassium (K) is being tested, the specimen cannot be chilled for more than 2 hours, because this causes K to leak out of the cells, causing a false elevation.
- Specimens for testing electrolytes (including potassium) should not be chilled.
- Specimens that require chilling are:

ammonia	lactic acid
blood gases	parathyroid hormone
catecholamine	pyruvate
gastrin	renin

Conversely, some tests require maintenance at normal body temperature (37°C) until tested. These include:

cold agglutinins	cryofibrinogen

Some analytes are **photosensitive**, or sensitive to light, and they should be wrapped with aluminum foil or placed in an amber specimen container to shield the specimen from light. Tubes should be kept closed at all times. Photosensitive analytes include:

bilirubin	folate
vitamins A, B_{12}, and B_6	**porphyrins**
beta-carotene	

Centrifugation refers to specimen handling and processing during centrifugation, in which the specimen is spun rapidly to separate cells from the liquid portion of blood.

The manufacturer's specifications generally indicate the speeds and times of centrifugation.

Blood specimens should be allowed to clot before centrifugation.

Tubes should be centrifuged with closures in place.

The centrifuge should have a top that secures appropriately.

Because centrifuges generate internal heat, they should be temperature controlled.

Specimens should not be centrifuged more than once; and specimens that contain separation devices *should never* be recentrifuged.

Many types of gel and non-gel devices are available to enable a barrier to form between the serum/plasma and the blood clot/cells during centrifugation. They all have a particular viscosity

(Continued)

TABLE ■ 5-2	**Basic Rules of Thumb**
CLSI Summary of Recommendations for the Handling and Processing of Blood Specimens (*continued*)	and specific gravity that is between those of the clot/cells and the serum/plasma. They may be incorporated into the tube as an additive, or they may be added just before centrifugation. Whatever the case, the manufacturer's directions should be followed. **Postcentrifugation** refers to specimen handling/processing after centrifugation and prior to removal of serum or plasma. Serum or plasma should be physically separated from cells as soon as possible and no more than 2 hours after the time of collection.

Evidence suggests that separated serum/plasma should remain at 22°C for no more than 8 hours. If testing cannot be completed within 8 hours, the sample should be refrigerated (2–8°C).
If testing is not completed within 48 hours, the separated serum/plasma should be frozen at or below −20°C unless the assay-specific directions indicate an alternative method of storage.

- Serum/plasma should not be repeatedly frozen and thawed.
- Frost-free freezers are not suitable for storage because of dehydration effects and temperature variances.
- Serum/plasma may be left in contact with a gel barrier or separator device as recommended by their respective manufacturers.
- The tube should be stored in an upright position with a secure closure.

Serum/plasma and whole blood should be kept covered at all times to avoid contamination, evaporation, changes in concentration, accidental spills, and/or the creation of aerosols.
Plunger-type filters are sometimes used to separate serum/plasma from the clot/cells before or after centrifugation. Consult the manufacturer's instructions for details and limitations of use.

SPECIMEN TRANSPORTATION GUIDELINES

Every health care facility has a specific protocol for specimen transportation and processing. Most laboratories require the use of a leak-proof plastic bag for enclosing and transporting the primary specimen tube (i.e., the blood samples taken directly from the patient). This bag protects the health care worker from exposure to pathogenic (disease-producing) microorganisms from leakage or spillage during specimen transportation.

The transport bag may have a pouch on the outside for the laboratory request slip, which eliminates the potential for contamination (Figure 5-3 ■). If possible, the blood specimens in evacuated tubes and microcollection tubes should be maintained in a vertical position with the tube cap or closure on top, to promote complete clot formation and to reduce the possibility of agitating the sample which may cause hemolysis. Handling blood specimens in a gentle manner also reduces the chances of hemolyzing the specimens.

For transportation of specimens from remote ambulatory sites, including home health collections, consider the following guidelines:

■ Follow the same handling guidelines set out in standard precautions.

■ Use the same safety equipment that is used in a hospital environment (e.g., closed venipuncture system, gloves, disposable laboratory coat, plastic blood collection tubes, and a biohazardous disposal container).

■ Transport all blood collection equipment and specimens in an enclosed or lockable container to avoid spills in case the transport automobile is in a collision. The container should have a biohazard warning label on it and notification procedures in case

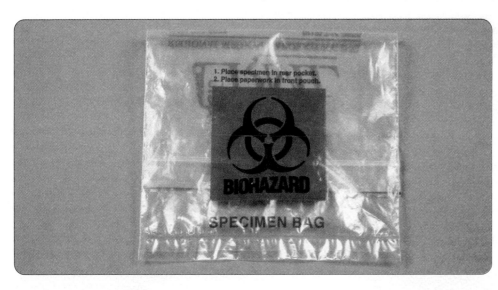

Clinical Alert ❗

Glycolytic action (the breakdown of glucose) from the blood cells interferes with the laboratory analysis of glucose, calcitonin, aldosterone, phosphorus, and some enzymes. Also, rough handling and agitation of the specimen can have an effect on hematology and coagulation tests (e.g., platelet activation and shortened clotting times).[3] Because of these interfering factors, the blood samples should be transported to the clinical laboratory *as soon as possible* after the time of collection so that the sample can be processed appropriately and serum or plasma can be separated from the blood cells. The serum or plasma that is separated from the cells must be handled according to specified testing procedures, but in general, serum can remain at room temperature for testing, be refrigerated, be stored in a dark place, or be frozen, depending on the prescribed laboratory method.

of an accident. Cold packs should be used in the container for transport during hot weather, or, conversely, the vehicle should be heated in freezing weather.

■ For home collection, be extra careful to dispose of waste properly and to place blood specimens in leak-proof plastic bags in an upright position inside a labeled transport container.

CHILLED SPECIMENS

As mentioned in Table 5-2, for special types of blood specimens, chilling is required. If a health care worker is requested to transport an arterial specimen for blood gas analysis, it should be in an airtight heparinized syringe and placed in a mixture of ice and water (Figure 5-4 ▦). The airtight container and the ice water decrease the loss of gases from the specimen. It is important to use ice water rather than solid chunks of ice; otherwise, parts of the specimen may freeze and hemolysis will result. Speed in specimen transportation is essential to prevent the loss of blood gases. Thus specimens that may require chilling are:[3]

blood gases/pH

gastrin

ammonia

lactic acid

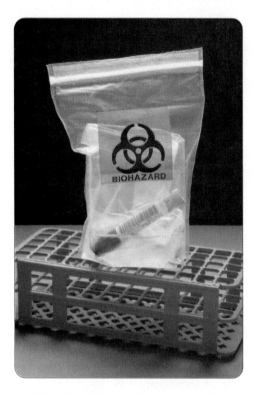

FIGURE ■ 5-4 Chilled Specimen Ready for Transportation to the Laboratory

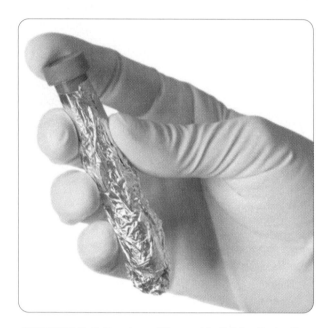

FIGURE ■ 5-5 Specimen Wrapped in Foil for Protection from Light

catecholamine

parathyroid hormone

PROTECTING SPECIMENS FROM LIGHT

Some chemical constituents in blood, such as bilirubin, are **photosensitive** (light sensitive) and decompose if exposed to light. Thus, blood collected for light-sensitive chemical analysis should be protected from bright light with an aluminum foil wrapping around the tube (Figure 5-5 ■) or an amber-colored transport bag. Light-sensitive constituents include the following:[3]

bilirubin

vitamins A and B_6

beta-carotene

folate

porphyrins

MICROBIOLOGICAL SPECIMENS

Blood, sputum, and urine specimens for microbiological culture need to be transported to the laboratory as quickly as possible, so that the specimens can be transferred to culture media and/or the urine analyzed. This enhances the likelihood of detecting pathogenic bacteria. Specimens for blood cultures can also be collected directly into culture media, which minimizes possible contamination and speeds contact with the culture media.

WARMED SPECIMENS

Some specimens require keeping the temperature at 37°C, normal body temperature, until the test is performed. These tests include cold agglutinins and cryofibrinogen. These blood specimens require a regulated heat source for transportation and handling purposes.

Specimen Delivery Methods

In larger facilities, the laboratory is most often the department responsible for the delivery of blood specimens to the location where they will be analyzed. However, other types of specimens, such as urine and sputum, are commonly delivered by transportation or nursing staff members. Whatever the site, guidelines should be available for the safe and efficient delivery of specimens; these may include a schedule of pick-ups, how to deliver STAT specimens, where to place specimens, how to "log in" specimens, how to store specimens and for how long, and similar procedures. There are a variety of methods to transport specimens:

Courier services are used for off-site areas such as reference laboratories, blood drawing stations, or remote clinics. Again, considerations prior to and during transportation should include adequate packaging and handling. This is especially true in hot or cold temperatures.

Hand delivery often involves the use of a log sheet to document the receipt of each specimen. In a hospital setting, the blood collection trays or carts are typically arranged to hold numerous specimens awaiting delivery to the laboratory. All specimens should be secured using test tube racks, a holder for microscopic slides, plastic holders, cups, and/or a leak proof container for ice water.

Pneumatic tube systems are used to transport specimens, patient records, messages, letters, bills, medications, x-rays, and laboratory test results. The CLSI reports that many studies have documented the validity of laboratory results after specimen transport through a pneumatic tube and suggest that the tests most affected (lactate dehydrogenase, potassium, plasma hemoglobin, and acid phosphatase) are compromised because of the disruption of red cells. Also, if samples must be kept at body temperature (e.g., testing for cryoglobulins and cold agglutinins), they should not be transported in a pneumatic tube system.[3] However, the majority of analytes are not usually affected, so this is an efficient means of specimen transport. It is recommended that blood collection tubes be placed in the pneumatic tube with shock-absorbent inserts padding the sides and with the tubes separated from one another, to prevent spillage or breakage. Clear plastic liners are also commercially available, so that if leaks do occur, they are visible and are contained to prevent contamination of the tube system, the carrier, and the personnel handling the specimens. Gloves should always be worn when loading or unloading specimens from the transport tube container, because they may be contaminated with biohazardous specimen leakage that is not visible to the naked eye.

Transportation by automated vehicles uses a small motorized and/or computerized container car attached to a network of track that is routed to appropriate sites in the laboratory and nursing stations.

Specimen Storage

Each laboratory should have specific criteria for keeping specimens stable during storage and for determining time and temperature requirements for testing procedures. Test results may exhibit significant changes caused by time delays. Even though some analytes may be stable for longer periods, CLSI suggests that cells be removed or separated from serum or plasma within 2 hours of collection. The results of some laboratory tests change significantly if the cells remain in contact with the plasma or serum, yet some may remain stable for longer time periods.

Specimen Rejection

Because a test result is only as good as the specimen it is performed on, there are occasions when a specimen (e.g., blood or urine) must be rejected. This is an uncomfortable situation, because it means that the patient may have to undergo another venipuncture or another trip to the clinic. Box 5-3 indicates important criteria for specimen rejection.

When a problem arises, the health care worker who drew the specimen and a supervisor should try to solve the problem initially. Errors should be acknowledged and documented with corrective actions. Other personnel may be involved as needed. Honesty and ethical communication are mandatory.

Clinical Alert ❗

If a specimen is not acceptable for testing, it should be disposed of properly, a request for a new specimen must be initiated by an authorized individual, documentation should note the situation, and the patient's physician should be notified.

BOX 5-3   **Criteria for Specimen Rejection**

Anticoagulated tube that contains blood clots

The requisition form and the specimen label do not match

Excessive delays in processing the specimen

Hemolyzed blood specimen (except for tests in which hemolysis does not interfere with the analysis)

Improper specimen transport temperature or storage

Improper blood collection tube (the correct additive is a requirement for specific tests)

Improper blood volume (too much or too little) in the collection tube (this can affect the blood to additive ratio)

Lipemic blood specimen (cloudy or milky appearance of serum due to ingestion of fatty foods)

Nonfasting blood specimen (unless appropriately noted)

Use of outdated supplies to collect the specimen (e.g., the expiration date has passed)

Variation in patient's posture (hormone values change based on whether the patient is sitting or reclining)

Timed specimens drawn at the wrong time

Unlabeled specimen tubes

Contaminated urine specimen

Self Study

Study Questions

For the following questions, select the one best answer:

1. Medical records serve what purpose?

   a. coordination of care
   b. maintain technical skills
   c. provide competency statements
   d. document certification

2. Bar codes can be used for which type of information?

   a. identification of blood cells
   b. patient identification numbers
   c. designation of right from left
   d. inventory of patients' belongings

3. What is the most error-free method for requesting a laboratory test?

   a. hand-written requisition
   b. computerized method
   c. verbal method
   d. verbal STAT method

4. A specimen should be protected from light for which of the following determinations?

   a. bilirubin concentration
   b. hemoglobin level
   c. glucose level
   d. blood cultures

5. A specimen should be chilled for which of the following analyses?

   a. complete blood count (CBC)
   b. bilirubin level
   c. blood gases
   d. glucose level

6. Normal body temperature (in degrees Centigrade) is:

   a. 25
   b. 37
   c. 98
   d. 100

7. Room temperature (in degrees Centigrade) is:

   a. 25
   b. 37
   c. 98
   d. 100

8. Thermolabile means sensitivity to:

   a. latex products
   b. temperature changes
   c. light
   d. seasonal allergies

9. Photosensitivity means sensitivity to:

   a. latex products
   b. temperature changes
   c. light
   d. seasonal allergies

10. Approximately how long does it take a normal blood specimen (without an anticoagulant or clot activator) to clot?

    a. 1–5 minutes
    b. 6–10 minutes
    c. 30–60 minutes
    d. >120 minutes

Case Study

Blood specimens for 12 patients were received via the pneumatic tube system in a large hospital laboratory within 15 minutes of each other. All specimens had been collected by a new phlebotomist. Six of the patients' specimens showed hemolysis and could not be used for laboratory analysis.

Questions

1. What is a likely cause of the hemolysis?

2. What should be done next?

Self Assessment

Check Yourself

Designing a Mock Requisition Form

Design a requisition form that includes all of the appropriate information for a laboratory test. With a peer, practice giving instructions on how to complete the form. Practice your communication techniques by double-checking that they completely understand. Ask them specific questions about parts of the requisition that might be hard to remember filling out.

Designing a Mock Specimen Label

Working with a partner, design a specimen label that includes all of the appropriate information for a specimen to be received in the clinical laboratory. Consider spacing and ease of compliance with all the required information. Discuss the various uses of these labels and what could happen if the information is incomplete. Practice writing your initials so that they are readable.

Competency Checklist: Specimen Transportation

This checklist can be completed as a group or individually.

(1) Completed (2) Needs to improve

_____ 1. List five essential items that should be on laboratory requisitions and specimen labels.

_____ 2. List 3 methods that are used to transport specimens.

_____ 3. Describe 3 examples of why a specimen might be unsuitable for laboratory testing.

_____ 4. Describe the 3 phases of processing and centrifugation of a sample.

_____ 5. Describe 3 reasons that specimens should be kept covered at all times.

References

1. Fiesta, J: *20 Legal Pitfalls for Nurses to Avoid.* Allentown, PA: Delmar Publishers, 1994.

2. College of American Pathologists (CAP) Commission on Laboratory Accreditation: Laboratory General Checklist. Available at: www.cap.org. Accessed 7/13/2006.

3. Clinical and Laboratory Standards Institute (CLSI): *Procedures for the Handling and Processing of Blood Specimens: Approved Guideline,* 3rd edition, volume 24, number 38, H18-A3. Wayne, PA: CLSI, 2004.

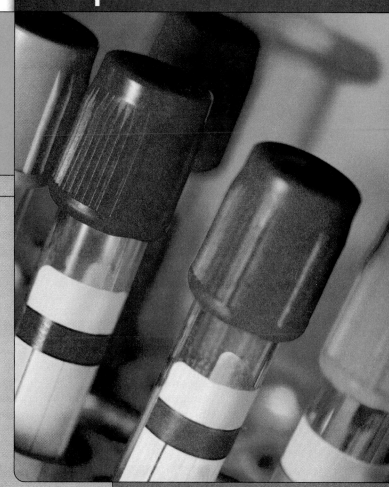

Chapter 6

Blood Collection Equipment

CHAPTER OBJECTIVES

Upon completion of Chapter 6, the learner should be able to do the following:

1. Describe the latest phlebotomy safety supplies and equipment.

2. Identify the various supplies that should be carried on a specimen collection tray when a skin puncture specimen must be collected.

3. Describe the differences between the venipuncture and skin puncture equipment and supplies.

4. Identify the types of safety equipment needed to collect blood by venipuncture and skin puncture.

KEY TERMS

acid citrate dextrose (ACD)

anticoagulants

capillary tubes

citrates

disposable sterile lancet

ethylene diaminetetraacetic acid
   (EDTA)

gauge number

heparin

holder (adapter)

latex allergy

lithium iodoacetate

microcontainers

Introduction to Blood Collection Equipment

Health care workers involved in blood collection use many types of supplies and safety equipment in the collection and transport of blood specimens. Blood collection devices with safety features decrease needlestick injuries. The collection equipment is used for venipuncture (blood collection from a vein), skin puncture (blood collection from a finger and/or an infant's heel), and arterial puncture (blood collection from an artery). Venipuncture equipment includes vacuum tubes and safety-needle collection devices that allow the blood collector to collect a patient's blood, plus a tourniquet to assist in locating a vein, supplies to cleanse the puncture site, labeling supplies, gloves, and special trays for the transport of the blood specimens. Box 6-1 lists the equipment used in routine venipuncture procedures.

Venipuncture Equipment

Venipuncture with a **vacuum (evacuated) tube** (VACUTAINER), as shown in Figure 6-1 ■, is the most direct and efficient method for obtaining a blood specimen. The vacuum tube system requires an evacuated tube, a special needle, and a special safety plastic **holder (adapter)** (Figure 6-2 ■) that covers the needle after blood collection. One end of the double-pointed needle enters the vein, the other end pierces the top of the tube, and the tube's vacuum aspirates the blood. The needle and/or plastic holder that covers the needle

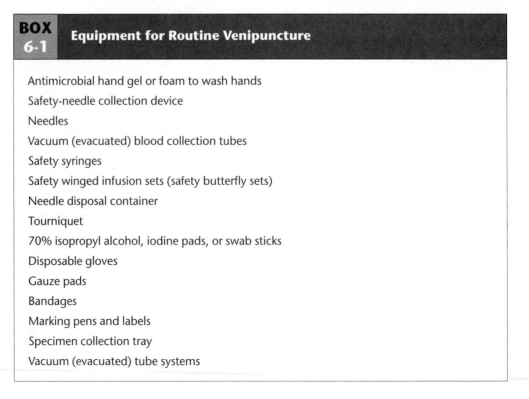

BOX 6-1   **Equipment for Routine Venipuncture**

Antimicrobial hand gel or foam to wash hands

Safety-needle collection device

Needles

Vacuum (evacuated) blood collection tubes

Safety syringes

Safety winged infusion sets (safety butterfly sets)

Needle disposal container

Tourniquet

70% isopropyl alcohol, iodine pads, or swab sticks

Disposable gloves

Gauze pads

Bandages

Marking pens and labels

Specimen collection tray

Vacuum (evacuated) tube systems

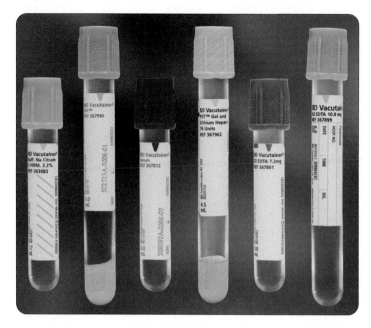

FIGURE ■ 6-1 Vacuum Tubes

Courtesy of BD VACUTAINER Systems, Preanalytical Solutions, *Franklin Lakes, NJ.*

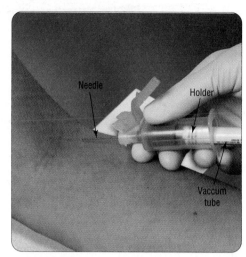

FIGURE ■ 6-2 Vacuum (Evacuated) Tube Holder System and Parts

Courtesy of BD VACUTAINER Systems, Preanalytical Solutions, *Franklin Lakes, NJ.*

after venipuncture have safety devices to protect the health care worker from a needlestick injury. State and federal laws require these "safety-engineered devices."

Blood Collection Tubes and Additives

Blood collection tubes are available in different sizes, in safety-engineered plastic, to reduce risk of tube breakage and blood spill. Glass collection tubes are not desirable because the risk of exposure to bloodborne pathogens (disease-causing organisms) is increased due to possible breakage. The two criteria used to describe vacuum tube size are: (1) the external tube diameter and length plus (2) the maximum amount of specimen to be collected into the vacuum tube. The smaller sizes (e.g., 13 mm external diameter × 75 mm length) are useful for collecting 2 mL of blood from pediatric (child or baby) and geriatric (elderly) patients and can be purchased with different types of additives (i.e., **anticoagulants**), as well as being chemically clean or sterile. Each vacuum tube top is color-coded according to the additive contained within the tube (see Table 6-1 ■).

Many tubes are designed to be used directly with the chemical, hematological, or microbiological instruments. In these cases, the tube of blood is identified by its bar code and is pierced by the instrument probe, and some blood sample is aspirated (pulled) into the instrument for analyses.

Traditionally, in most clinical laboratories, serum and plasma have been used to perform various assays. More recently, though, heparinized whole blood has become the specimen of choice for several clinical chemical laboratory instruments used in STAT (immediate) situations. Using whole blood as a specimen decreases the time involved in acquiring the test result, because centrifugation is not required before laboratory testing.

Many coagulation factors are involved in blood clotting, and coagulation can be prevented by the addition of different types of anticoagulants.[1] These anticoagulants often contain preservatives that can extend the metabolism and life span of the red blood cells (RBCs) after blood collection. Another major use of anticoagulants and preservatives is in

TABLE ■ 6-1

Specimen Type and Collection Vacuum Tubes

Specimen Type	Collection Tubes (Top Color/Type)	Additive
Clotted blood/serum	Gray and red	Polymer barrier
	Yellow and red	Polymer barrier
	Gold	Polymer barrier
	Red	None
	Orange	Thrombin
	Yellow and gray	Thrombin
	Brown	Polymer gel
Whole blood/plasma	Green and gray	Polymer barrier and lithium **heparin**
	Green (yellow top)	Polymer barrier and lithium heparin
	Light green	Polymer barrier and lithium heparin
	Light blue	Trisodium citrate
	Lavender (purple)	EDTA (K_3), EDTA (K_2), or EDTA (Na_2)
	Gray	**Sodium fluoride** and potassium oxalate
	Green	Lithium heparin
	Green	Sodium heparin or ammonium heparin
	Royal blue	Sodium heparin or EDTA (Na_2) sterile tube for toxicology and nutritional studies
	Pink	Blood bank (EDTA)
	Tan	EDTA (K_2) tube for lead testing
Clotted blood/serum	Royal blue	No additive; but sterile tube for trace elements, toxicology, and nutritional studies
	Brown	No additive or sodium heparin, but lead-free glass and sterile for lead determinations
Whole blood	Lavender (purple)	EDTA (K_3), EDTA (K_2), or EDTA (Na_2)
	Green	Lithium heparin, sodium heparin, or ammonium heparin
	Black	Sodium citrate
	Yellow	Sodium polyanetholesulfonate (SPS) or **acid citrate dextrose (ACD)**

the collection of plasma for laboratory analysis. Specific anticoagulants or preservatives must be used depending on the test procedure ordered. Anticoagulants cannot be substituted for one another. Coagulation of blood can be prevented by the addition of anticoagulants such as **oxalates**, **citrates**, **ethylene diaminetetraacetic acid (EDTA)**, or heparin. Oxalates, citrates, and EDTA prevent the coagulation of blood by removing calcium and forming insoluble calcium salts. These three anticoagulants cannot be used in calcium determinations; however, citrates are frequently used in coagulation blood studies. EDTA is used for platelet counts and platelet function tests. Fresh EDTA-anticoagulated blood allows preparation of blood smears for differential (diff) counts because cell sizes are not affected. Heparin is used in assays such as ammonia and plasma hemoglobin, and it prevents blood clotting by inactivating the blood-clotting chemicals thrombin and factor X. Pediatric tubes are available from manufacturers for patient blood collections in which it is anticipated that a "smaller amount of blood" will be collected. These tubes provide accurate laboratory results even though a smaller amount of blood is collected.

Clinical Alert !

Two important things to remember when using vacuum blood collection tubes:

1. These tubes have been designed for a certain amount of blood to be collected into the tube by vacuum in relation to the amount of prefilled anticoagulant in the tube.
2. If an insufficient amount of blood is collected in the anticoagulated tube, the laboratory test results may be wrong because of the incorrect amount of blood mixed with anticoagulant, and the sample should not be used for testing.

GRAY-TOPPED TUBES

Gray-topped vacuum tubes usually contain (1) potassium oxalate and sodium fluoride, (2) sodium fluoride and EDTA, (3) sodium fluoride, or (4) **lithium iodoacetate** and heparin (see Box 6-2). This type of collection tube is primarily used for glucose (sugar) tests. The terms *antiglycolytic agent* and *glycolytic inhibitor* are the terms for this tube's additive because it prevents glucose breakdown.

GREEN-TOPPED TUBES

The anticoagulants sodium heparin, ammonium heparin, and lithium heparin are found in green-topped vacuum tubes. These tubes are used in various laboratory assays requiring plasma or whole blood, which are mainly chemical tests.

Lithium heparin tubes are used for many assays, including:

- glucose;
- blood urea nitrogen (BUN);
- ionized calcium;
- creatinine; or
- electrolyte studies.

However, this anticoagulant is not suitable for tests involving the measurement of lithium or folate levels. Similarly, sodium heparin tubes should not be used for assays that measure the sodium concentration.

BOX 6-2 **Contraindications for Gray-Topped Tubes**

Because sodium fluoride destroys many enzymes, the gray-topped tube should *not* be used in blood collections for enzyme determinations that include:

- creatine kinase (CK);
- alanine aminotransferase (ALT);
- aspartate aminotransferase (AST); or
- alkaline phosphatase (ALP).

Likewise, potassium oxalate destroys blood cell features. Thus, gray-topped tubes should not be used for hematological studies because blood cells are identified and counted in these tests.

Green-topped vacuum tubes should not be used for collections for blood smears. When used for cytogenetic studies, these tubes must be sterile.

PURPLE (LAVENDER)-TOPPED TUBES

The purple-topped vacuum tubes (which contain EDTA) are used for most hematological procedures as well as for blood-banking procedures. These tubes are also used for molecular diagnostic testing. EDTA does not alter the size of the cells, so it is ideal as an anticoagulant when blood is collected for cell counts and differentials (Box 6-3).

LIGHT BLUE–TOPPED TUBES

Many coagulation procedures, such as prothrombin time (PT) and activated partial thromboplastin time (APTT), are done on blood collected in light blue–topped vacuum tubes, which contain sodium citrate. Tubes must be filled, or coagulation results will be inaccurate, which could lead to the wrong treatment for the patient. Sodium citrate buffers coagulation factors, making it the best anticoagulant for coagulation testing. Patients with high hematocrit levels must have special tubes prepared to maintain a proper ratio of anticoagulant to blood.

RED-TOPPED, ROYAL BLUE–TOPPED, BROWN-TOPPED, AND TAN-TOPPED TUBES

The red-topped tubes are tubes without anticoagulant for the collection of serum to be used in chemical and serological tests. Thus, the collected blood will clot in this tube. The red-topped glass tubes have no additives and are recommended for blood collections to be used in blood-bank testing. The red-topped plastic tubes have a clot activator and are not recommended for blood-banking procedures. The collected blood in these plastic tubes with clot activators must be gently inverted to ensure mixing of the clot activator with the blood. The blood should clot within 60 minutes. The royal blue–topped tubes are used to collect samples for nutritional studies, therapeutic drug monitoring, and toxicological studies. The royal blue–topped tube is the "trace element" tube. The brown-topped tube contains heparin or no additive and is used for testing blood lead values. The tan-topped tube is also used for lead testing, and it contains EDTA.

BLACK-TOPPED TUBES

From certain manufacturers, a black-topped tube containing sodium citrate is available for blood collections used to determine the erythrocyte sedimentation rate (ESR).

YELLOW-TOPPED TUBES

Sterile blood specimens are ordered for blood cultures when the patient is suspected of having septicemia (bacteria in the bloodstream). A major problem with collecting blood for culture is that the patient's sample can become contaminated with microorganisms

BOX 6-3	Purple-Topped Tubes

If a purple-topped tube is underfilled, the patient can possibly have

- inaccurate blood cell counts,
- inaccurate hematocrit test results, and
- inaccurate staining on differential blood smears.

from the skin. Thus, the blood must be collected in a sterile container (vacuum tube, vial, or syringe) under aseptic conditions. (See Chapter 11 for blood culture collections.) The additive SPS is in the yellow-topped tubes for blood culture specimen collections in microbiological tests. Also, as shown in Figure 6-3 ■, blood can be collected directly into vacuum vials that contain culture media.

Note that tubes containing ACD may also have a yellow top. These tubes are used for specialty blood banking, such as HLA typing, DNA, and paternity testing.

SERUM SEPARATION TUBES (MOTTLED-TOPPED, SPECKLED-TOPPED, AND GOLD-TOPPED TUBES)

Another tube is the serum separation tube, such as the VACUETTE serum tube (Figure 6-4 ■) and the BD VACUTAINER Plus SST tube. These tubes must be gently inverted with the blood to ensure mixing of the clot activator. These tubes contain a polymer barrier in the bottom of the tube. During centrifugation, the polymer barrier forms a barrier between the serum and blood cells. Blood clotting occurs within 30 minutes.

PINK-TOPPED TUBES

Pink-topped tubes contain EDTA and are used for blood-bank collections.

MOLECULAR DIAGNOSTICS TUBES

Special sterile vacuum tubes for molecular diagnostic studies are available that contain different additives (e.g., sodium citrate and sodium heparin) as required for the different testing procedures. Manufacturers use tops of different color for these tubes.

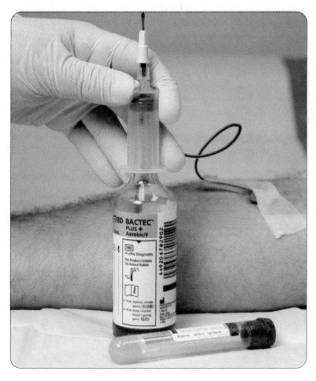

FIGURE ■ 6-3 Collecting Blood for Culture Using the BD BACTEC Culture Vial

Courtesy of BD (Becton-Dickinson and Company), Sparks, MD.

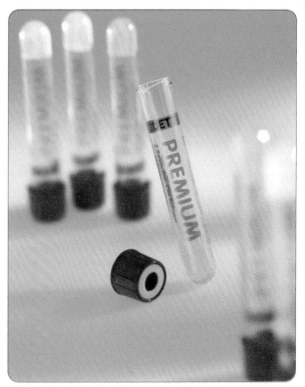

FIGURE ■ 6-4 VACUETTE Serum Tube

Courtesy of Grenier Bio-One, Kremsmunster, Austria.

Safety Syringes

Some patients' veins are too fragile for blood collection with vacuum tubes, so safety syringes are generally used for the collection process.[2] Syringes are hazardous and pose an increased risk of accidental needlesticks.

Syringes are sometimes used for collecting blood from central venous catheter (CVC) lines. Major syringes consist of the needle, safety cover, hub, barrel, and plunger (Figure 6-5 ■). The barrel and the plunger are made to fit together tightly so that when the plunger is in the barrel and drawn back, a vacuum is created. To fit properly, the needle and syringe must be compatible and are attached at the hub. This vacuum allows blood or other fluids to be aspirated, or sucked, into the barrel as the plunger is pulled back. The barrel of the syringe has graduated measurements in milliliter (mL) or cubic centimeter (cc) increments. For specimen collection purposes, 5- to 20-mL syringes are most often used. In addition, the health care worker should ensure that the syringe is the correct size for the amount of blood to be collected.

A safety syringe shielded-transfer device (Figure 6-6 ■) must be used to avoid possible exposure to the patient's blood.[3] The plunger must not be pushed down as the tubes are being filled from the syringe because doing so is extremely hazardous. Also, pushing

FIGURE ■ **6-5**

Example of a Safety Syringe

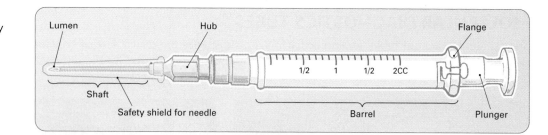

FIGURE ■ **6-6** BD SafetyGlide Needle and BD Blood Transfer Device

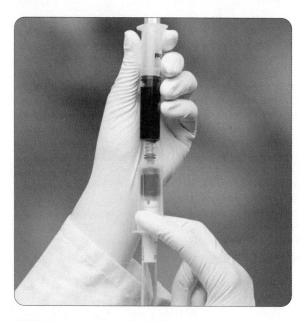

Courtesy of BD VACUTAINER Systems, Preanalytical Solutions, *Franklin Lakes, NJ.*

the plunger may damage cellular components and cause hemolysis because of the forceful expulsion of blood. The syringe needle should be shielded after blood collection, removed, and discarded in a sharps disposal container.[4] The BD blood-transfer device is attached to the syringe, and a vacuum tube is inserted into the transfer device. The blood is transferred from the syringe to the tube using the tube's vacuum. Specialized tubes and bottles that fit the adapter are also available for blood culture collection.

Clinical Alert ❗

- Safety engineering controls (needlestick protection) and safe work practices must be used when collecting blood with a syringe.
- Avoid the use of syringes in blood collection if at all possible.
- Needleless safety blood-transfer devices must be used to transfer the blood from the syringe to the vacuum tube.

Safety Needles/Holders

The gauge and length of a needle used on a syringe or a vacuum tube is selected according to the specific task. The **gauge number** indicates the diameter of the needle; the smaller the gauge number, the larger the needle diameter and higher the flow rate (Box 6-4).

For example, larger (18-gauge) needles are used for collecting donor units of blood (450 mL or less), whereas smaller (21- and 22-gauge) needles are used for collecting specimens for laboratory assays. When blood is collected from children, a 21- to 23-gauge needle is usually used with a tuberculin, or 3-mL, syringe or with a winged infusion set. The gauge number indicates the diameter of the needle; the smaller the gauge number, the larger the needle diameter and higher flow rate. The length of the needle depends on the depth of the vein to be punctured. Needles are usually available as either 1 or 1.5 inch.

Needles are sterilized and packaged by vendors in sealed shields that maintain sterility. These sealed shields are packaged in individual containers that are color coded according to the gauge size of the needles and must be twisted apart before the needles are used in blood collection.

The needle attaches to the safety holder/adapter, or syringe, at its hub. For example, the BD Eclipse safety-shielding blood needle attaches to a holder (Figure 6-7 ▪). The BD Eclipse shield is activated immediately after the blood collection tubes are filled and the needle is removed from the vein. When the thumb pushes forward on the shield, as shown in Figure 6-7, an audible click indicates that the safety shield is locked in place. This single-use adapter provides immediate containment of a used needle.

Another protective holder that provides effective, immediate containment of a used needle is the Venipuncture Needle-Pro (Figure 6-8 ▪). After removing the needle from the patient's vein, the health care worker activates the needle guard by holding the tube holder and pressing the needle guard against a hard surface so that the guard swings over the needle. Once engaged, both ends of the needle are covered, protecting the blood collector from an accidental needlestick.

BOX 6-4	**Needle Sizes Used for Blood Collection**

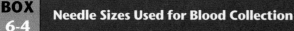

- Larger (16- to 18-gauge) needles are used for collecting donor units of blood (e.g., 450 mL).
- Smaller (21- and 22-gauge) needles are used for collecting specimens for laboratory assays.

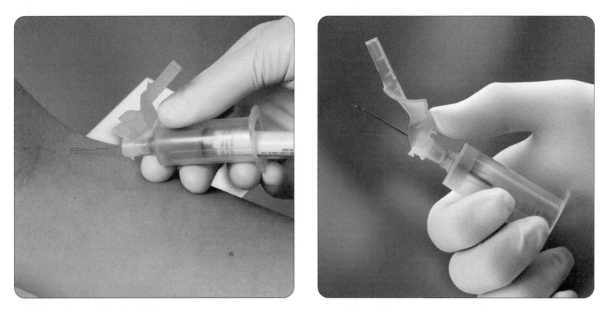

FIGURE ■ 6-7 BD Eclipse Blood Collection Needle Attached to a Holder

Courtesy of BD VACUTAINER Systems, Preanalytical Solutions, Franklin Lakes, NJ.

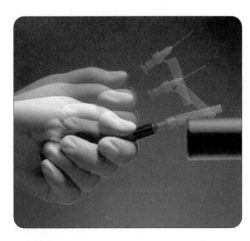

FIGURE ■ 6-8 Venipuncture Needle-Pro Needle Protection Device

Courtesy of Portex, Inc., Keene, NH.

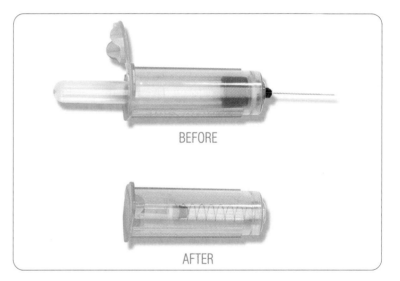

FIGURE ■ 6-9 Vanishpoint Blood Collection Tube Holder

Courtesy of Retractable Technologies, Little Elm, TX.

The Vanishpoint blood collection system features a blood collection tube holder and a small tube adapter. The needle is automatically retracted from the patient when the end cap is closed after the last tube has been removed. It virtually eliminates exposure to the contaminated needle and the possibility of needlestick injury (Figure 6-9 ■).

Another vacuum tube assembly developed to prevent needlestick injuries is the PUNCTUR-GUARD Blood Collection Needle. PUNCTUR-GUARD is actually two needles, one inside of the other. The internal "needle" is hollow and has a flat, or blunt, end. This blunt needle is recessed inside of the outer sharp needle. When blood collection is performed, the sharp needle accesses the vein. Blood is collected into vacuum tubes. Once the last tube is filled, the health care worker activates the safety feature, while the needle is still in the patient's vein. Activation of the safety feature advances the inner blunt needle forward, past the sharp tip of the outer needle. Because it occurs in the vein, the patient does not feel the change.

The VACUETTE QuickShield Safety Tube Holder is used to prevent accidental needle-stick injuries during venous blood collection (Figure 6-10 ■). It can be used in conjunction with VACUETTE blood collection needles. The device is used by pressing the protective cover over the needle with the aid of a stable surface and then disposing of the needle and holder into a sharps disposal container.

Sarstedt, Incorporated, offers the S-Monovette Blood Collection System (Figure 6-11 ■), which is an enclosed multiple-sampling blood collection system that collects blood using either an aspiration or vacuum principle of collection. Using the aspiration procedure replaces syringe draws for patients with difficult veins and can prevent uncomfortable resticks. All tubes are plastic with screw caps, which minimizes the risk of breakage and aerosol formation when caps are removed. Each needle has an integral holder that does not require assembly before use and cannot be disassembled. Thus, it prevents reuse of the holder.

For any of these blood collection needle and tube holder devices, disposing of the tube holder while it is still attached to the needle ensures that the tube-puncturing needle remains protected during and after disposal.[4] This safety method significantly reduces the risks of needlestick injuries and blood exposure from the tube-puncturing needle to automatically retract into it after blood collection.

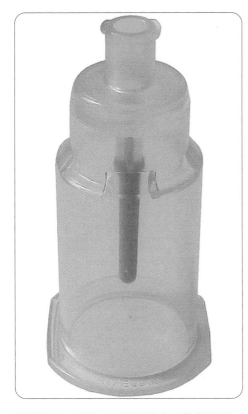

FIGURE ■ **6-10** VACUETTE QUICKSHIELD Safety Tube Holder

Courtesy of Greiner Bio-One GmbH, Kremsmuenster, Austria.

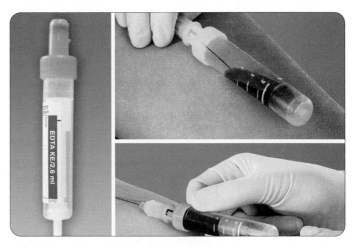

FIGURE ■ **6-11** Sarstedt S-Monovette Venous Blood Collection System

Courtesy of Sarstedt, Inc., Newton, NC.

Needles

The tip of each needle should be checked for damage. A blunt or bent tip can be harmful to the patient's vein and may result in failure to collect blood.

Multiple-sample needles are used with vacuum collection tubes and the holder to allow for multiple tube changes without blood leakage within the plastic holder. The multiple-sample needle has a plastic cover over the tube-top puncturing portion of the needle; this cover creates a leakage barrier.

It is important to use needles with holders or syringes that are compatible with the needle to avoid the possibility of leaking blood and blood exposure.

THE BUTTERFLY NEEDLE (BLOOD COLLECTION SET)

The butterfly needle, also called a blood collection set or winged infusion set, is the most commonly used intravenous device. It is a stainless steel beveled needle and tube with attached plastic wings on one end and a Luer fitting attached to the other. The most common butterfly needle sizes are 21 and 23 gauge, and the length of these needles range from 1/2 to 3/4 inches long. The smaller angle of insertion can occur with the shorter needle. The butterfly needle is sometimes used in the collection of blood from patients who are difficult to stick by conventional methods (e.g., elderly persons, patients with cancer, and children).

> **Clinical Alert** !
>
> The safety device *must* be activated on the butterfly needle after venipuncture to avoid needlestick injury.

Numerous types of safety butterfly needles are available and must be used according to OSHA regulations. These safety needles each have a shield that automatically covers the contaminated needle point upon withdrawal from the patient's vein. One example is the Kendall MONOJECT ANGEL WING blood collection set (Figures 6-12A ■ and 6-12B ■). It has a stainless steel safety shield that automatically resheaths the needle during withdrawal from the patient.

BD VACUTAINER Systems *Preanalytical Solutions* has the BD VACUTAINER Push Button Blood Collection Set (see Figure 6-13 ■), which provides immediate protection against needlestick injury when it is properly activated within the vein and in accordance with the BD directions.

Greiner Bio-One manufactures the VACUETTE safety blood collection set (Figure 6-14 ■). It is a winged needle device with a safety shield. Bio-Plexus produces the PUNCTUR-GUARD winged set for blood collection. The safety device uses an internal hollow blunt built within the sharp outer needle. When the blood samples have been withdrawn, the "internal blunt" is activated before the needle is removed from the vein, thus reducing exposure to a sharp contaminated needle. Terumo Medical Corporation manufactures the Surshield Safety Winged Blood Collection Set (Figure 6-15 ■), a safety-engineered butterfly device for blood collection or IV insertion. No matter what type of safety blood collection set is used, it is important to use a Luer adapter (fitting) from the same manufacturer, to avoid possible blood leakage and exposure.

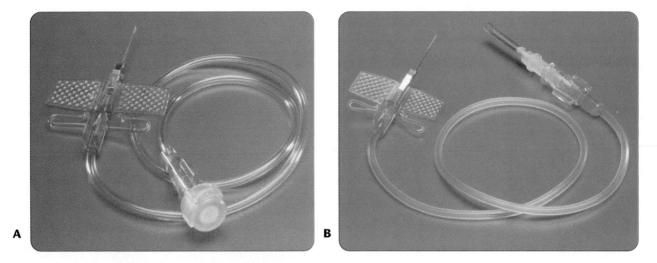

FIGURE ■ 6-12 ANGEL WING Blood Collection Set with (A) Female and (B) Male Luer
Courtesy Tyco Healthcare Group, LP.

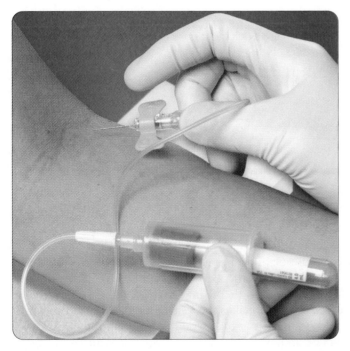

FIGURE ■ 6-13 Blood Collection with BD VACUTAINER Push Button Blood Collection Set
Courtesy of BD VACUTAINER Systems, Preanalytical Solutions, *Franklin Lakes, NJ.*

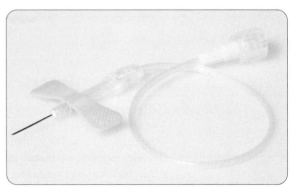

FIGURE ■ 6-14 VACUETTE Safety Blood Collection Set
Courtesy of Greiner Bio-One, Kremsmunster, Austria.

NEEDLE AND OTHER SHARPS DISPOSAL

Needles, syringes, and lancets (sterile, disposable sharp devices used in skin puncture) must be discarded in rigid, leakproof, plastic containers, reducing the possibility of needle sticks. Each unit is usually orange or red and is disposable as biohazardous waste (Figure 6-16 ■).

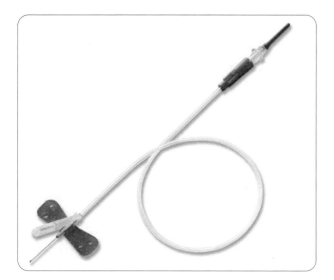

FIGURE ■ 6-15 Surshield Safety Winged Blood Collection Set
Courtesy of Terumo Medical Corp., Somerset, NJ.

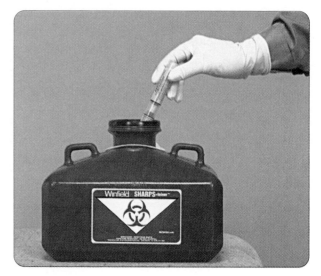

FIGURE ■ 6-16 Sharps Disposal Container with the Required Biohazard Sign

Several sizes of sharps disposal containers are available for use at the bedside, on the cart, in isolation, and on home health care trays. Before beginning a blood collection procedure, note the location of the nearest sharps container.

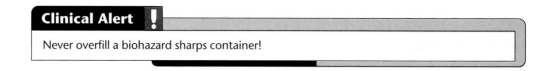

Clinical Alert

Never overfill a biohazard sharps container!

Tourniquets

The tourniquet is a key to successful venipuncture: it provides a barrier to slow down venous flow. Tourniquets are used in specimen collection to apply enough pressure to the arm to slow the return of venous blood to the heart. This slowing of venous return causes pooling of blood in the veins, which makes the veins more visible and easier to feel and find. A tourniquet should not restrict arterial blood flowing into the arm. Blood should enter the arm at a normal rate and, with the use of a tourniquet, return to the heart at a slower rate. If the tourniquet is too tight, all blood flow will cease, making it difficult to collect.

Tourniquets that are usually used include the pliable strap, the Velcro type, and the blood pressure cuff. The blood pressure cuff can be used successfully when veins are difficult to find. Another type of tourniquet is the Seraket, which uses a seat-belt design. It allows the health care worker to release the venous pressure partially by using a lever that releases some pressure, but not all. Thus, if the health care worker needs to tighten the tourniquet again, the lever can be used to adjust the tourniquet. Because errors in laboratory test results can occur from prolonged tourniquet pressure, the Seraket provides a solution to this problem. One drawback of this type of tourniquet, however, is the difficulty in cleaning and decontaminating it if it is soiled with blood between each patient use.

Velcro-type tourniquets are popular because they are easy to apply and comfortable for the patient. Alternatively, because of major concern for infection control in health care institutions, many facilities now use a disposable natural latex tourniquet strap to help prevent cross-contamination. Many patients are allergic to latex; thus, other types of tourniquets must be available to use to avoid an allergic reaction. Nonlatex disposable tourniquets are now available as a good option for the blood collector and patient. If the tourniquets used in the health care facility are not disposable, they must be wiped between each patient with 70% isopropyl alcohol and disinfected with a chlorine bleach dilution of 1:10 if contaminated with blood or other body fluids.

Gloves for Blood Collection

Safety guidelines have been established for health care workers to help them prevent the possibility of acquiring infections, such as hepatitis or those associated with AIDS. These guidelines include the use of gloves during collection of blood from patients (Figure 6-17 ■). It is recommended that health care workers use non latex gloves (see Chapter 4 for **latex allergic** reactions). Also, health care workers should not use gloves with talc powder containing calcium, because tubes of patients' blood may become contaminated with this powder, and such contamination can result in falsely elevated calcium values.

Gloves should be changed after each patient's blood collection.

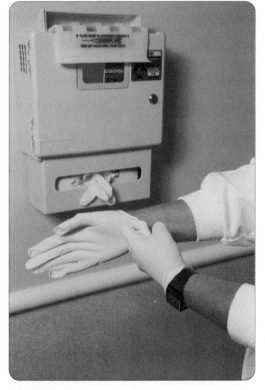

FIGURE ■ 6-17 Use of Gloves

Clinical Alert !

- Change gloves between patients' blood collections.
- Do not wash, disinfect, or reuse the gloves.

Antiseptics, Sterile Gauze Pads, and Bandages

The health care worker needs antiseptics, **sterile gauze pads**, and bandages for blood collection by either venipuncture or microcollection. Therefore, 70% isopropyl alcohol preparation and iodine swab sticks or pads (for blood cultures) are essential items for blood collection. In home health care and other ambulatory health care environments where soap and water may not be available, a waterless antiseptic agent (Figure 6-18 ■) should be carried with other blood collection items and used before and after blood collection.

Microcollection Equipment

Usually, skin puncture blood-collecting techniques are used on infants, because venipuncture is excessively hazardous. The maximum volume of blood that generally can be collected from an infant at any one time is approximately 2.5 mL. Larger volumes are obtained from older children and adults.

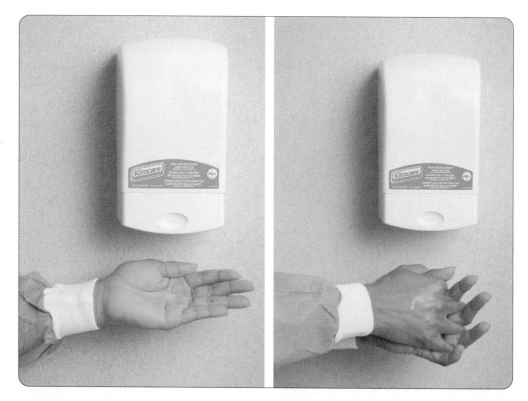

FIGURE ■ 6-18 Waterless Antiseptic Agent

Waterless antiseptic agents can be mounted in wall dispensers or carried with other blood collection supplies in travel-size containers

LANCETS AND TUBES

For infants, the Clinical Laboratory Standards Institute recommends a penetration depth of less than 2.0 mm on heel sticks to avoid penetrating bone. The BD Quikheel lancet (Figure 6-19 ■) is available for two different incision depths, depending on the needs of the infant. The teal-colored Quikheel Infant lancet has a preset incision depth of 1.0 mm and a width of 2.5 mm. The purple-colored Quikheel Preemie lancet has a preset incision depth of 0.85 mm and a width of 1.75 mm. This lancet blade retracts permanently after activation, to ensure safety to the health care worker.

The BD Genie lancet (Figure 6-20 ■) is another safety-engineered device for skin puncture blood collection. The Genie lancet is available in an assortment of puncture widths and depths, as well as in a needle lancet for glucose testing.

Clinical Alert !
■ **Disposable sterile lancets** that are retractable to avoid bloodborne pathogen exposure should be used to puncture the skin for skin puncture collections.
■ Surgical blades should not be used for skin puncture because of the hazard to the patient and health care worker.

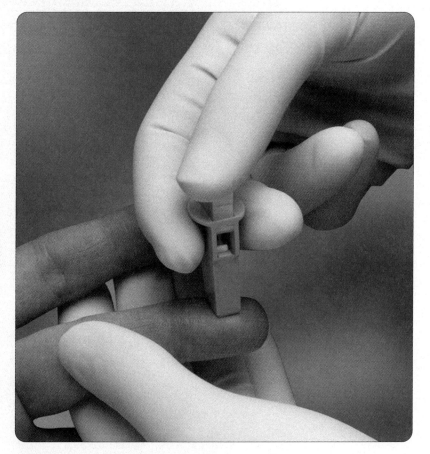

FIGURE ■ **6-20** BD GENIE LANCET

Courtesy of BD VACUTAINER Systems, Preanalytical Solutions, *Franklin Lakes, NJ.*

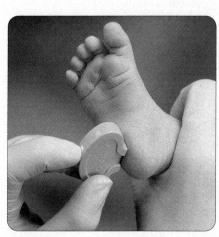

FIGURE ■ **6-19** BD Quikheel Lancet

Courtesy of BD VACUTAINER Systems, Preanalytical Solutions, *Franklin Lakes, NJ.*

ITC produces fully automated, single-use, automatically retracting, disposable devices that provide safety both for the neonate and for the health care worker (Figure 6-21 ■). The Tenderlett incises 1.75 mm deep, Tenderlett Jr. incises 1.25 mm deep, and Tenderlett Toddler incises only 0.85 mm deep. The retracting blade of each of these devices eliminates potential injury from an exposed blade contaminated with blood.

Another safety device for microcollection is the MONOJECT Monoletter Safety Lancet (Figure 6-22 ■) for fingerstick collections. The Greiner Bio-One lancet (Figure 6-23 ■) is a safety microcollection device available for various puncture depths.

A laser-based device that is FDA approved for blood collection is the Lasette. The laser penetrates to a depth of 1 to 2 mm and a width of 250 μm. This is a smaller puncture hole than other devices make.[5] To collect a reliable small-volume blood sample, it is important to use properly designed blood microcollection tubes that are made of plastic for safety.

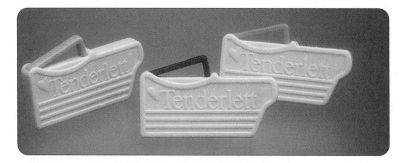

FIGURE ■ 6-21 Tenderlett Automated Skin Incision Device

Courtesy of ITC, Edison, NJ.

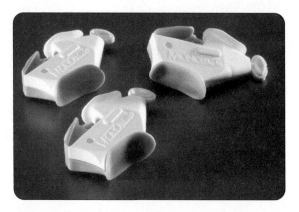

FIGURE ■ 6-22 MONOJECT Monoletter Safety Lancet

Courtesy Tyco Healthcare Group, LP.

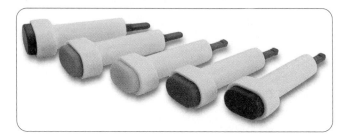

FIGURE ■ 6-23 Greiner Bio-One Lancets for Microcollection

Courtesy of Greiner Bio-One, Kremsmunster, Austria.

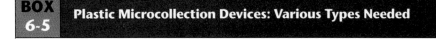

BOX 6-5	**Plastic Microcollection Devices: Various Types Needed**

- Serum or plasma separator devices in different color codes (same colors as for vacuum color-topped tubes described earlier according to additives, e.g., purple contains EDTA)
- Disposable plastic calibrated microcollection tubes
- Plastic microhematocrit tubes
- Microdilution systems (e.g., BD Unopette)

The **microcontainers** recommended for use for skin puncture collections are listed in Box 6-5.

Microhematocrit **capillary tubes** are disposable narrow-bore pipettes that are used for packed red cell volume (hematocrit) in microcentrifugation. These plastic tubes have colored bands; a red band indicates a heparin-coated tube, and a blue band indicates no anticoagulant. Plastic microcollection containers available for general laboratory collections (e.g., chemistry and immunology) are usually color-coded according to the established protocol for blood collection vacuum tube tops. Thus, purple- or lavender-topped tubes contain EDTA, green-topped tubes contain heparin, red-topped tubes have no additive, and gray-topped tubes have sodium fluoride to inhibit blood enzymes that destroy glucose.

Tyco Healthcare Group, LP, manufactures the Samplette micro-blood collector, which is offered with a full range of anticoagulants and serum and plasma separation gels. One of its collectors is an amber capillary blood separator that provides protection for light-sensitive analytes (e.g., bilirubin).

Electrolytes and general chemistry analytes are some of the tests that can be collected in the BD Microtainer tube, which has its own capillary blood collector, self-contained serum separator, and Microgard closure, which is safety engineered to reduce the risk of tube leakage and specimen splatter. Each tube is imprinted with two markings, a minimum 250-microliter line and a maximum 500-microliter line, to assist in collecting appropriate volumes (Figure 6-24 ■).

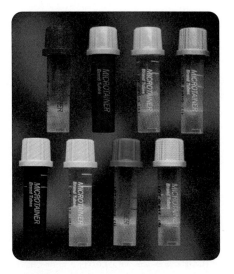

FIGURE ■ 6-24 BD Microtainer Tube

Courtesy of BD VACUTAINER Systems, Preanalytical Solutions, *Franklin Lakes, NJ.*

Alternatively, two or more capillary tubes can be used for electrolyte and general chemistry collection. One advantage of these tubes is that if blood hemolyzes in one capillary tube, another capillary tube containing the patient's sample can be used for the chemical analyses.

The Microvette capillary blood collection system is another microcollection system that is offered with a full range of anticoagulants and serum separation gel. This system can be used to collect, store, and separate samples in the same unbreakable, disposable container.

RAM Scientific, Incorporated, has developed an unbreakable plastic capillary-receptacle system called the SAFE-T-FILL capillary blood collection system. The device consists of a plastic capillary inserted into a microtube receptacle (Figure 6-25 ■). With the attached receptacle, blood flows directly to the bottom of the tube. This system makes the blood drawing safe and clean. The capillary can then be removed, and the tube is closed with the appropriate color-coded cap.

For most chemical assays using the various types of microcollection devices, lithium and ammonium salts of heparin are the anticoagulants of choice for microcollections. They have rarely been reported to interfere with the determination of electrolytes and most other chemical assays.

Another type of microcollection device is the Unopette, shown in (Figure 6-26 ■). This device serves as a collection and dilution unit for blood samples and, thus, increases the speed and simplicity of laboratory procedures. These devices are prefilled with specific amounts of diluents or reagents, or both, for different types of laboratory assays. Some of the more common procedures in which Unopette devices are used include the WBC count, RBC count, platelet count, and RBC fragility.

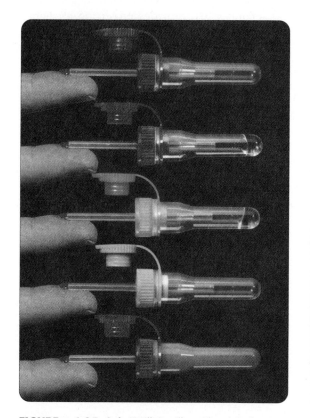

FIGURE ■ 6-25 Safe-T-Fill Capillary Blood Collection Device

Courtesy of Ram Scientific, Inc., Needham, MA.

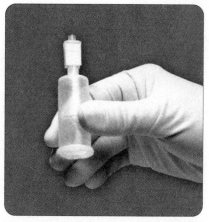

FIGURE ■ 6-26 Unopette, a Collection and Dilution Unit for Blood Samples

Courtesy of BD VACUTAINER Systems, Preanalytical Solutions, *Franklin Lakes, NJ.*

The standard Unopette system indicates:

1. a disposable, self-filling diluting pipette consisting of a straight, thin-walled, uniform-bore, plastic capillary tube fitted into a plastic holder, and

2. a plastic reservoir containing a premeasured volume of reagent for diluting.

Specimen Collection Trays

The health care worker collecting blood specimens needs a specimen tray (Box 6-6 and Figure 6-27 ■) to take on blood-collecting rounds. The tray is usually made of plastic (preferably latex-free) and must be made of a plastic that can be sterilized. The tray should

BOX 6-6	**Items to Carry on a Blood Microcollection Tray**

1. Seventy percent isopropyl alcohol and iodine or Betadine pads
2. Marking pens for labels
3. Microcollection blood serum separator tubes
4. Capillary whole blood cell collectors with 0.23 mg of EDTA
5. Safety lancets for skin puncture
6. Sterile gauze pads or bandages
7. Unheparinized plastic microcollection tubes
8. Heparinized plastic microcollection tubes (250, 400, and 500 μL)
9. Heparinized Natelson tubes (75 μL)
10. Unopette devices for collection and dilution procedures
11. Disposable gloves
12. Appropriate warming device
13. Thermometer
14. Biohazardous waste containers for sharps
15. Glass microscope slides
16. Capillary safety tube sealer
17. Antimicrobial hand gel or foam to wash hands without water and soap

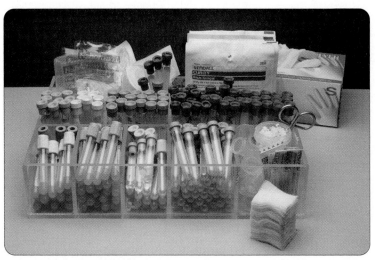

FIGURE ■ 6-27 Specimen Collection Tray

include all necessary collection equipment. For example, when working in a children's hospital, the tray must contain microcollection equipment, such as that described earlier. For home health care providers and reference laboratory couriers, the necessary collection supplies, equipment, and collected blood must be carried in an enclosed container with the biohazard symbol shown on the outside. It should be lockable to protect the contents from tampering or accidental contamination. It also should have a tight seal to reduce the risk of infection from bloodborne pathogens due to spills or accidents.

Health care workers who collect blood from adults usually have the following equipment on their trays or in their safety container for travel for home health care:

1. Marking pens or pencils
2. Vacuum tubes containing the anticoagulants designated in the clinical laboratory blood collection manual
3. Safety holders for vacuum tubes
4. Safety needles for vacuum tubes and syringes
5. Safety syringes
6. Tourniquet (nonlatex)
7. Safety blood collection sets (butterfly needle assembly)
8. Seventy percent isopropyl alcohol, iodine pads, or swab sticks
9. Sterile gauze pads
10. Bandages
11. Biohazardous waste containers for used needles, holders, and lancets
12. Safety lancets for skin puncture
13. Unopette devices for finger-stick blood collection
14. Microcollection blood serum and plasma separator tubes
15. Microcollection capillary whole blood collectors with 0.23 mg of EDTA (200 micro L)
16. Disposable gloves
17. Cloth towel or washcloth
18. Thermometer
19. Antimicrobial hand gel or foam to wash hands without water and soap

Self Study

Study Questions

For the following questions, select the one best answer.

1. The yellow-topped vacuum collection tube has which of the following additives?

   a. lithium heparin
   b. trisodium citrate
   c. sodium polyanetholesulfonate (SPS)
   d. EDTA

2. The butterfly blood collection set is frequently used with the needle gauge size of:

   a. 23
   b. 20
   c. 19
   d. 18

3. Which of the following anticoagulants is found in a royal blue–topped blood collection tube?

   a. no additive
   b. lithium heparin
   c. 3.2% sodium citrate
   d. ammonium heparin

4. Lithium heparin is a suitable anticoagulant for collecting blood to run which of the following tests?

   a. erythrocyte sedimentation rate
   b. zinc level
   c. glucose level
   d. lithium level

5. Which of the following is a blood microcollection system?

   a. Microtome
   b. BD Eclipse
   c. RAM SAFE-T-FILL
   d. VACUETTE QUICKSHIELD

6. A blood cell count requires whole blood collected in a:

   a. green-topped tube
   b. purple-topped tube
   c. yellow-topped tube
   d. light blue–topped tube

7. Specimens for which of the following tests must be collected in light blue–topped blood collection tubes?

   a. PT and APTT
   b. glucose
   c. trace elements
   d. ESR

8. Blood collection for blood-banking procedures can be collected in which of the following tubes?

   a. pink-topped tubes
   b. black-topped tubes
   c. royal blue-topped tubes
   d. light blue–topped tubes

9. A prefilled device used as a collection and dilution unit is the:

   a. MONOJECT tube
   b. BD Unopette
   c. Sarstedt S-Monovette Blood Collection System
   d. RAM SAFE-T-FILL

10. Which of the following anticoagulants is recommended for blood smear preparations?

    a. lithium heparin
    b. sodium heparin
    c. EDTA
    d. SPS

Case Study

Ms. Perez is a diabetic and has come to the health care facility to have her blood glucose (sugar) level checked. In addition, the physician has ordered an AST to be run on her blood.

Questions

1. Which blood collection tube should be used to obtain the blood for the glucose level?

2. Can the blood from the same tube collected for the glucose be used to obtain a result for the AST?

Self Assessment

Check Yourself

Identifying the Proper Equipment for Blood Collection

1. Describe three examples of the combined safety needles/holders for venipuncture and three examples of microcollection lancets. For the microcollection lancets, identify the maximum incision depth that should occur for neonates, children, and adults.

2. Based on your educational readings and/or experience, what do you recommend should be carried on the phlebotomy tray for the type (elderly, healthy adults, children, etc.) of patients from whom you collect blood.

3. Describe two blood collection tubes that have been made to collect blood for lead values and explain the difference between the two tubes.

Competency Checklist

This checklist can be completed as a group or individually.

(1) Completed (2) Needs to improve

_____ 1. Correctly identifies blood collection tubes according to additive and color of top.

_____ 2. Identifies safety devices for venipuncture collection.

_____ 3. Lists blood collection equipment necessary for collection from a newborn infant.

References

1. Clinical and Laboratory Standards Institute (CLSI): *Tubes and Additives for Venous Blood Specimen Collection; Approved Standard,* 5th ed. (H1-A5). Wayne, PA: CLSI, 2003.

2. Rossen J, Stoker R: *The Compendium of Infection Control Technologies.* Palm City, FL, 2005.

3. Pugliese G, Salahuddinm, eds.: *Sharps Injury Prevention Program: A Step-By-Step Guide.* Chicago: American Hospital Association, 1999.

4. Occupational Safety and Health Administration (OSHA), US Dept. of Labor: OSHA Safety and Health Information Bulletin (SHIB): *Re-Use of Blood Tube Holders.* October 15, 2003.

5. News & Views: Lasers to replace lancets? *Lab Med* 1997;28(11):689.

Additional Resources

1. International Sharps Injury Prevention Society. www.isips.org

2. Premier Safety Institute. www.premierinc.com/SAFETY

3. Kohn LT, Corrigan JM, Donaldson MS, eds: Institute Of Medicine. *To Err Is Human: Building A Safer Health System.* Washington, DC: National Academy Press, 2000.

4. Shelton P, Rosenthal K: Sharps injury prevention: select a safer needle. *Nurs Management* 2004;35(6):25–31.

Preanalytical Complications in Blood Collection

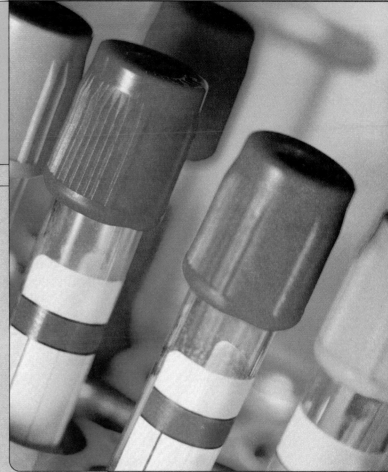

Upon completion of Chapter 7, the learner should be able to do the following:

1. Describe preanalytical complications related to blood collection procedures.

2. Explain how to prevent and/or handle complications in blood collection.

3. List at least five factors about a patient's physical disposition (i.e., make-up) that can affect blood collection.

4. List examples of substances that can interfere in clinical testing of blood analytes and describe methods used to prevent these interferences.

5. Describe how allergies, a mastectomy, edema, and thrombosis can affect blood collection.

6. List preanalytical complications that can arise with test requests and identifications.

7. Describe complications associated with tourniquet pressure and fist pumping.

8. Identify how the preanalytical factors of syncope, petechiae, neurological complications, hemoconcentration, hemolysis, and intravenous therapy affect blood collection.

9. Describe methods used to prevent these interferences.

Chapter 7

KEY TERMS

basal state

fasting

hematoma

hemoconcentration

hemolysis

lipemic

mastectomy

obesity

occluded veins

petechiae

sclerosed veins

syncope

thrombi

turbid

Overview

Preanalytical variables that are important to health care workers involved with blood collection are shown in Box 7-1.

As mentioned in other chapters, preanalytical variables are particularly critical to health care workers, because most of them can be controlled. Often when a blood collection error occurs it could have been prevented by taking precautions (i.e., proper ID check of patient). Occasionally, however, patient complications during or after the blood collection procedure are unavoidable. If so, the health care worker must be knowledgeable about methods that will decrease the negative impact of the complication to the patient, to the quality of the blood sample, to the health care worker, or to all three. This chapter covers patient complications and preanalytical variables that are reported most often.

Patient Complications Affecting Blood Specimens

Blood specimens used to determine the amount of the patient's glucose, cholesterol, triglycerides, electrolytes, proteins, and so on, should be collected when the patient is in a **basal state**—that is, in the early morning, approximately 12 hours after food intake. The results of laboratory tests on basal state specimens are most constant. However, several factors—including diet, exercise, emotional stress, **obesity**, menstrual cycle, pregnancy, diurnal variations, posture, tourniquet application, and chemical constituents (alcohol or drugs)—can cause changes in the basal state. Health care workers need to have a general understanding of these possible patient changes and their effects on laboratory testing.

DIET

To ensure that the patient is in the basal state, the physician must require the patient to fast overnight. The term **fasting** refers to no food or drinks (except water). The required time period necessary for fasting depends on the test procedures to be performed. Before collecting a specimen, the health care worker should ask the patient whether he or she had anything to eat or drink. The amounts of blood analytes significantly change after meals and, thus, are not correct for many clinical chemistry tests. If the patient has eaten or had anything other than water to drink recently but the physician still needs the test, the word "nonfasting" must be written on the requisition and/or directly on the specimen.

When giving instructions to the patient to fast for blood tests, it is important to gain the patient's cooperation by using professional behavior. Inadequate patient instructions can cause mistakes in specimen collection. Casual instructions are apt to be taken lightly by the patient or even forgotten. If asked to explain fasting restrictions to a patient, the instructions should be thorough and clear, with emphasis on the important points of the

BOX 7-1	**Variables Important in Specimen Collection**

- Patient assessment and physical disposition
- Test requests
- Specimen collection
- Specimen transport
- Specimen receipt in the laboratory

procedure. Some patients assume that the term fasting refers to abstaining from (i.e., avoiding) food and water. Abstaining from water can result in dehydration, which can cause errors in test results. Thus, the health care worker must ensure that the patient understands all the requirements. Written instructions are also helpful, if available.

If a procedure involves some discomfort or inconvenience, the patient should be informed. For example, if blood is to be collected for timed blood glucose levels, cholesterol levels, and/or triglyceride levels, the patient needs to fast for 8 to 12 hours. The health care worker can inform the patient that several specimens will be collected at timed intervals and that he or she may drink water, but that coffee, tea, and chewing gum should be avoided because they may cause an error in the lab results.

OBESITY

More than one-half of adult patients in the United States are overweight. Obese patients generally have veins that are difficult to visualize and/or palpate. (Refer to Chapter 8 to view examples of different arm veins.) If the vein is not entered when first punctured, the health care worker must be careful not to probe (i.e., dig) excessively with the needle, because doing so destroys red blood cells (RBCs) and causes errors in blood test results. Usually the patient him- or herself knows where the "best site" is for venipuncture, so it is helpful to check with the patient before selecting the site.

DAMAGED, SCLEROSED, OR OCCLUDED VEINS

Obstructed, or clogged, veins do not allow blood to flow through them; **sclerosed**, or hardened, veins are a result of inflammation and disease. Patients' veins that have been repeatedly punctured often become scarred and feel hard when the arm is palpated to find a venipuncture site. Because blood is not easily collected from these sites, they should be avoided.

ALLERGIES

Some patients are allergic to iodine, alcohol, or other solutions used to cleanse a puncture site. If a patient states that he or she is allergic to a solution, all efforts should be made to use another cleansing agent. (Chlorohexidine has been reportedly used as an alternative to cleanse the skin. After application, it can be wiped off with sterile water.)[1] In addition, some patients are allergic to latex. Latex-free tourniquets, gloves, and bandages must be used for patients who have this allergy. (See Chapter 4 for more information about latex allergy.)

MASTECTOMY

Patients who have undergone a **mastectomy** (i.e., surgical removal of the breast) often have resulting lymphedema (increased lymph fluid) on the side of the surgery. The fluid in the area may make the patient more prone to infections; therefore, the arm and area around the arm on the side of the mastectomy should be protected from cuts, scratches, burns, and blood collection.

EDEMA

Some patients develop edema (i.e., an abnormal accumulation of fluid in the tissues) because of reasons other than a mastectomy (e.g., heart failure, renal failure, inflammation, malnutrition, and bacterial toxins). This swelling can be localized or spread out over a larger area of the body. The health care worker should avoid collecting blood from these sites, because veins in these areas are difficult to palpate or locate, and the specimen may become

> **Clinical Alert** !
>
> Venipuncture and/or skin puncture should never be performed on the same side as that of a mastectomy (unless *written* approval by the physician is obtained), because the patient is more susceptible to infection, and some analytes in the blood may be altered. Also, the pressure from the tourniquet could lead to injuries in a patient who has had this type of surgery. If the patient has had a double mastectomy, fingersticks are better sites for blood collection. However, the physician should provide written permission for this blood collection to occur.

contaminated with fluid. Again, consultation with the physician is sometimes needed to determine whether and where a blood specimen should be taken.

THROMBOSIS

Thrombi are solid masses derived from blood constituents that reside in the blood vessels. A thrombus may partially or fully occlude (close) a vein or artery, and such occlusion will make venipuncture more difficult.

> **Clinical Alert** !
>
> **Burned or Scarred Areas**
>
> Areas that have been burned or scarred should be avoided during phlebotomy. Burned areas are very sensitive and susceptible to infection, and veins under scarred areas are difficult to palpate. Collecting specimens from these sites can be very painful.

VOMITING

Sometimes the thought or sight of blood before or during blood collection leads to vomiting. If this reaction occurs, have the patient take deep breaths and use a cold compress on his or her head. Also, the patient's physician needs to be informed about this complication.

Complications Associated with Test Requests and Identification

IDENTIFICATION DISCREPANCIES

Improper identification is the most dangerous and costly error a health care worker can make, because it can be life-threatening. Identification should include a match between the patient's identification, his or her verbal confirmation, and the test requisition. At least two patient identifiers are necessary to avoid an identification error. Bed labels, water pitchers, or door charts should not be used as a patient identifier. Even armbands are not completely reliable (Refer to Chapter 8 for more details on identification procedures.)[2] Sometimes a phlebotomist is the first to detect a discrepancy between a name on the requisition and the name that the patient states or the name on the armband. In these cases, the discrepancy should be reported to a supervisor and/or nurse and may result in the prevention of other errors related to that patient. These discrepancies must be resolved before the collection of any samples.

TIME OF COLLECTION

Timing factors can affect test results. In some cases, such as testing drug levels, the timing of the collection must coincide with when the dosage was given. Early morning specimens are most commonly requested in hospital settings, because a fasting specimen is preferred (given that reference ranges are based on fasting specimens). If a health care worker is running late, the specimen might be collected after an inpatient has eaten breakfast and would require a special notation about his or her "nonfasting" condition.

REQUISITIONS

Checking the requisition to match the laboratory tests requested with the appropriate type of collection tube is essential to minimize the amount of blood collected from each patient. Too much blood loss because of excessive specimen removal can result in anemia.

Complications Associated with the Specimen Collection Procedure

TOURNIQUET PRESSURE AND FIST PUMPING

Laboratory test results can be falsely elevated or decreased if the tourniquet pressure is too tight or is maintained for too long. The pressure from the tourniquet causes biological analytes to leak from the tissue cells into the blood, or vice versa. For example, plasma, cholesterol, iron, lipid, protein, and potassium levels will be falsely elevated if the tourniquet pressure is too tight or prolonged. These falsely elevated results may be seen with as short as a 3-minute application of the tourniquet (the recommended time for tourniquet application is no longer than 1 minute at a time).[3] In addition, some enzyme levels can be falsely elevated or decreased because of tourniquet pressure that is too tight or prolonged. Also, pumping of the fist before venipuncture should be avoided, because it leads to an increase in the plasma, potassium, lactate, and phosphate concentrations.

FAILURE TO DRAW BLOOD

Several factors may cause the health care worker to "miss the vein." These factors include not inserting the needle deep enough, inserting the needle all the way through the vein, holding the needle bevel against the vein wall, or losing the vacuum in the tube (as demonstrated in Figure 7-1 ■). During needle insertion, the gloved index finger can be used to help locate the vein. The needle may need to be moved or withdrawn somewhat and redirected. The only acceptable redirections are backward and forward in a relatively straight line. In an elderly (geriatric) patient, the vein may be "tough" during needle entry, and it may roll; such rolling can cause the needle to slip to the side of the vein instead of properly puncturing it. Thus, the health care worker must securely anchor the vein before blood collection, to prevent rolling. If the vein rolls, it is the fault of the blood collector, because the anchoring technique used on the vein was not sufficient. Do not blame the patient.

On occasion, a blood collection vacuum tube will have no vacuum because of a manufacturer's error, the age of the tube, or tube leakage after a puncture. Therefore, an extra set of tubes should be readily available in case this should happen during venipuncture. Also, needles for evacuated tube systems have been known to unscrew from the barrel during venipuncture. If this happens, the tourniquet should be released immediately and the needle removed from the arm as the safety device is activated over the needle, to avoid a needlestick to the blood collector.

FAINTING (SYNCOPE)

Syncope is the sudden loss of consciousness caused by a lack of oxygen to the brain that results in an inability to stay in an upright position. Patients usually recover their orientation quickly, but injuries (e.g., abrasions and cuts) often result from falling to the ground. Syncope may be caused by a variety of things, including low blood glucose levels, heart

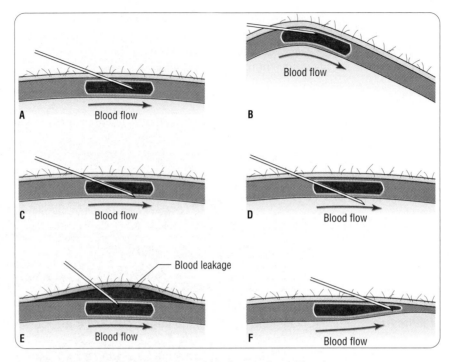

FIGURE ▪ 7-1 Needle Positioning and Failure to Draw Blood

A. Correct insertion technique; blood flows freely into needle. B. Bevel on the vein upper wall does not allow blood to flow. C. Bevel inserted into the vein's lower wall does not allow blood to flow. D. Needle inserted too far. E. Needle partially inserted, which causes blood leakage into tissue. F. Collapsed vein

Clinical Alert ❗

If a patient faints during or after the procedure, the health care worker should try to end the venipuncture procedure immediately and make sure that the patient does not fall or become injured. Sometimes controlling the situation is difficult because of the patient's physical size; however, the health care worker should use common sense about the safest position for a patient. If a patient has fainted and is in a secure position, the health care worker should quickly request assistance from the nursing staff or a physician. A patient who has fainted should recover fully before being allowed to leave and should be instructed not to drive a vehicle for at least 30 minutes. Patients often think too soon that they have recovered, but when they try to stand up, they collapse again, risking injury. An incident report must be filed with the health care facility regarding the fainting incident and any injuries resulting from the fall, the immediate precautions taken, and what instructions were provided, to the patient to prevent the possibility of long-term complications (e.g., a car accident after the fainting incident).

ailments, rapid breathing, mental conditions, or medications. Many patients become dizzy and faint ("get weak in the knees") at the thought or sight of blood. Also, patients who have donated blood recently and/or fasting patients frequently become faint. Therefore, the health care worker should be aware of the patient's condition throughout the collection procedure. This can be done by asking ambulatory patients whether they tend to faint or have ever previously fainted during blood collections. If so, they should be moved from a seated position to a lying position. Even for an ambulatory patient without a history of fainting, it is still extremely important to use a blood collection chair with a "locked" armrest to avoid the possibility of a fall if he or she faints. If a seated patient feels faint, the needle should be removed, the patient's head should be lowered between the legs, and the patient should breathe deeply. If possible, the health care worker should ask for help and move the patient to a lying position. Talking to patients can often reassure them and distract their attention from the blood collection procedure. Bed-bound patients also faint during blood collection, although rarely. In any case, the health care worker should stay with the patient for at least 15 minutes until he or she recovers or until a nurse or physician takes over. A wet towel gently applied to the forehead or a glass of juice or water may help the patient feel better.

HEMATOMAS

When the area around the puncture site starts to swell, usually blood is leaking into the tissues and causes a **hematoma**. A hematoma can occur when the needle has gone completely through the vein, the bevel opening is partially in the vein, or not enough pressure is applied to the site after puncture. This swelling results in a large bruise after several days (Figure 7-2 ■). If a hematoma begins to form, the tourniquet and the needle should be removed immediately, and pressure should be applied to the area for approximately 2 minutes. If the bleeding continues, a nurse should be notified.

PETECHIAE

Petechiae, small red spots appearing on a patient's skin, indicate that minute amounts of blood have escaped into outer skin layers. This complication may be a result of a blood clotting abnormality such as thrombocytopenia—that is, a low platelet count—and should be a warning that the patient's puncture site may bleed excessively. Petechiae also occur during illnesses with fever.

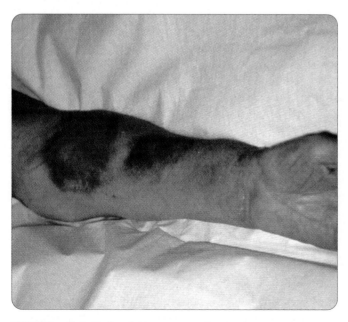

FIGURE ■ 7-2 Patient's Hematoma after Venipunctures

Source: Johnson & Johnson Medical Division, Ethicon, Inc., One Johnson & Johnson Plaza, New Brunswick, NJ 08901 1997. Used with permission of the copyright owner.

EXCESSIVE BLEEDING

Most patients stop bleeding at the venipuncture site within a few minutes. Patients receiving anticoagulant therapy and/or high dosages of arthritis medication or other medication, however, may bleed for a longer period. Often, elderly patients are receiving these medications and must be watched carefully for excessive bleeding. Also, coagulation abnormalities can cause excessive bleeding. Thus, anytime a venipuncture is performed, pressure must be applied to the venipuncture site until the bleeding stops.

> **Clinical Alert !**
>
> The health care worker must not leave the patient until the bleeding stops or a nurse takes over to assess the patient's situation. In rare instances, the health care worker may accidentally puncture an artery instead of a vein. An artery has pulsating pressure that causes the blood to squirt out in pulses. These cases require that pressure be applied as quickly as possible to stop the bleeding and that a nurse and/or supervisor be notified as soon as possible.

NEUROLOGICAL COMPLICATIONS

If the health care worker accidentally inserts the needle all the way through the vein, he or she may hit the nerve below the vein. If this happens, the patient will most likely have a sharp, electric tingling (and painful) sensation that radiates down the nerve. The tourniquet should be released immediately, the needle removed, and pressure held over the blood collection site. An incident report on the occurrence should be completed and given to the supervisor.

> **Clinical Alert !**
>
> A rare but serious complication that may occur during blood collection is a seizure (a sudden attack or convulsion). Try to keep the patient from hitting things. If a patient begins to have a seizure, the health care worker should immediately release the tourniquet, remove the needle, move the patient to a lying position if they have not fallen already, attempt to hold pressure over the blood collection site, and call for help from the nursing station. No attempt should be made to place anything in the patient's mouth unless the health care worker is experienced and authorized to do so.

HEMOCONCENTRATION

Hemoconcentration, the increase in red blood cells, and other cells and solids in the blood is caused from loss of fluid in the surrounding tissues around the venipuncture site. These may be due to several factors, including prolonged (i.e., longer than 1 minute) tourniquet application; massaging, squeezing, or probing a site; long-term intravenous (IV) therapy; and sclerosed or **occluded veins**. All of these practices and/or sites for venipuncture should be carefully avoided.

INTRAVENOUS THERAPY

Every time a catheter (IV) is used, vein damage occurs. Circulatory blood is rerouted to branching veins and can result in hemoconcentration. As a consequence, patients on IV therapy for extended periods often have veins that are palpable and visible but damaged or occluded (blocked). An arm with the IV line should not be used for venipuncture, because the specimen will be diluted with IV fluid. Instead, the other arm or another site should be considered. Alternatively, sometimes the nurse or the physician can disconnect the IV fluid and collect blood from the line that is already inserted. In this situation, the first few milliliters of the specimen should be discarded to remove the IV fluid, and a note should be made on the laboratory requisition that this step was performed.

HEMOLYSIS

Hemolysis results when RBCs are lysed (i.e., destroyed), hemoglobin is released, and serum or plasma, which is normally straw colored, becomes tinged with pink or red. If a specimen is grossly hemolyzed, the serum or plasma appears very dark red. Hemolysis can be caused by improper phlebotomy techniques, such as using a needle that is too small, expelling the blood vigorously into a tube, shaking or mixing tubes vigorously, performing blood collection before the alcohol has dried at the collection site, or pulling a syringe plunger back too fast (although syringes are not recommended for routine use). Hemolysis may also be the result of physiological abnormalities (e.g., sickle cell diseases, exposure to drugs or toxins, artificial heart valves, some infections).[4] Hemolysis due to poor technique or sample handling causes falsely increased results for many analytes, including potassium, magnesium, iron, lactate dehydrogenase, phosphorus, ammonia, and total protein. Hemolysis also shows falsely decreased RBC counts, hemoglobin, and hematocrit. These problems can easily be prevented with appropriate handling. The health care worker should document the fact if he or she notices that a specimen is hemolyzed.

COLLAPSED VEINS

Veins collapse when blood is withdrawn too quickly or forcefully during venipuncture, especially when blood is being collected from smaller veins (see Figure 7-1F) and/or the veins of geriatric patients. Thus, the health care worker should use a smaller blood collection tube and/or a smaller needle size during the collection process for patients with smaller veins and/or geriatric patients. A collapsed vein should not be probed with the needle. The health care worker will notice that the tube is filling properly, but then the blood entering the tube starts to slow and stops flowing. A smaller tube size should be used for the remainder of the blood collections. If the problem is not resolved, then the patient should be recollected using a syringe because the health care worker can control the force of vacuum exerted on the vein.

TURBID OR LIPEMIC SERUM

After the cells have settled or have been separated from the serum or plasma, it is normally clear, light yellow, or straw colored. **Turbid** serum or plasma appears cloudy or "milky" and can be a result of bacterial contamination or high lipid levels in the blood. Turbidity is primarily caused by ingestion of fatty substances, such as meat, butter, cream, and cheese. If a patient has recently eaten fatty substances, he or she may have a temporarily elevated lipid level, and the serum will appear **lipemic**, or cloudy. Because lipemic serum or plasma does not represent a basal state and may indicate some chemical abnormalities, documentation about the appearance of the serum or plasma may be useful to the physician.

IMPROPER COLLECTION TUBE

Learn which common laboratory tests require which collection tubes. However, there are so many possible laboratory tests and tubes available that you should also be familiar with how and where to seek information (electronically via laboratory reference manual, etc.) about test and tube requirements that you are unfamiliar with. An example of a blood specimen collected in the wrong tube would be as follows: green-topped tubes containing lithium heparin are not suitable for a patient's lithium studies because laboratory values will be falsely high, suggesting that the patient has a toxic level of lithium when he or she really does not.

Self Study

Study Questions

The following questions may have more than one answer.

1. Which of the following is the likely cause of hemoconcentration?

   a. long-term IV therapy
   b. lysing of the RBCs
   c. excessive needle probing
   d. bacterial contamination

2. Which of the following is a solid mass derived from blood constituents and can block a vein (or an artery)?

   a. hemolyzed RBC
   b. hemolyzed WBC
   c. glucose
   d. thrombus

3. If blood is to be collected for a timed blood triglyceride–level determination, the patient must fast for how long?

   a. 4–6 hours
   b. 6–8 hours
   c. 8–12 hours
   d. 14–16 hours

4. Syncope refers to:

   a. hemoconcentration
   b. edema
   c. fainting
   d. scarring at the venipuncture site

5. If the tourniquet is applied for longer than 3 minutes, which of the following analytes will most likely become falsely elevated?

   a. glucose
   b. bilirubin
   c. potassium
   d. lithium

6. To ensure that the patient is in the basal state for laboratory testing,

   a. the patient must sleep for at least 8 hours
   b. the physician must require the patient to fast overnight
   c. the physician must require the patient to fast and not drink water overnight
   d. the patient must rest for at least 10 hours and not drink water or eat any food

7. What cleansing agent can be used for a patient's venipuncture site if the patient is allergic to iodine and alcohol?

   a. sterile water
   b. phenol
   c. chlorohexidine
   d. chlorophenol

8. Small red spots on a patient's skin due to a blood clotting abnormality is referred to as:

   a. hemoconcentration
   b. petechiae
   c. hemolysis
   d. syncope

9. Sclerosed veins are a result of:

   a. hemolysis
   b. hemoconcentration
   c. inflammation
   d. syncope

10. A hemolyzed specimen can lead to falsely increased results for:

    a. RBC count
    b. hematocrit
    c. hemoglobin
    d. potassium

Case Study

Dorothy, a new health care worker at the Westward Ambulatory Clinic, had a requisition to collect a fasting blood specimen from Mrs. Gonzalez, who had come to the laboratory area at 9 A.M. for the specimen collection. Dorothy followed through with the necessary protocol to check Mrs. Gonzalez's identification and to prepare for the blood

collection. During her preparation for blood collection, she asked Mrs. Gonzalez whether she had eaten anything since the night before. Mrs. Gonzalez stated that she had not had any food since 7 P.M. the night before. Dorothy also should have asked when Mrs. Gonzalez had last had anything to drink.

Question

1. How should Dorothy proceed with the fasting blood specimen for the blood glucose test?

Self-Assessment

Check Yourself

Ready to Give Patient Instructions for Fasting Blood Specimens

Write out the instructions you would give to a patient who needs to fast before a blood collection procedure. Try to think of all the most unusual questions that the patient might ask about eating or drinking.

Practice giving the instructions to a friend or coworker. Practice your communication techniques by double

checking that they completely understand; ask them specific questions about their comprehension of the fasting process; and ask them to give a friendly and constructive critique of your instructions.

Competency Checklist: Preanalytical Complications in Blood Collection

This checklist can be completed as a group or individually.

(1) Completed (2) Needs to improve

_____ 1. List five factors about a patient's physical disposition that can affect blood collection.

_____ 2. List 3 examples of substances that can interfere in clinical testing of blood analytes.

References

1. Ernst, D: Iodine disinfectant for infants, tips from the clinical experts. *Med Lab Obs* July 2003:54, www.mlo-online.com.

2. Kahn, S: Specimen mislabeling: a significant and costly cause of potentially serious medical errors. http://www.bloodgas.org. April, 2005. Last accessed on 06/27/06.

3. Statland, BE, Winkle, P, Bokelund, H: Factors contributing to intraindividual variation of serum constituents: effects of posture and tourniquet application on variation of serum constituents in healthy subjects. *Clin Chem* 1974;20:1513.

4. Arzoumanium L: BD Tech Talk. *What Is Hemolysis: What Are the Causes.* Vol. 2, No 2: 10/2003.

Additional Resources

1. Weight Watchers: Welcome brochure. Woodbury, NY: Weight Watchers. Available at: www.weightwatchers.com. Accessed November 10, 2006.

2. Guder, WG, Narayanan, S, Wisser, H, et al.: *Samples: From the Patient to the Laboratory.* Munich, Germany: Git Verlag Publishers, 1996.

3. McGlasson, DL: Laboratory variables that may affect test results in prothrombin times (PT)/international normalized ratios (INR). *Lab Med* 2003;34(2):124–9.

4. Clinical and Laboratory Standards Institute (CLSI). *Procedures for the Collection of Diagnostic Blood Specimens by Venipuncture.* Approved Standard 5th ed. (H3-A5). Wayne, PA: CLSI, 2003.

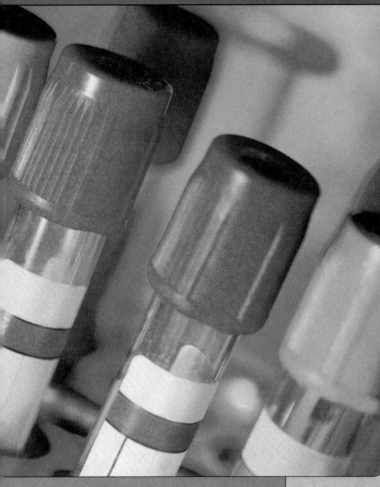

Chapter 8

Venipuncture Procedures

CHAPTER OBJECTIVES

Upon completion of Chapter 8, the learner should be able to do the following:

1. Describe the patient identification process.
2. List supplies used in a typical venipuncture procedure.
3. Describe hand hygiene and gloving procedures before and after venipuncture.
4. Identify the most appropriate sites for venipuncture.
5. Describe how to apply a tourniquet to a patient's arm and its effects on the venipuncture process.
6. Describe the decontamination process for a venipuncture and for blood cultures.
7. Describe the detailed steps of a venipuncture procedure.
8. Describe the "order of draw" for collection tubes.
9. Describe the importance of timed, fasting, and STAT specimens.
10. Describe at least three potential causes of phlebotomy complications during a venipuncture procedure.

KEY TERMS

butterfly system
Clinical and Laboratory Standards Institute (CLSI)
decontaminated
evacuated tube system
hand hygiene
physician–patient relationship
specimen rejection
STAT
syringe method
therapeutic drug monitoring (TDM)
timed specimen
tourniquet
winged infusion system

Blood Collection Process

There are essential steps that are part of every successful blood collection procedure. Figure 8-1 ▦ is a flow chart that demonstrates the basic venipuncture process. In some cases, steps may occur simultaneously (e.g., checking the patient's physical condition while confirming the identification); in others, a problem may arise that prevents the health care worker from going further in the procedure (e.g., the verbal identity of the individual does not match the written documentation or the supplies needed for the venipuncture have expired). Each step of the patient encounter must be evaluated carefully in a detailed manner, with care taken not to omit any of the essential components.[1,2]

1. Prepare yourself by decontaminating hands and reviewing laboratory test orders.
2. Approach, identify, and position the patient comfortably.
3. Assess the patient's physical disposition, including diet and/or whether the patient is sensitive to latex.
4. Select and prepare equipment and supplies.
5. Find a suitable puncture site.
6. Prepare/decontaminate the puncture site.
7. Choose a venipuncture method.
8. Collect the samples in the appropriate tubes and in the correct order.
9. Discard contaminated supplies.
10. Label the samples.
11. Assess the patient to ensure bleeding has stopped.
12. Decontaminate hands.
13. Manage and document any special circumstances that occurred during the phlebotomy procedure.

EXERCISING STANDARD PRECAUTIONS

Precautionary measures such as **hand hygiene** and the use of gloves should be considered routine procedures and are covered in Chapter 4: Safety and Infection Control. These procedures are vital to the well-being of the patient and the health care worker and must be practiced continuously. Hand hygiene and gloving procedures are most commonly done as soon as the health care worker is in visual contact with each patient, *before* beginning the procedure. This gives the patient a visual assurance of cleanliness and reinforces a safety-conscious gesture for both the patient and the health care worker. A clean, pressed uniform or "scrubs" with a laboratory coat is comfortable attire and instills a sense of professionalism and hygiene, which is gratifying to patients and promotes a safer work environment. Glove removal and hand hygiene should be again performed *after* each patient encounter. Refer to Procedures 4-1, 4-2, and 4-3 for hand hygiene and gown, mask, and gloving techniques.

Because human skin and nails are colonized with microorganisms, the transmission of pathogens can occur easily from a health care worker to a patient. Health care workers who have direct patient contact should not wear artificial nails, and natural nails should be less than one quarter of an inch long.[3] Refer to Figure 8-4 ▦. Adherence to hand hygiene techniques (handwashing or use of alcohol-based hand rubs) has been shown to significantly reduce outbreaks of infections, including antimicrobial-resistant infections (e.g., methicillin-resistant *Staphylococcus aureus*, MRSA).[3]

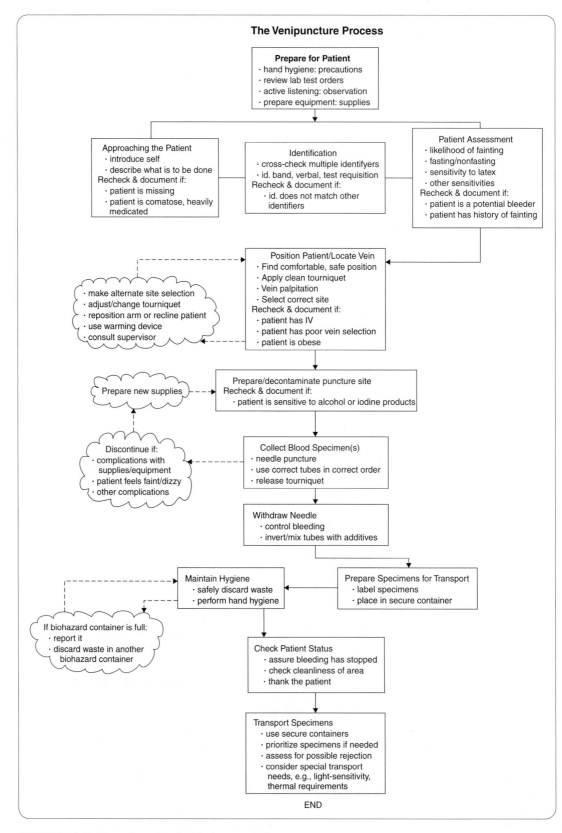

FIGURE ■ 8-1 Flow Chart for the Venipuncture Process

Mentally Preparing for the Patient Encounter

RATIONALE

To help the health care worker mentally focus on the importance of the individual patient and prepare for that specific venipuncture procedure.

EQUIPMENT

- Phlebotomy supplies
- Personal protective equipment (PPE) (gloves, clean uniform, laboratory coat, etc.)
- Test requisitions
- Writing pen
- Bar code reader/scanner (if applicable)

PREPARATION

(1) Prepare and assemble PPE, phlebotomy supplies, test requisitions, writing pen, and appropriate patient information before the patient encounter and prior to the venipuncture process.

(2) Identify the patient properly.

(3) Wash or sanitize your hands with an alcohol hand rinse, then put on gloves.

PROCEDURE

(4) The health care worker needs a positive, professional appearance (neat and clean) and temperament (optimistic and open-minded) before beginning the patient encounter. Take a deep, cleansing breath before beginning (Figure 8-2 ■). As you do this, focus on the individual patient and the requests for that particular patient. Use the cleansing breath to center your attention on the upcoming venipuncture task as you temporarily remove yourself from other distracting factors in the workplace (e.g., TV noise, telephones, and other conversations). Use your keen observations to determine any special circumstances or needs that the patient may have.

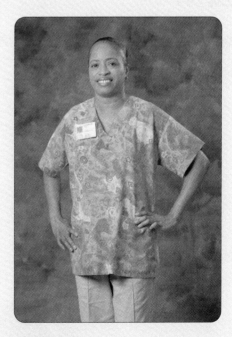

FIGURE ■ 8-2

(continued)

5 Arrange and check phlebotomy supplies, test requisitions, writing pen, and appropriate patient information before beginning the patient encounter and venipuncture process (Figure 8-3 ■).

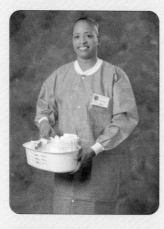

FIGURE ■ 8-3

6 If the patient information is incomplete on test requisitions, the health care worker may not be able to identify the patient correctly, or he or she may not know in which tubes to collect the blood. In such cases, obtain assistance from a laboratory supervisor or a nurse before collecting the sample.

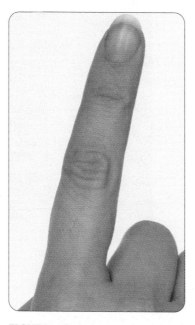

FIGURE ■ 8-4 Appropriate Length of Fingernails for Health Care Workers Who Have Direct Contact with Patients

> ### Clinical Alert ❗
>
> Remember that the use of gloves does not eliminate the need for hand hygiene, nor does good hand hygiene eliminate the need for gloves. Hands should be **decontaminated** before and immediately after specimen collection procedures, and new gloves should be used for each patient. These are requirements for proper technique.
>
> Be familiar with policies regarding precautions for handling blood and body fluids. *All specimens should be treated as if they are hazardous and infectious*, according to the standard precautions described in detail in Chapter 4.

Assessing, Identifying, and Approaching the Patient

TEST REQUISITIONS

Laboratory test requests are usually transmitted electronically or as a paper requisition. Electronic (computer-generated) requests contain the same required information as paper requisitions. The health care worker should be familiar with both types.

> ### Clinical Alert ❗
>
> If the health care worker does not understand the test ordered, a supervisor, laboratory technologist, or nurse should be consulted *before* the procedure. Knowing which tests are requested helps the health care worker to prepare the patient appropriately and collect the specimen in the appropriate tubes and in the correct order. Failure to do so results in preanalytical errors, misleading test results, and repeated venipunctures.

PATIENT IDENTIFICATION PROCESS

Positive patient identification is the most crucial responsibility for which a health care worker is held accountable. The Joint Commission recommends using "at least two patient identifiers (neither to be the patient's room number) whenever taking blood samples or administering medications or blood products."[4] Patient identification errors can occur at the time of phlebotomy or as the specimen is being prepared for testing—for example, after centrifugation when the specimen is divided into aliquots. The process of identifying patients varies slightly on the basis of the patient's location (inpatient or outpatient or emergency room), the type of patient (pediatric or adult), whether the patient is conscious or unconscious, and the available information at the time (armband or picture identification).

> ### Clinical Alert ❗
>
> If there is a discrepancy in the identification process, the specimen should not be obtained until identity can be verified. Discrepancies should be reported immediately. Identification errors can be life-threatening for the patient and pose significant liability to both the health care worker who makes the error and the health care facility that employs him or her. Never base identity on records or charts placed on the patient's bed or equipment. Identity errors occur because of inaccurate requisitions, mixed-up paperwork, or failure to follow identification procedures. All discrepancies should be reported to a supervisor.

The Basics of Patient Identification

RATIONALE

To use appropriate patient identifiers whenever taking blood samples.

EQUIPMENT

Not applicable

PROCEDURE

Patient identification involves *at least 3 steps:*

1. After greeting a conscious patient (Figure 8-5 ■), ask the patient to state and spell his or her full name and identification number or birth date. (You may also request the patient's address.) For example: "Hello, sir, could you please verify your name and identification number? Could you please spell your last name for me?"

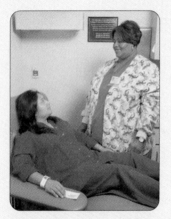

FIGURE ■ 8-5

2. Compare the information stated with the information on the laboratory test requisitions (Figure 8-6 ■).

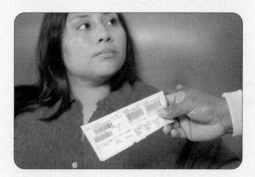

FIGURE ■ 8-6

3. Confirm the information (from steps 1 and 2) with another source of reliable, verifiable identification (e.g., printed identification number, hospital identification bracelet, driver's license, nurse, and parent) (Figure 8-7 ■). If all three steps indicate the same identity, proceed with the rest of the specimen collection procedure.

Refer to Chapter 5 for more information about requisitions.

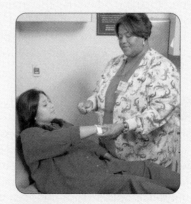

FIGURE ■ 8-7

BOX 8-1	Advances in Identification Systems

Bar codes are quick, accurate, cost-effective, and widely used for patient and specimen identification and tracking. Wireless technology such as radio frequency identification (RFID), which uses radio waves to transmit data, is also being used for patient identification and tracking specimens. Some hospitals have also incorporated a small picture of the patient into his or her armband as an additional visual verification step.

Inpatient Identification

Hospitalized patients (except those just entering an emergency room) must wear an identification bracelet indicating the first and last names and a designated hospital number (sometimes called a unit number). Hospital identification numbers provide a unique number for each patient and help hospital personnel to distinguish between patients with the same first and/or last names (Box 8-1).

Information on the identification bracelet may also include the patient's room number, bed assignment, and physician's name. A three-way match should be made with the identification bracelet, the test requisition, and the patient's statement of his or her name, birthday, or address.

Clinical Alert ⚠

There are special cases that involve patients with severe burns or in isolation, in which the identification is attached to the patient's bed rather than the arm. These are the only circumstances in which a health care worker may use a bed-labeled identification tag to confirm identity. This step should be followed up by a nurse's confirmation and appropriate documentation.

Identification of Patients Who Are Sleeping

A patient who is sleeping should be awakened and have the patient identity verified before blood is collected. Verbal information should be compared with the information on the requisition and the identification bracelet.[2]

Clinical Alert ⚠

The health care worker should *not* ask, "Are you Ms. Doe?" because an ill patient on medication may mistakenly utter something, nod, or answer yes. Therefore, the best tactic is to ask, "What is your name?" or "Please state your name and birthday," and let the patient reply. The patient must be correctly identified by his or her identification bracelet. If the patient does not have an identification bracelet, the nurse responsible for the patient must be asked to make the identification. The name of the nurse should be noted.

Patients who are semiconscious, comatose, mentally incompetent, or sleeping may jerk unexpectedly during the blood collection process, particularly as the needle is inserted into the arm.[2] If the patient cannot be awakened, seek assistance from an authorized health care worker during the procedure to help secure the patient's arm.

Identification of Patients Who Are Unconscious, Mentally Incompetent, or Do Not Speak the Language

A nurse, relative, or friend may identify patients who are unconscious, mentally incompetent, or comatose or who cannot speak the health care worker's language by providing the patient's name, address, and identification number, and/or birth date. Again, this information should be compared with the information on the requisition to confirm identity. Any discrepancy should be reported to a supervisor.[1,2]

Identification of Infants and Young Children

It is preferable to use the same identification procedures for both children and adults; however, it is not always practical. A nurse or relative may identify an infant or child by providing the name, address, and identification number, and/or birth date.

Emergency Room Patient Identification

Patients often come to the emergency room (ER) unconscious and/or unidentified. The **Clinical and Laboratory Standards Institute (CLSI)** suggests that a temporary master identification (e.g., hospital number attached to the patient's body by wristband or other suitable device) may be provided until a positive identification can be made.

Outpatient/Ambulatory Patient Identification

Ambulatory patients are normally called to a blood collection area from a waiting room. Thus, ambulatory patient identification takes more time, because the patients have to walk into the specimen collection area then show some form of identification (e.g., ID card or driver's license) before any specimens are collected. If the patient has the card available, positive identification can occur in the same manner as with hospitalized patients. Again, the identification process should involve the three-way match: verbally asking for name, address, and/or birth date, confirmation with the test requisitions, and a form of ID.

PHYSICAL CLUES FOR ASSESSMENT OF THE PATIENT

As mentioned previously, factors related to the physical or emotional disposition of the patient may affect the blood collection process, so be keenly aware and be able to prepare more adequately for the venipuncture. The health care worker can get clues about the patient's disposition by being observant and alert and by listening carefully—for example, if there is an empty food tray by the patient's bedside, it is likely that the patient has eaten recently, and a notation about the nonfasting condition should be made after confirming the observation with the patient. The following statement might confirm it with the patient, "Mr. Jones, it looks like you might have finished your breakfast recently, could you tell me when you last ate or drank anything?" A clue about something unusual may come after talking to the patient or after the identification process has taken place. In the case of ambulatory patients, it is important to know if they have fainted during prior venipunctures. A simple question may evoke more information. For example, "Mr. Jones, have you ever fainted during or after a blood-collection procedure?"

APPROACHING THE PATIENT

Several professional and courteous behaviors and phrases can help make the patient–health care worker encounter a smooth interaction (Box 8-2). The first of these is a polite knock (no banging) on the patient's door before entering the patient's room. The health care worker should introduce him- or herself and state which department he or she is from—e.g., the laboratory—and that he or she has come to collect a blood sample. Sometimes,

BOX 8-2	Typical Health Care Worker–Patient Interaction

The following scenario is one example of a health care worker and patient interaction just before the blood collection. It begins when the health care worker politely knocks on the patient's door and slowly enters the room.

Health care worker: Good morning. I am Ms. Smith from the laboratory, and I have come to collect a blood sample.

Pause to give the patient an opportunity to speak. If the lights are off or dimmed, explain that you need to turn the lights on. Doing so gives the patient a moment to adjust to the idea of bright lights if he or she has been asleep.

Health care worker: Could you please spell your name and state your identification number?

Patient: I am John Jones. J-O-H-N J-O-N-E-S. Zero, three, one, seven.

Health care worker: May I please see your identification (ID) armband?

Check the armband against laboratory requisitions and the patient's verbal identification. If all three match, proceed.

Health care worker: This will take only a few minutes.

Patient: Will it hurt?

Health care worker: It will hurt a little, but it will be over soon. Please allow me to look at your arm veins. I am going to palpate the area to feel for a vein. Is that okay with you?

Patient: No problem, it's okay.

Proceed with the remainder of the procedure, maintaining a highly professional atmosphere and a respectful attitude. Ascertain whether the patient has been fasting.

Health care worker: Mr. Jones, when was the last time you ate or drank anything?

Do not use the term *fast* because some patients may not understand it completely.

Patient: Last night when I had dinner.

As supplies are being readied, the health care worker could demonstrate that she is opening a new needle. She should also inquire about latex sensitivity if using latex products (gloves or tourniquet).

Health care worker: Mr. Jones, naturally I'll be using a new tourniquet and needle to collect your blood sample. Have you ever fainted during or after a blood collection procedure?

Patient: No, never.

Health care worker: Okay then, please hold still while I check for a vein, and then I'll collect the specimen. You will feel a needle prick.

At the end of the procedure, say the following:

Health care worker: Let me check your arm one more time. Thank you, Mr. Jones.

the health care worker may need to explain to the patient that the physician ordered the laboratory test or tests. The health care worker may also need to explain the procedure as supplies are being set up or as gloves are put on. During setup, the specimen collection tray should not be placed on the patient's bed, because it is not a stable surface, or on the patient's eating table, because of possible contamination of items or other specimens on the tray. As supplies are being readied and the vein is being palpated, the health care worker may try to alleviate some of the patient's fears. It may be reassuring to purposefully show the patient that the supplies are "new" and "unused."

Clinical Alert ⚠

If a physician, clergy, or nurse is consulting with the patient, the specimen collection procedure should be delayed until the consultation is completed. The **physician–patient relationship** has priority over a phlebotomy procedure unless the request is for a timed or STAT specimen. In this case, ask for permission to proceed.

When friends or relatives are in the room, politely explain to the patient that a specimen is needed and ask whether the guests would mind leaving the room temporarily. The patient may also give permission for the guests to stay during the venipuncture procedure.

Equipment Selection and Preparation

SUPPLIES FOR VENIPUNCTURE

Being prepared means having all supplies readily available. Supplies for venipuncture differ according to the method used (i.e., **evacuated tube system** or winged infusion/ **butterfly system** or **syringe method**) and the tests that have been ordered. Supplies common to most methods of blood collection are the following:

- Laboratory requisitions or labels
- Marking pens
- Gloves
- Nonlatex tourniquets
- Alcohol pads/skin disinfectants
- 2 iodine-tincture scrub swab sticks or chlorohexidine gluconate swab sticks for blood cultures
- Safety needles with single-use, evacuated tube holders and winged infusion sets
- Safety syringes and syringe transfer devices
- Blood collection tubes
- Plastic capillary tubes with tube sealer
- Nonlatex bandages and sterile gauze pads
- Glass microscope slides
- Puncture-proof sharps container

Supplies should be readily available and selected just prior to the procedure (Figure 8-8 ■). Supplies are discussed in more detail in Chapter 6.

POSITIONING OF THE PATIENT AND VENIPUNCTURE SITE SELECTION

It is important to make the patient comfortable and safe and to choose the least hazardous site for blood collection by skin puncture or venipuncture. Health care workers should know about useful devices and the positions and locations of veins, refer to Figures 8-9 ■ through 8-14 ■.

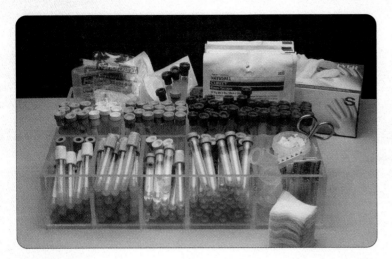

FIGURE ■ 8-8 Well-Stocked Phlebotomy Tray

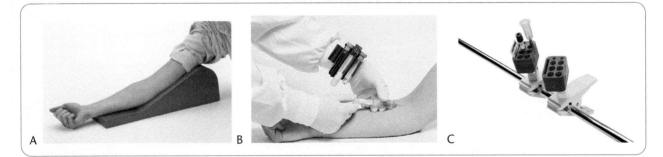

FIGURE ■ 8-9 Devices to Assist in Positioning the Patient and Supplies. A. A phlebotomy wedge is used to stabilize and cushion the arm in a comfortable position. B. This tube holder fits on the health care worker's wrist to keep blood collection tubes immediately available during and after the procedure. C. This tube holder provides a temporary and easy-to-access device that holds the tubes in an upright position

Courtesy of MarketLab: www.marketlabinc.com.

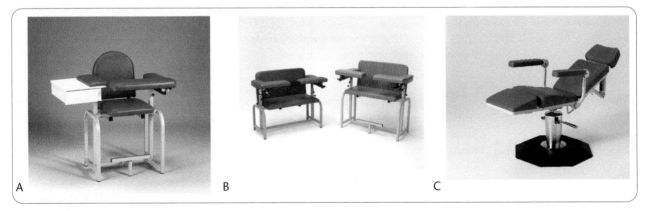

FIGURE ■ 8-10 Blood Collection Chairs. A. Extra-tall chairs are advantageous for the health care worker, because they eliminate "stooping over" a chair during the procedure. They should be used for patients who have greatest mobility and are not likely to lose balance or who have trouble getting in or out of the chair. B. Extra-wide chairs for large and/or obese patients. C. Recliner-style chair

Courtesy of Clinton Industries, Inc., and MarketLab: www.marketlabinc.com.

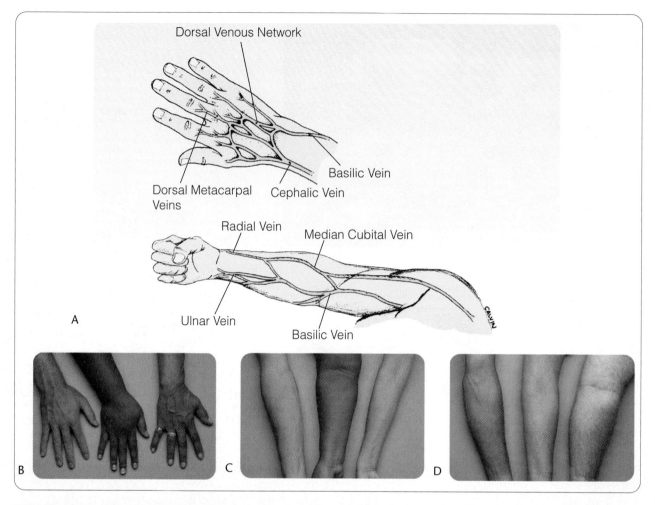

FIGURE ■ **8-11** Individual Vein Variations in the Hand and Arm. Visible vein patterns are dramatically different among individuals. Learn to visualize but, more importantly, feel the veins before venipuncture. A. A typical human arm labeled with prominent veins. B. Dorsal hand veins show up in different locations and in varying degrees of visibility in three hands. The first is a young adult white male; the other two are African American females, one young adult and one middle-aged. Note the variability in skin tones as well. C. These arms are all of adults of different ages with varying skin tones, muscle mass, fatty tissue, and bone structure. D. Note that in the arms with more muscle mass and fatty tissue, the veins are hardly visible at all. In all cases, rely on feeling the vein rather than seeing it.

The most common sites for venipuncture are in the antecubital area of the arm just below the bend of the elbow, because this is where the median cubital, cephalic, and basilic veins lie close to the surface of the skin and are most prominent. The common choices for vein selection are:

1. Median cubital (sometimes called the median vein)—most commonly used vein for venipuncture because it is the easiest to obtain blood from and has been reported to be less painful.[5]

2. Cephalic vein—on the outer edge (thumb side) of the arm.

3. Basilic vein—on the inside edge (pinkie side) of the antecubital fossa area; it is in close proximity to the median nerve and the brachial artery so the other choices are usually preferable.

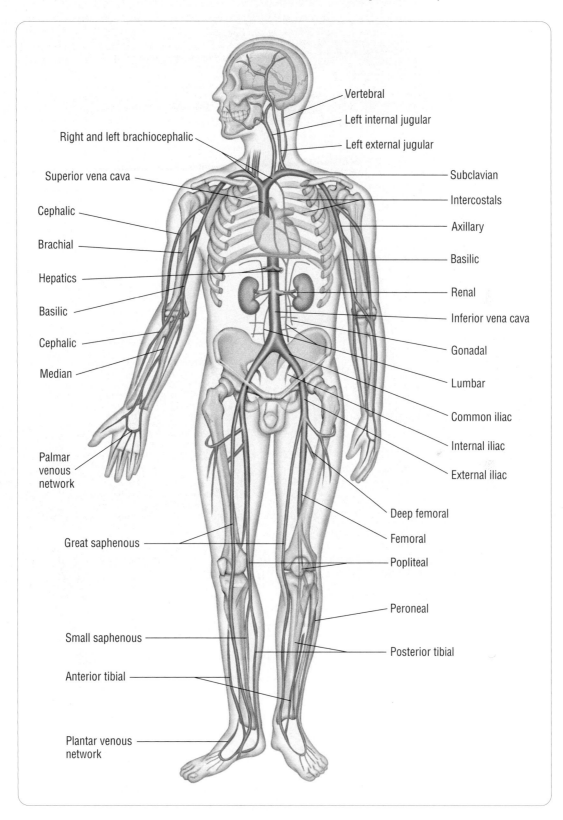

FIGURE ■ 8-12 An Overview of the Venous System

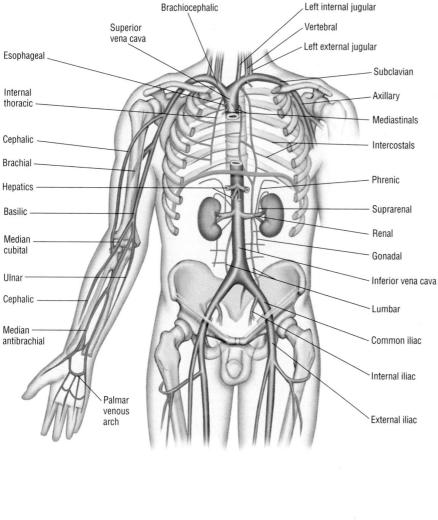

Esophageal

Internal thoracic

Cephalic

Brachial

Hepatics

Basilic

Median cubital

Ulnar

Cephalic

Median antibrachial

Palmar venous arch

Superior vena cava

Brachiocephalic

Left internal jugular

Vertebral

Left external jugular

Subclavian

Axillary

Mediastinals

Intercostals

Phrenic

Suprarenal

Renal

Gonadal

Inferior vena cava

Lumbar

Common iliac

Internal iliac

External iliac

FIGURE ■ 8-13 Venous Drainage of the Abdomen and Chest

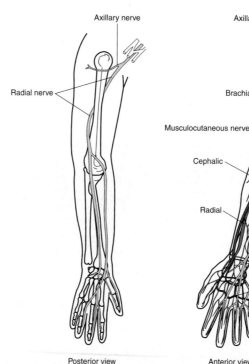

FIGURE ■ 8-14 Veins, Arteries, and Nerves of the Arm

Axillary nerve

Radial nerve

Posterior view

Right subclavian

Axillary nerve

Axillary

Brachial

Musculocutaneous nerve

Cephalic

Radial

Radial nerve

Median nerve

Basilic

Ulnar nerve

Ulnar

Median of forearm

Deep palmar venous arch

Superficial palmar venous arch

Anterior view

Clinical Alert ❗

Serious damage can occur if a nerve is accidentally punctured, probed, or nicked during the venipuncture procedure. If the patient complains of severe pain during the procedure, the needle must be removed *immediately* and the procedure discontinued. Assistance should be sought from a nurse or supervisor. Only a physician can evaluate whether or not nerve damage has occurred. Nevertheless, the incident should be documented. Figure 8-14 depicts the proximity of nerves in relation to the veins.

    Arteries do not feel like veins and should not be confused. Arteries pulsate, are more elastic, and have a thick wall. Accidental arterial puncture may result in excessive bleeding and hematoma (bruising caused by localized bleeding) formation. If the health care worker believes that he or she has punctured an artery, the needle should be removed immediately, and direct pressure should be applied to the site for at least 5 minutes or until bleeding has stopped.[1] A supervisor or nurse should be notified.

Clinical Alert ❗

Reasons for not using the patient's arm veins include the following:

- Intravenous (IV) lines in both arms
- Burned or scarred areas
- Areas with a hematoma
- Cast(s) on arm(s)
- Thrombosed veins (thrombosed veins lack resilience, feel much like a rope cord, and roll easily)
- Edematous arms (swollen area because of excessive amounts of tissue fluids)
- Mastectomy on one side only (use of the arm on the unaffected side is acceptable for venipuncture)
- Mastectomy on both sides (Neither arm should be used because of fluid accumulation. However, if *no other puncture sites are available*, blood can be collected without using a tourniquet, and a notation about this situation should be documented. In some hospitals, a doctor's authorization is required before collecting blood in this situation.)

Palpating the entire antecubital area enables the health care worker get an idea of the size, angle, and depth of the vein. The patient can assist in the process by making a fist and keeping it tightly closed. Veins may also be used for transfusion, infusion, and therapeutic agents, so sometimes physicians request that veins have restricted use ("reserved") for those purposes only.

    Alternative sites for blood collection when the antecubital area cannot be used are hand veins and, in some cases, foot veins and/or a capillary or fingerstick specimen. Veins on the dorsal side of the hands or wrists (i.e., the back side) are acceptable venipuncture sites if the median cubital, cephalic, or basilic veins are inaccessible. Veins in the wrist or ankle tend to move, or roll aside, as the needle is inserted; therefore, it may be helpful to have the patient extend the foot or hand into a position that helps hold the vein taut (see Figure 8-15 ■). Venipuncture in small veins is facilitated by the use of a 21- to 23-gauge safety butterfly needle and by carefully anchoring/positioning the vein before needle insertion.

    Ankle and foot veins (on the dorsal, or upper, side) should be used *only* if arm veins have been determined to be unsuitable and if the health care worker has been authorized to do so. Arm veins are sites preferred over foot or ankle veins, because coagulation and

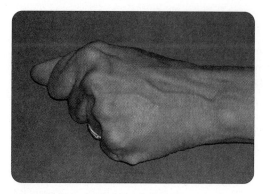

FIGURE ■ 8-15 Dorsal Hand Veins. Hand veins are more prominent if the hand is held taut

Clinical Alert !

For hand vein punctures, the posterior, or dorsal (the back of the hand), opposite of the wrist should be used. Do *not* use the anterior side or the palmar venous network in the wrist, because nerves are easily injured by needle probing in this area (Figure 8-16 ■).

vascular complications tend to be more troublesome in the lower extremities. Thus, foot and ankle veins should not be used for cardiac or diabetic patients. Some hospitals do not allow the use of the lower extremities (foot and ankle) for blood-sampling sites. Other hospitals allow sampling from these sites only after permission has been granted by the patient's physician and after the health care worker has been properly trained. If allowed, a smaller needle is again recommended.

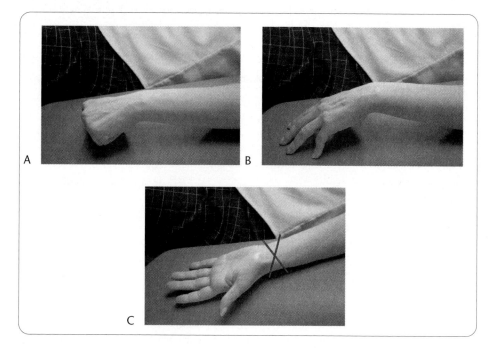

FIGURE ■ 8-16 Dorsal Side of the Wrist

WARMING THE PUNCTURE SITE

Warming the puncture site helps facilitate phlebotomy by increasing arterial blood flow to the area. Several warming devices are available commercially that are quick and easy to activate and provide localized heat to the potential venipuncture area. Another method is to use a clean towel or a washcloth heated to about 42°C. When the warm towel is wrapped around the site for 3 to 5 minutes, the skin temperature can increase several degrees. The wrap can be encased in a plastic bag to help retain heat and keep the patient's bed dry. The health care worker may leave the warm wrap on the patient while he or she collects specimens from other patients, and then return to the original patient after several minutes.

TOURNIQUET APPLICATION AND PUNCTURE SITE DECONTAMINATION

A **tourniquet** (preferably single-use, latex-free) or blood pressure cuff makes veins more prominent and easier to puncture by causing venous filling. The tourniquet slows down blood flow toward the heart so that it gathers in the veins.[1] A soft rubber tourniquet about 1 inch (2.5 cm) wide and about 15 to 18 inches (45 cm) long is most comfortable for patients, affordable, and easy to use, and it comes in a variety of colors. Practices differ slightly on the use of a tourniquet. Experienced health care workers are often able to find a puncture site by palpating the antecubital area without a tourniquet, then applying the tourniquet just before the needle puncture. However, less experienced health care workers are encouraged to take their time in finding a suitable puncture site, so it may be necessary to apply the tourniquet while palpating the antecubital area, then release the tourniquet for a short period of time, then reapply it before the needle puncture.

Procedure 8-3   Use of a Tourniquet

RATIONALE

Tourniquet application causes veins to fill with blood, thereby assisting in location of a suitable venipuncture site and enabling easier blood flow once the needle has been inserted.

EQUIPMENT

- Latex-free clean tourniquet
- Gloves
- Alcohol-based hand disinfectants

PREPARATION

(1) Identify the patient properly.

(2) Wash or sanitize your hands using appropriate agents, dry them, then put on gloves.

(continued)

PROCEDURE

3 Use a clean latex-free tourniquet (Figure 8-17 ■).

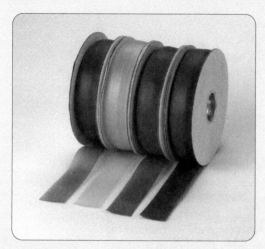

FIGURE ■ **8-17** *Courtesy of MarketLab: www.marketlabinc.com.*

4 Stretch the ends of the tourniquet around the patient's arm about 3 inches (7.6 cm) above the venipuncture area (antecubital area). Hold both ends of the tourniquet in one hand while the other hand tucks in a section next to the skin and makes a partial loop with the tourniquet (Figure 8-18 ■).

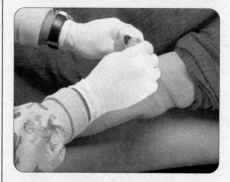

FIGURE ■ **8-18**

5 The tourniquet should be tight but not painful to the patient. Do *not* leave it on for more than 1 minute. Do *not* place it over sores or burned skin; however, depending on the policies of each health care facility, it may be placed over a hospital gown sleeve or a piece of gauze.

6 When it is time to release the tourniquet, the partial loop should allow for easy release by the health care worker. (For patient comfort and to obtain a good specimen, do not leave it on the patient's arm while readying supplies to perform the initial puncture, especially if the process takes longer than 1 minute. If there is a time delay, reapply the tourniquet.) Release it *after* the needle puncture, when blood has begun to flow into the collection tubes. During the venipuncture, release the tourniquet with one hand, because the other hand will be holding the needle and tubes.

7 Once released, it can remain loosely on the arm or surface of the work area (e.g., bed or blood collection chair) until the procedure is completed (Figure 8-19 ■).

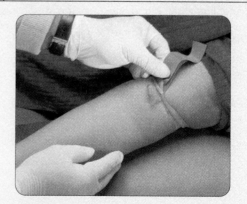

FIGURE ■ **8-19**

Clinical Alert !

A tourniquet should not be left on for more than 1 minute because it becomes uncomfortable and causes hemoconcentration—that is, increased blood concentration of large molecules, such as proteins, cells, and coagulation factors. The patient may be asked to make a fist and hold it, because excessive clenching also results in hemoconcentration. If no vein becomes apparent, or "pops up," the patient may be asked to dangle the arm for 1–2 minutes to allow blood to fill the veins to capacity, then the tourniquet may be reapplied and the area palpated again. The health care worker should never stick a vein unless it can be felt. It is better to defer the patient to someone else who can search for the vein than to take a blind chance.

Procedure 8-4   Decontamination of the Puncture Site

RATIONALE

To provide a clean decontaminated area of the skin in which to make the needle puncture.

EQUIPMENT

- Gloves
- Gauze pad soaked in 70% isopropanol (isopropyl alcohol) or a commercially packaged alcohol pad

PREPARATION

(1) Identify the patient properly.

(2) Wash or sanitize your hands using appropriate agents, dry them, then put on gloves.

PROCEDURE

(3) Once the site is selected, decontaminate it with a gauze pad soaked in 70% isopropanol (isopropyl alcohol) or with a commercially packaged alcohol pad.

(4) Rub the site with the alcohol pad, working in concentric circles from the inside out. If the skin is particularly dirty, repeat the process with a new alcohol pad (Figure 8-20 ▪).

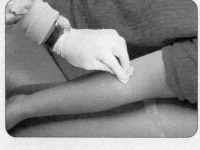

FIGURE ▪ **8-20**

(continued)

Decontamination of the Puncture Site *(continued)*

(5) Decontaminate your own gloved finger if you intend to palpate the site again. Air-dry the site or dry it with sterile gauze (Figure 8-21 ■).

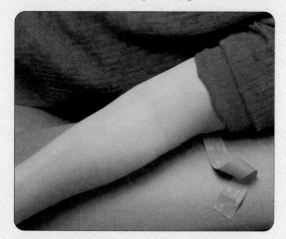

FIGURE ■ **8-21**

(Iodine preparations are primarily used for drawing blood for blood gas analysis and blood cultures. Follow the manufacturer's directions for appropriate decontamination results. However, most procedures include a 60-second alcohol scrub, followed by a second scrub for 30–60 seconds with iodine tincture, then iodine removal with a sterile gauze or alcohol pad. For some patients, iodine causes skin irritation. For patients who are allergic to both iodine and/or alcohol, chlorohexidine has been reported as an alternative skin decontaminant with removal of excess solution using sterile saline.[6])

Clinical Alert ❗

The decontaminated area should never be touched with any nonsterile object. The alcohol should be allowed to dry (for approximately 30–60 seconds), or it should be wiped off with sterile gauze after the site is prepared; otherwise, the puncture site will sting, and the alcohol may cause hemolysis and/or interfere with test results, such as blood alcohol levels. Blowing on the site to hasten the drying process is not advised, because doing so may recontaminate the site.

Venipuncture Methods

EVACUATED TUBE SYSTEM AND WINGED INFUSION SYSTEM, OR BUTTERFLY METHOD

CLSI recommends that venipuncture specimens be collected with a system that enables blood to flow directly into the tubes.[1] Evacuated tube systems and **winged infusion systems** are widely available, equipped with safety devices and comply with this recommendation. Procedure 8-5 demonstrates a basic venipuncture technique.

Health care workers should note that although the procedural steps for the puncture are the same for the evacuated tube system and the winged-infusion system, there may be different steps to follow as the tubes are actually filled. Because the tubing from the winged infusion system contains air, it will under fill the first evacuated tube by 0.5 mL, which affects the additive-to-blood ratio. Therefore, a red-topped nonadditive tube should be filled before any tube with additives. After the first tube, the order of the tube draw should be the same as other methods. When tubes for coagulation are the only ones to be collected, it is suggested that a "dummy" tube be collected and discarded. This fills the tubing with blood so that the correct additive-to-blood ratio is obtained for the following coagulation tube. When using the winged infusion system, each tube should be held horizontally or slightly downward to keep the additive at the bottom of the tube. This avoids

Performing a Venipuncture

RATIONALE

To provide a safe, effective, and efficient method to obtain a blood specimen.

EQUIPMENT

- Personal protective equipment (PPE) (gloves, clean uniform, laboratory coat, etc.)
- Laboratory requisitions or labels
- Marking pens
- Nonlatex tourniquet
- Alcohol pads/skin disinfectants
- 2 iodine-tincture scrub swab sticks or chlorohexidine gluconate swab sticks for blood cultures
- Safety syringes and syringe transfer devices
- Safety needles with single-use, evacuated tube holders and winged infusion sets
- Blood collection tubes
- Plastic capillary tubes with tube sealer
- Nonlatex bandages or sterile gauze pads
- Glass microscope slides
- Puncture-proof sharps container
- Test requisitions
- Writing pen
- Bar code reader/scanner (if applicable)

PREPARATION

1. After greeting and identifying the patient, decontaminate hands and don gloves.

2. Assemble equipment in the presence of the patient. Offer to answer any questions for the patient (Figure 8-22).

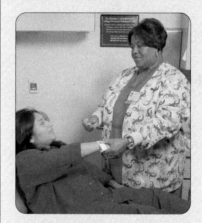

FIGURE ■ 8-22

PROCEDURE

3. Prepare equipment according to the manufacturer's instructions, including attaching a needle onto the appropriate holder. For an evacuated tube system, the most commonly used, the safety needle is screwed directly onto the tube holder.

(For a safety winged-infusion or butterfly apparatus, the smaller needle [1/2–3/4 inch in length and 21–23 gauge in diameter] comes attached to a thin tubing with a Luer adapter that, in turn, must be attached to a tube holder.)

(continued)

④ Position the patient's arm slightly bent, in a downward but comfortable manner. Apply the tourniquet and check for potential sites by palpating the vein. Feel for the median cubital vein first (it is usually bigger and anchored better), the cephalic vein (depending on its size) is the second choice (it does not roll and bruise as easily as the basilic), and the basilic vein is third choice. If a suitable vein is not felt, remove the tourniquet and try the other arm. Remember, do not leave the tourniquet on for more than 1 minute. Choose a vein that feels the fullest. If necessary, warm the site or lower the arm further in a downward position to pool venous blood (Figure 8-23 ■).

⑤ Select the site and decontaminate the patient's skin with an alcohol pad in a circular motion from inside to outside (Figure 8-24 ■). Allow it to air dry, and do not blow on it. (The tourniquet can be removed during this step and reapplied when the site is dry.) Ask the patient to "please close your fist," to make veins more prominent and easier to puncture. Avoid vigorous hand exercise or "pumping," because it affects some laboratory values. Never say that "this will not hurt"; simply mention to the patient that he or she will "feel a stick" or say, "Please remain still while I begin the procedure, you will feel a slight prick." Be mindful that from this step forward a patient may feel faint and/or lose consciousness.

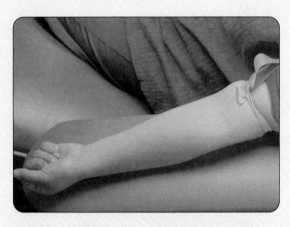

FIGURE ■ **8-23**

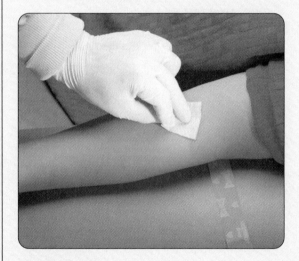

FIGURE ■ **8-24**

⑥ Remove the needle cap carefully so as not to touch anything that would contaminate it. If it does touch any surface that is not sterile, replace it with a new needle assembly and discard the old one. Hold the needle assembly in one hand while the thumb of the other hand anchors the vein 1 to 2 inches below the puncture site. (Some health care workers use the thumb and forefinger of the "free hand" to

anchor the vein. Others place the last three fingers of the "free hand" under the elbow to steady the arm even more.) Position the needle so that it is parallel or running in the same direction as the vein. Insert the needle quickly, with the bevel side up, and at a 15- to 30-degree angle with the skin. A slight "pop" should be felt as the needle enters the vein (Figure 8-25 ■).

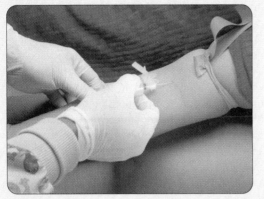

FIGURE ■ 8-25

7 Press the evacuated tube gently onto the sheathed needle. Blood should begin to flow. If blood does not flow, palpate gently above the puncture to feel for the vein and possibly reorient the needle slightly. Do not probe!

8 As the blood begins to flow, instruct the patient to open his or her fist and release the tourniquet. (The tourniquet can be left on until after the tubes have filled if it appears that blood flow is slow; however, always remove it before withdrawing the needle.) Carefully push an evacuated tube into the holder so that the tube closure is punctured by the inside needle and blood can enter. Orient the tube in a downward position to avoid any possibility of backflow (Figure 8-26).

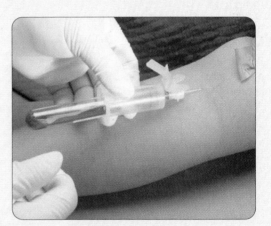

FIGURE ■ 8-26

9 Allow the blood to flow into the tube until it stops so that the proper dilution of blood to additive can occur. Watch carefully to see when the blood flow ceases. If multiple sample tubes are to be collected, remove each tube from the holder with a gentle twist-and-pull motion and replace it with the next tube. (During tube transfer, be mindful of these key issues: hold the needle apparatus firmly and motionlessly so that the needle remains comfortable and in the vein during tube changes, follow the correct order of draw, and remember that blood stops flowing between tube changes because of the inner needle design, which allows a sleeve to block flow if it is not in use.) Experienced health care workers can gently mix/invert a full tube in one hand while holding the needle apparatus and waiting for another tube to fill. Some health care workers switch hands to use a dominant hand during tube exchange. Whatever the case, find the approach that is most reliable and comfortable for both patient and health care worker.

(continued)

(10) When all tubes have been filled and removed from the holder, withdraw the needle, move it away from the patient, and hold a gauze pad over the site (Figure 8-27 ■).

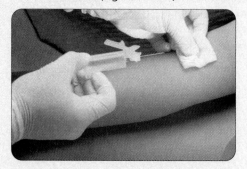

FIGURE ■ **8-27**

(11) Immediately activate the safety device according to the manufacturer's instructions. This may involve resheathing/covering the needle once it has been withdrawn or rotating a device that renders the needle blunt before withdrawal from the vein. Instruct the patient to apply pressure to the site using the gauze. (If necessary, continue gentle inversion of the specimen tubes for complete mixing of additives with the blood. Remember: do not shake the tubes. Dispose of the entire needle apparatus. Do *not* disassemble it prior to disposal.

(12) Apply pressure until the bleeding has stopped.(Figure 8-28 ■). Keep an eye on the patient for signs of syncope. Label specimens appropriately (patient's first and last name, identification number, date, time of collection, and health care worker's initials).

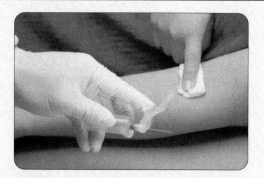

FIGURE ■ **8-28**

AFTER THE PROCEDURE

(13) Dispose of contaminated supplies and equipment.

(14) Double-check to make sure that the bleeding has stopped and apply a bandage, if appropriate.

(15) Wash or sanitize your hands.

(16) Thank the patient for cooperating and depart with *all* specimens and *all* remaining supplies (Figure 8-29 ■). Do not leave anything at the patient's bedside.

(17) Deliver the sample immediately to the laboratory.

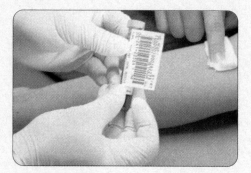

FIGURE ■ **8-29**

Clinical Alert !

A safety winged infusion system, butterfly needle assembly, or scalp needle set can be used for certain patient populations or for particularly difficult venipunctures. This type of method may be useful in the following circumstances:

- Patients with small veins
- Pediatric or geriatric patients
- Patients having numerous needlesticks (e.g., cancer patients)
- Patients in restrictive positions (e.g., traction and severe arthritis)
- Patients who are severely burned
- Patients with fragile skin and veins
- Patients who specifically request it because they feel it is less painful
- Short-term infusion therapy

the transfer of additives from one tube to the next. It is also suggested that small evacuated collection tubes (i.e., 13 × 75 mm or 4 mL) be used with winged infusion sets to avoid collapsing fragile veins. If using a syringe attached to the Luer adapter, a small syringe, such as 5 or 10 mL, should be used for the same reason. The 23-gauge needle is the best choice for small veins, including infants. A 25-gauge needle has a smaller diameter but may lead to hemolysis as the specimen is withdrawn.

Health care workers should be extra cautious as the butterfly needle apparatus is removed from the patient, because it tends to hang loose on the end of the tubing and may sometimes recoil unexpectedly. Therefore, the safety device that is built into the system should be activated immediately. Use of winged infusion or butterfly systems requires training and practice, but they are widely used because patients report that they are less painful than other methods. Use of this system may be more hazardous for health care workers than the use of conventional needles. Failure to activate the safety devices correctly as described by the manufacturers may result in a higher incidence of needlestick injuries.

Procedure 8-6

Syringe Method

RATIONALE

Syringes are *not* routinely used for venipuncture because of many safety concerns, issues of accidental cross-contamination of anticoagulants if the blood specimen is injected into multiple evacuated tubes using the same needle and syringe, and potential clotting in the syringe. However, use of a blood transfer device can minimize these problems. There are also circumstances when a syringe is helpful, such as for veins that collapse easily. Syringes are helpful in this case because the pressure withdrawing the blood can be more easily and gently controlled.

EQUIPMENT

- Personal protective equipment (PPE) (gloves, clean uniform, laboratory coat, etc.)
- Laboratory requisitions or labels
- Marking pens
- Nonlatex tourniquet
- Alcohol pads/skin disinfectants

(continued)

- 2 iodine-tincture scrub swab sticks or chlorohexidine gluconate swab sticks for blood cultures
- Safety syringes and syringe transfer devices
- Safety needles with single-use, evacuated tube holders and winged infusion sets
- Blood collection tubes
- Plastic capillary tubes with tube sealer
- Nonlatex bandages or sterile gauze pads
- Glass microscope slides
- Puncture-proof sharps container
- Test requisitions
- Writing pen
- Bar code reader/scanner (if applicable)

PREPARATION

1 After greeting and identifying the patient, decontaminate hands and don gloves.

2 Assemble equipment in the presence of the patient. Offer to answer any questions for the patient.

PROCEDURE

3 Prepare equipment according to the manufacturer's instructions. Use a syringe with a safety device.

4 Before the needle is inserted, move the plunger back and forth to allow for free movement and to expel all air.

5 Use the same approach to needle insertion as that used for the evacuated tube method.

6 Once the needle is in the vein, draw back the syringe plunger slowly until the required amount of blood is drawn. (It may be helpful to turn the syringe slightly so that the graduated markings are visible.)

7 Take care not to accidentally withdraw the needle while pulling back on the plunger, and do not pull hard enough to cause hemolysis (i.e., rupture of the cells) or collapse of the vein.

8 After releasing the tourniquet and collecting the appropriate amount of blood, withdraw the entire needle assembly quickly and activate the safety device immediately, depending on the manufacturer's specifications.

9 Remove the needle or winged collection set and discard it appropriately.

Clinical Alert !

Do not panic if blood does not flow immediately after the puncture is made. The following suggestions may help:[1]

- Recheck the needle placement and vein by palpating above the needle insertion site.
- Change the needle position *slightly, but do not probe;* that is, pull *gently* outward or push *gently* forward or rotate slightly so that the bevel is positioned correctly in the vein. These should be minute movements so as to minimize the risk of complications.
- Attempt the collection from another site but do not make more than two attempts.

10 Immediately fill the evacuated tubes for testing using a blood transfer device (Figure 8-30 ■).

11 Fill the tubes until flow stops; there is no need to push the plunger to expel blood.

12 Fill the tubes in the same order as that for the evacuated tube method.

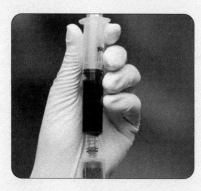

FIGURE ■ 8-30 Blood Transfer Device

Courtesy of BD VACUTAINER Systems, Preanalytical Solutions, Franklin Lakes, NJ.

AFTER THE PROCEDURE: BANDAGE FOR THE PUNCTURE SITE

13 Apply a dry, sterile gauze pad with pressure to the puncture site for several minutes or until bleeding has ceased. If the patient has a free hand, ask them to apply the pressure. Keep the patient's arm straight, slightly bent at the elbow, or elevated slightly above the heart. Apply a bandage and instruct the patient to leave it on for at least 15 minutes (Figure 8-31 ■).

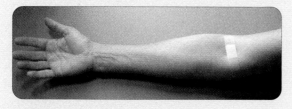

FIGURE ■ 8-31 Applying a Bandage

14 If the patient continues to bleed, apply pressure yourself until the bleeding stops. Then apply a gauze bandage and instruct the patient to leave it on for at least 15 minutes. If the patient continues to bleed, notify a nurse and/or supervisor.

15 Discard all disposable or contaminated equipment into appropriate containers. Paper and plastic wrappers can be thrown into a wastebasket. Needles and lancets should not be thrown into a wastebasket, however, but into a sturdy, puncture-proof, disposable container to be autoclaved or incinerated (Figure 8-32 ■). Any items that have been contaminated with blood should be disposed of in biohazardous disposal containers as explained in the universal precautions. (Refer to Chapter 4, "Safety and Infection Control," and Chapter 6, "Blood Collection Equipment.")

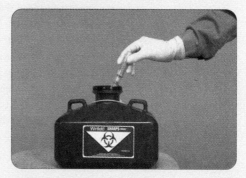

FIGURE ■ 8-32 Needle Disposal

(continued)

Syringe Method *(continued)*

16 Wash or sanitize your hands.

17 Thank the patient for cooperating and depart with *all* specimens and *all* remaining supplies. Do not leave anything at the patient's bedside.

18 Deliver the samples immediately to the laboratory.

Clinical Alert !

Use Once and Discard Immediately

Needles, lancets, syringes, and other bloodletting devices—collectively called *sharps*—that are capable of transmitting infection from one person to another should be used only *once*, then immediately discarded. Sharps must be discarded in puncture-resistant containers that are easily accessible, located in areas where they are commonly used, and have proper warning labels. Blood tube holders should be used only once because of the potential needlestick hazards associated with the double-ended needle at and after disposal. Shearing or breaking of contaminated sharps is illegal and strictly prohibited. Bending, recapping, or removing contaminated needles is not acceptable practice.

BOX 8-3 Order of Draw for Blood Collection Tubes

Collect blood in multiple evacuated tubes that contain various additives. Collecting blood in the correct order reduces the chances of erroneous laboratory test results due to additive carry-over and cross contamination from one tube to the next.

During the actual venipuncture process of filling tubes with blood, the Clinical and Laboratory Standards Institute (CLSI) recommends the following specific order (order of draw) when collecting blood in multiple tubes (either glass or plastic) via the evacuated method or the syringe transfer method (Box 8-4):[1]

1. Blood culture tubes (yellow closure) or blood culture vials. Blood cultures are always drawn first after special skin decontamination procedures, to decrease the possibility of bacterial contamination.
2. Coagulation tube (sodium citrate) (light blue closure).
3. Serum tube, with or without clot activator, with or without gel (red or speckled closure). (Glass, nonadditive serum tubes can be filled before the coagulation tube. However, plastic serum tubes containing a clot activator may interfere with coagulation tests.)
4. Heparin tube (green closure) with or without gel plasma separator.*
5. EDTA tube (purple/lavender closure) used for routine hematology tests.
6. Glycolytic inhibition tube (potassium oxalate/sodium fluoride or lithium iodoacetate/heparin) (gray closure).

*A Tip Worth Remembering: If laboratory test requests require blood cultures (yellow), serum tubes (red), and heparin tubes (green), remember this phrase related to traffic lights: "yellow light, red light, green light, go." Even though it does not account for all tubes, it helps with the order of draw in these cases.

BOX 8-4	Other Issues Related to Filling the Blood Collection Tubes

- During the venipuncture procedure, care should be taken that the additive or anticoagulant present in one tube does not come into contact with the multisample needle as the tubes are changed. To minimize the transfer of anticoagulants from tube to tube, holding the tube horizontally or slightly downward during blood collection is recommended. If an anticoagulant is inadvertently carried into the next tube, it may cause erroneous test results.
- Be attentive to the "fill" rate and volume in each tube. Evacuated tubes with anticoagulants must be filled for the proper mix of blood with the anticoagulant: i.e., the blood-to-additive ratio.
- Although the use of a syringe should be restricted to special cases, occasionally a large volume (more than 20 mL) of blood needs to be drawn using a syringe. Closures on the tubes should not be removed, and a safety syringe–shielded transfer device should be used to transfer the blood into the tubes.

ORDER OF TUBE COLLECTION

Multiple blood assays are often ordered on patients. A specified "order of draw" (Figure 8-33 ■ and Box 8-3) reduces the effects of additive carry-over and cross-contamination from one tube to the next. Carry-over of additives can cause erroneous laboratory results.

SPECIMEN IDENTIFICATION AND LABELING

Completed labels should be firmly attached to the patient's specimens in the presence of the patient.[4] Labels must accompany all blood specimens (Boxes 8-5 and 8-6).

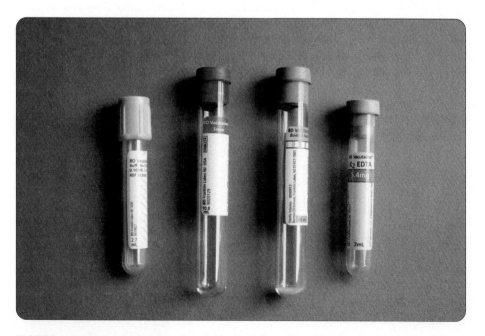

FIGURE ■ 8-33 Example of Various Tubes and Sizes Placed in the Correct Order of Draw. (Note that not all tubes are included in this example.)

Clinical Alert

Special Considerations for Coagulation Testing[1,7,8,9]

- The coagulation specimen should be the second or third tube drawn when multiple tubes are collected.
- Whenever coagulation tests (prothrombin time [PT] and partial thromboplastin time [PTT]) are the sole tests ordered, accurate results can be obtained using one tube. (Until recently, most phlebotomy practices have required that at least one other tube of blood be drawn and discarded before the coagulation test specimen, so as to diminish contamination with tissue fluids that could initiate the clotting sequence.) Each health care worker should use the procedure adopted by his or her own facility. However, if coagulation studies are the *only* tests ordered, and a *winged infusion (butterfly) system* is to be used for collection, a "discard" tube should be collected before drawing the citrate tube. This is the only way to rid the specimen of the air in the winged infusion tubing. If this air in the "dead space" enters the citrate tube, it causes an inaccurate blood-to-citrate ratio.
- Because coagulation tests require a specific plasma concentration of sodium citrate, "overfilling" the tube may cause artificial results or falsely short clotting times.
- If a tube is "underfilled," the opposite occurs, and artificial results indicate falsely prolonged clotting times.
- Immediately after collection, coagulation tubes should be mixed gently to prevent clotting in the tube. However, an excessive number of inversions or vigorous mixing can lead to platelet activation and shortening of clotting times when tested.

BOX 8-5 Labels for Blood Specimens

Specimens should be labeled (using adhesive and/or bar coded labels) immediately at the patient's bedside or ambulatory setting, before leaving the patient. Laboratory procedure manuals should contain explicit instructions about labeling requirements. Supervisors should spend ample time not only training new employees in correct identification and labeling practices but also observing as they perform the steps.

The health care worker may write directly on the container. Commercial collection tubes may have affixed blank labels for this purpose. Similarly, hospitals often use computer-generated labels for collection tubes; however, capillary tubes, microcollection tubes and vials, or other containers without labels must be identified, either by labeling them directly with a permanent felt-tipped pen, wrapping an adhesive label around them, or placing them into a larger labeled test tube for transport. In some cases, small computerized adhesive labels with printed information are available with and detachable from the requisition form.

Specimen labels should consistently include the following information:[1,2]

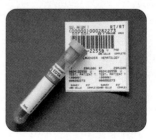

1. Patient's full name
2. Patient's identification number
3. Date of collection
4. Time of collection
5. Health care worker's initials
6. Patient's room number, bed assignment, or outpatient status (optional)

| **BOX 8-6** | **Ideas for Improving Venipuncture Practices** |

All members of the health care team should strive to improve phlebotomy practices. A few suggestions for improving efficiency and quality include:

- Coordination of laboratory requests among *all* staff physicians and nurses working with the patient, to reduce duplicate and triplicate laboratory orders.
- Possible modifications to laboratory testing panels and better education of physicians to be aware of all the tests on each laboratory panel.
- The laboratory could be notified when multiple timed tests are ordered. For example, if a patient needs a hemoglobin test at 2:00 P.M. and a glucose test at 3:00 P.M., coordinating the times and drawing both specimens during one venipuncture may be possible.
- Reassessment of STAT test orders to make sure that they are clinically necessary.
- **Therapeutic drug monitoring** (i.e., timed laboratory analysis of serum drug levels to determine adequate dosing) should be coordinated among laboratory, nursing, and pharmacy personnel.
- The laboratory should be aware of patient transfers.
- The number of times that a patient can be punctured should be monitored. (Generally, a health care worker should not puncture a patient more than twice before calling for a second opinion.)
- The number of times that a patient can be punctured in one day should be coordinated and minimized.
- The total volume of blood that can be drawn daily from a patient, especially for infants, children (Appendix 4), and critically ill patients must be monitored.
- Health care workers should restrict discussion about a patient's clinical information to very basic facts about the tests that have been ordered. It should be emphasized that the patient's physician ordered the tests and can answer questions about them in more detail.
- Procedures for documenting a patient's refusal to have blood collected should be established. All patients have a right to refuse treatment. Explain to the patient that laboratory results are used to help the physician make an accurate diagnosis, establish proper treatment, and monitor the patient's health status and that the patient's cooperation would be greatly appreciated. If the patient continues to refuse, remain professional and acknowledge his or her right to refuse. Documentation of the refusal should be made and the patient's physician notified.
- Guidelines for **specimen rejection** (i.e., criteria that relate to the suitability of a specimen for testing or when it may not be used) should be periodically reviewed.

Clinical Alert ❗

Tubes should not be prelabeled, because if they are then not used, they may be erroneously picked up and used for another patient. Also, a different health care worker may complete the venipuncture if the initial health care worker is unsuccessful. In that case, the prelabeled tubes may display the initials of the first health care worker and, therefore, be inaccurate. In addition, if the prelabeled tubes are not used, tearing off the old or unused label may be difficult because of the adhesive; thus, either a new label (from a different patient) would have to be placed on the tube with a partially torn label or the unused tube would have to be discarded. Either option is unsatisfactory, messy, and wasteful.

Clinical Alert !

Before leaving the patient, be cognizant of the following issues.

- The health care worker should always make sure the bleeding has stopped, decontaminate hands, thank the patient, and ensure that all the information on the label is complete and correct before leaving the patient's hospital room or before drawing blood from another clinic outpatient.
- The date and time are necessary information, because physicians need to know exactly when the specimen was drawn so that they may correlate results with any medications given or with changes in the patient's condition. Requisition forms only indicate the date and time when a laboratory test was ordered, rather than the date and time when it was collected.
- The health care worker's initials are necessary to help clarify questions about the specimen or patient if any arise during laboratory processing or testing.
- All supplies and equipment must be removed from the patient's bedside.

Procedure 8-7

Leaving the Patient

RATIONALE

To assure that the patient is no longer bleeding and has no further complications related to the venipuncture procedure.

EQUIPMENT

- Nonlatex bandages
- Pen
- Alcohol-based hand rub or soap/water
- Biohazard containers
- Bar code scanner (if applicable)

PREPARATION

1 Scan surfaces for extraneous supplies.

2 Before leaving the room, wash or sanitize your hands.

PROCEDURE

Before leaving the patient's side, perform the following steps:

3 Check the puncture site to make sure that the bleeding stopped and that the patient does not feel faint if they are on foot.

4 Apply an adhesive bandage if the patient is agreeable.

5 Ensure that all tubes are appropriately labeled.

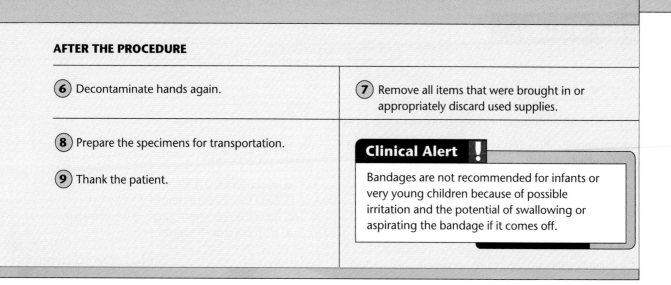

AFTER THE PROCEDURE

⑥ Decontaminate hands again.	⑦ Remove all items that were brought in or appropriately discard used supplies.
⑧ Prepare the specimens for transportation. ⑨ Thank the patient.	**Clinical Alert** ❗ Bandages are not recommended for infants or very young children because of possible irritation and the potential of swallowing or aspirating the bandage if it comes off.

Prioritizing Patients

During the course of a day's work at a busy hospital or clinic, a health care worker may have to make decisions about the order in which blood work is obtained. Priorities must be set and adhered to, whether they concern the order in which certain blood tests are drawn on a particular patient or which patients are to be drawn first from among a group. If these distinctions are not made properly, test results can be affected, and interpretation of the results may be difficult.

Timed specimens—If a test is ordered to be drawn at a particular time, e.g., glucose should be drawn 2 hours after a meal, the health care worker is responsible for drawing the blood as near to the requested time as possible. The glucose value in the blood is constantly changing, so the blood must not be drawn too early, which yields a falsely elevated result, or too late, which yields a falsely normal result. Timed specimens are also crucial for TDM. The laboratory results taken from blood samples for TDM are used in establishing a patient's drug dose.

STAT, or emergency, specimens—STAT specimens must be acted on immediately because the patient has a medical condition that must be treated or responded to as a medical emergency.

Self Study

Study Questions

The following questions may have more than one answer.

1. An unconscious emergency patient may be identified by which of the following means?

   a. a name on the patient's bed
   b. temporary identification label
   c. patient's backpack
   d. ER clerk

2. Identification procedures for outpatients may include asking for which of the following?

   a. photo identification
   b. birth date
   c. address
   d. identification by a family member

3. The most common sites for venipuncture are in which of the following areas?

   a. the dorsal side of the wrist
   b. the antecubital area of the arm
   c. the middle finger
   d. the earlobe

4. Applying a tourniquet is useful for:

   a. providing an indication of the size of the vein
   b. distracting the patient from the discomfort of the procedure
   c. providing an indication of the depth of the vein
   d. allowing blood to pool in the veins

5. What effect does warming the site have on venipuncture?

   a. prevents veins from rolling
   b. makes veins stand out
   c. causes hemoconcentration
   d. increases localized blood flow

6. How long should the tourniquet be placed around the patient's arm?

   a. approximately 4 minutes
   b. until the needle is removed
   c. until the entire venipuncture is completed
   d. no more than 1 minute

7. How many times should one patient be punctured during a procedure?

   a. only once
   b. no more than twice
   c. three times
   d. four times

8. Which of the following tubes should always be drawn first?

   a. blood culture
   b. lavender-topped tube
   c. light blue–topped tube
   d. red-topped tube

9. When should safety devices be activated during a venipuncture procedure?

   a. before beginning the procedure
   b. just before sticking the patient so that no one will get hurt
   c. immediately after withdrawal from the vein unless the manufacturer recommends otherwise
   d. just before putting it in the waste container

10. During a venipuncture procedure using evacuated tubes when should the tourniquet be released?

    a. before the blood flows into the tube
    b. after the blood flows into the tube
    c. before the needle is inserted
    d. after the needle has been withdrawn

Case Study

A health care worker was assigned to collect blood specimens from a hospitalized, comatose patient. The health care worker entered the hospital room to begin the identification process. The sign on the patient's bed indicated that the patient was Anne Bentsen; however, the laboratory requisitions were for Ann Beaumont. As the health care worker approached the patient to check for identification, she noticed that the patient had an IV in one arm and appeared to be asleep.

Question

1. What should the health care worker do to confirm the identification of the patient and to collect the blood specimen?

Case Study

The following laboratory tests were ordered for a patient who had recently had a mastectomy on her left side: PT and PTT, blood cultures, hemoglobin and hematocrit, electrolytes, and cell counts (WBC and RBC).

Questions

1. What site would be most appropriate for the venipuncture?

2. What would be the correct order of drawing the evacuated tubes during the venipuncture?

Self Assessment

Check Yourself

Patient Identification and Name Clarification

1. Patients frequently have the same or similar last name. Common ones are Smith, Jones, and Johnson. As a self-assessment exercise or with a partner, pretend you are tired and at the end of a busy work shift. Practice saying the names listed below and describe what you would do if any of these patients appeared for venipuncture at the same time:

   Betsy Johnson and Betty Johnston
   P. Garcia and J. C. Garza
   Jan Cheung and Jen Chang
   John Riley and Jon Reilly

2. Consider how important each step of the identification process is in these (and all) situations. Next, come up with a list of names that you are familiar with. "Tune-in" your eyes and ears to notice different spellings and verbal pronunciations of these names. Practice using phrases to request the exact spelling of a patient's name. Remember that language differences and/or accents may cause one name to sound like another, therefore resulting in misunderstandings. However, if the identification process is followed carefully and thoroughly, mistakes can be prevented. All discrepancies in the identification process should be reported to a supervisor.

Competency Checklist: Patient Identification

This checklist can be completed as a group or individually.

(1) Completed (2) Needs to improve

_____ 1. List three ways to confirm a patient's identity.

_____ 2. List 3 methods _that would not be reliable_ for confirming a patient's identity.

Competency Checklist: Preparing for the Patient Encounter

This exercise can be done during an actual patient encounter or as a mock encounter. If possible, record a video of the encounter to aid in the assessment critique.

(1) Completed (2) Needs to improve

_____ 1. The health care worker demonstrates a positive, professional appearance.

_____ 2. The health care worker demonstrates positive body language, including a pleasant facial expression and good posture before beginning the patient encounter.

_____ 3. The health care worker has protective equipment, phlebotomy supplies, test requisitions, writing pen, and appropriate patient information before beginning the venipuncture process.

_____ 4. The health care worker can describe what to do if he or she cannot identify the patient correctly or if information is incomplete.

Competency Checklist: Use of a Tourniquet and Site Selection

Practice on a partner several times before practicing on a patient.

(1) Completed (2) Needs to improve

_____ 1. A clean latex-free tourniquet is used by stretching the ends of the tourniquet around the patient's arm about 3 inches (7.6 cm) above the venipuncture area (antecubital area). The tourniquet is applied tightly but not painful to the patient. It is not left on more than 1 minute.

_____ 2. The antecubital area is palpated appropriately. (Not too hard, not too softly.)

_____ 3. Veins are located and identified appropriately. One or more options can easily be identified in the antecubital area.

_____ 4. When it is time to release the tourniquet, the partial loop should allow for easy release by the health care worker using only one hand, because the other hand will be holding the needle and tubes.

_____ 5. Next, practice applying the tourniquet on the lower arm to identify dorsal hand veins.

_____ 6. Palpate and identify the best option for venipuncture on the dorsal side of the hand.

_____ 7. Release the tourniquet during the appropriate time frame.

Competency Checklist: Decontamination of the Puncture Site

Choose a partner to work with. Your partner or supervisor can evaluate the extent to which the site is adequately decontaminated.

(1) Completed (2) Needs to improve

_____ 1. Once the site is selected, it is decontaminated with an alcohol-soaked gauze or a commercially packaged alcohol pad.

_____ 2. The site is rubbed with moderate pressure applied to the alcohol pad, working in concentric circles from the inside out.

_____ 3. Adequate time is allotted for the site to dry.

_____ 4. Practice decontaminating your gloved finger.

Competency Checklist: Performing a Venipuncture

The steps listed below are typical for either venipuncture system.

(1) Completed (2) Needs to improve

_____ 1. After greeting and identifying the patient, decontaminating hands, donning gloves, and preparing equipment in the presence of the patient, the health care worker offers to answer any questions for the patient.

_____ 2. The health care worker prepares equipment according to the manufacturer's instructions, including attaching a needle onto the appropriate holder.

_____ 3. The patient's arm is positioned properly.

_____ 4. A clean tourniquet is applied and potential sites are checked by palpating the vein.

_____ 5. If a suitable vein is not felt, the tourniquet is removed and applied to the other arm.

_____ 6. Practice warming the site or lower the arm further in a downward position to pool venous blood.

_____ 7. An appropriate site is selected and decontaminated with an alcohol pad in a circular motion from inside to outside. It is allowed to air dry.

_____ 8. The patient is asked to "please close your fist."

_____ 9. The patient is told that he or she will "feel a stick" or "please remain still while I begin the procedure, you will feel a slight prick."

_____10. The patient's arm is held below the site, pulling the skin slightly with the thumb.

_____11. The needle assembly and arm are held appropriately.

_____12. The needle is parallel to the vein and at the appropriate angle.

_____13. The patient is instructed to open his or her fist after blood begins to flow, and the tourniquet is released at the appropriate time.

_____14. Evacuated tubes are pushed into the holder in an appropriate manner.

_____15. Evacuated tubes are filled in the correct order and until the blood flow stops in each tube.

_____16. Each tube is removed from the holder with a gentle twist-and-pull motion and replaced with the next tube.

_____17. Tubes are gently mixed in one hand while holding the needle apparatus and waiting for another tube to fill.

_____18. When all tubes have been filled, the needle is withdrawn in an appropriate manner.

_____19. Bleeding is adequately controlled.

_____20. The safety device is activated according to the manufacturer's instructions.

_____21. The patient is instructed to apply pressure to the site using the gauze.

Competency Checklist: Order of Draw

The following cases indicate tests requested for laboratory evaluation. Practice numbering the tubes in the correct order of collection for a venipuncture:

(1) Completed (2) Needs to improve

_____ 1. Lavender closure used for hematology tests (CBC), yellow closure used for blood cultures, serum closure used for many chemistry tests.

_____ 2. Heparin (green), serum electrolytes (red speckled), coagulation (light blue)

_____ 3. blood cultures, coagulation, hematology

_____ 4. coagulation, serum protein

_____ 5. heparin, EDTA, serum cholesterol, coagulation

_____ 6. Using a butterfly method: coagulation, hematology

Competency Checklist: Leaving the Patient

This checklist can be completed as a group or individually.

(1) Completed (2) Needs to improve

_____ 1. The health care worker rechecks the puncture site to see whether the bleeding has stopped or the patient wants a bandage.

_____ 2. The health care worker asks whether the patient is feeling faint.

_____ 3. The health care worker labels all specimens appropriately.

_____ 4. Used supplies are discarded appropriately.

_____ 5. Hands are decontaminated after the procedure.

_____ 6. Specimens are readied for transport in a secure fashion.

_____ 7. The health care worker thanks the patient before leaving the room.

References

1. Clinical and Laboratory Standards Institute (CLSI), formerly the National Committee for Clinical Laboratory Standards (NCCLS): *Procedures for the Collection of Diagnostic Blood Specimens by Venipuncture*, Approved Standard, 5th Ed., document H3-A5. Wayne, PA: CLSI, 2003.

2. Clinical and Laboratory Standards Institute (CLSI), formerly the National Committee for Clinical Laboratory Standards (NCCLS): *Procedures and Devices for the Collection of Diagnostic Capillary Blood Specimens*, Approved Standard, document H4-A5. Wayne, PA: CLSI, 2004.

3. Centers for Disease Control and Prevention: Guideline for hand hygiene in health-care settings. MMWR Morb Mortal Wkly Rep 2002;51(16): www.cdc.gov/handhygiene/.

4. Joint Commission on Accreditation of Healthcare Organizations: 2007 National Patient Safety Goals, www.jcaho.org, 2007.

5. Jackson, S: Caution: Entering the danger zone, proper vein selection is key in successful venipunctures. *Advance for Medical Laboratory Professionals,* March 24, 2003:10.

6. Ernst, D: Iodine disinfectant for infants. *Medical Laboratory Observer,* July 2003: 54, www.mlo-online.com.

7. Lawrence, JB: Preanalytical variables in the coagulation laboratory. *Lab Med* 2003;1:34, 49–57.

8. Gottfried, EL, Adachi, MM: Prothrombin time and activated partial thromboplastin time can be performed on the first tube. *Am J Clin Pathol* 1997;107(6):681–3.

9. Adcock, DM, Kressin, DC, Marlar, RA: Are discard tubes necessary in coagulation studies? *Lab Med* 1997;28(8):530–3.

Additional Resources

1. American Society for Clinical Pathology: ASCP LABQ-P, continuing educational exercises for phlebotomy. http://www.ascp.org/education/selfStudyPublications/labQ/default.aspx, 2007.

2. Clinical and Laboratory Standards Institute (CLSI): consensus standards for all phases of specimen collection that assist with regulatory and accreditation requirements, and quality improvements. www.clsi.org, 2007.

3. Institute for Quality in Laboratory Medicine: www.iqlm.org, 2007.

4. The Joint Commissions: www. jcaho.org, 2007.

Chapter 9

Capillary Blood Specimens

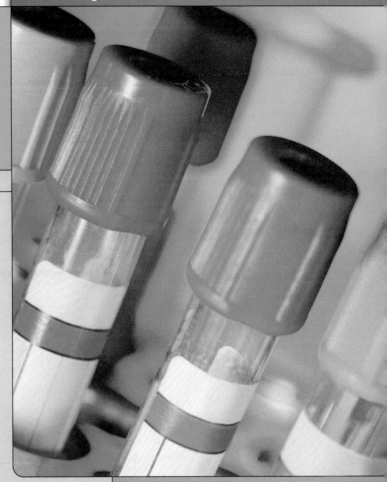

KEY TERMS

capillary action

capillary blood

cyanotic

dehydrated

differentials

feathered edge

interstitial (tissue) fluid

osteochondritis

osteomyelitis

peripheral circulation

Indications for Skin Puncture

Skin punctures are particularly useful for both adult and pediatric patients when small amounts of blood can be used for laboratory testing. It is crucial to withdraw *only the smallest amounts of blood needed* for laboratory testing from neonates, infants, and children so that the effects of blood-volume reduction are minimal. A 10-mL blood sample, which could be tolerated by most adults, would represent 5% to 10% of the *total* blood volume in a neonate's body.[1]

Clinical Alert ⚠

Venipuncture in children, especially infants, should be avoided when possible because of the risk of complications due to taking too much blood (iatrogenic hazards) or difficulties with the puncture site. These complications may include anemia, cardiac arrest, hemorrhage, damage to surrounding tissues or organs, infections, and injuries from restraining the child during the procedure.[1]

Skin punctures or "fingerstick" procedures are used if the following conditions occur in adult patients:[1]

- Severe burns
- Obesity
- Thrombotic tendencies
- Fragile veins (e.g., in geriatric patients)
- When veins are being "saved" for therapy (e.g., for cancer patients)
- Home testing (e.g., blood glucose monitoring)
- Point-of-care testing (POC)

Fingerstick procedures are not recommended if the following circumstances are present:

- Laboratory testing that requires large amounts of blood
- The patient has swollen fingers. If a fingerstick is performed, interstitial fluids may dilute the blood specimen
- The patient is **dehydrated** (lacking or loss of water from the body)
- A patient may have poor **peripheral circulation** (near the surface of the body)
- The following tests are ordered: coagulation studies (because of a dilution effect with interstitial fluid), blood cultures, and erythrocyte sedimentation rate (ESR) determinations

Composition of Capillary Blood

Capillary blood acquired by skin puncture is different from that of venous or arterial blood acquired by other methods. Capillary blood is more of a mixture, composed of blood from:

- arterioles
- venules

- capillaries
- intracellular and **interstitial (tissue) fluids** (fluids that form within tissue layers and gaps)

Generally speaking, there are slight differences in laboratory values of glucose, potassium, total protein, and calcium when serum or plasma have been compared with skin puncture blood. In all cases, except glucose, the values are lower in skin puncture blood.[1]

Collecting Diagnostic Capillary Blood Specimens

The first steps used for the venipuncture procedure also apply to skin puncture procedure (preparing oneself and supplies, identifying the patient, performing hand hygiene, and decontaminating the site). However, subsequent steps are slightly different (Figure 9-1■).

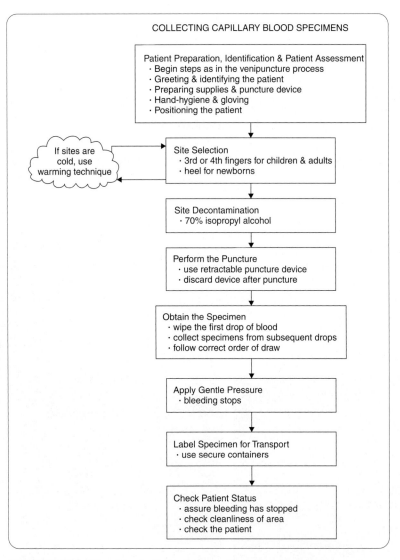

COLLECTING CAPILLARY BLOOD SPECIMENS

Patient Preparation, Identification & Patient Assessment
· Begin steps as in the venipuncture process
· Greeting & identifying the patient
· Preparing supplies & puncture device
· Hand-hygiene & gloving
· Positioning the patient

If sites are cold, use warming technique

Site Selection
· 3rd or 4th fingers for children & adults
· heel for newborns

Site Decontamination
· 70% isopropyl alcohol

Perform the Puncture
· use retractable puncture device
· discard device after puncture

Obtain the Specimen
· wipe the first drop of blood
· collect specimens from subsequent drops
· follow correct order of draw

Apply Gentle Pressure
· bleeding stops

Label Specimen for Transport
· use secure containers

Check Patient Status
· assure bleeding has stopped
· check cleanliness of area
· check the patient

FIGURE ■ 9-1 Flow Chart: Collecting Capillary Blood Specimens

Supplies for Skin Puncture

Supplies for skin puncture are available from many manufacturers (see Chapter 6) and depending on the actual tests that are ordered the supplies may differ, but the basic list includes the following (Figure 9-2 ■):

- Disposable gloves
- Automatic retractable safety puncture devices
- Disinfectant pads (70% isopropanol)
- Sterile nonlatex bandages and gauze pads
- Glass microscope slides
- Diluting fluids as required by manufacturers
- Plastic microcollection tubes
- Plastic-coated capillary tubes
- Capillary tube sealers or closures
- Laboratory request slips or labels
- A marking pen
- A puncture-proof biohazard discard container

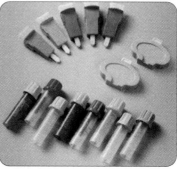

FIGURE ■ 9-2 Capillary Collection Supplies

Courtesy of BD VACUTAINER Systems, Preanalytical Solutions, Franklin Lakes, NJ.

Clinical Alert ❗

Glass capillary tubes should *not* be used, because they break easily and can cause injury. Use plastic capillary tubes instead.

SKIN PUNCTURE SITES

Skin puncture in adults and older children most often involves one of the fingers. The fleshy, central palmar surface of the distal phalanx (fingertip section) of the third (middle) finger or fourth (ring) finger of the nondominant hand is the preferred site for puncture. The puncture should be made at the thickest part of the finger (not the sides or extreme tip where the tissue is not as thick)[1] (Figure 9-3 ■).

For infants less than 1 year old, or neonates, the recommended site for skin puncture is the lateral or medial plantar surface of the heel.[1]

FIGURE ■ 9-3

Sites for Finger Puncture

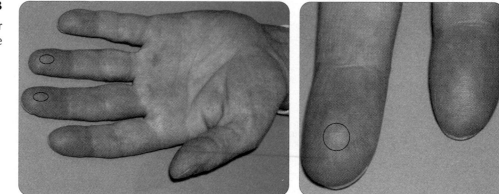

Clinical Alert !

The following sites are *not generally recommended* for routine skin punctures:[1]

- Earlobe (Even though the earlobe is still used by some, it is not a preferred site because of possible interference with pierced earrings; also, because of the site's close proximity to the eyes, a puncture device may cause undue anxiety to a patient)
- Central arch area of an infant's heel and posterior curve of the heel (because of the risk of injuring nerves, tendons, cartilage, and bone)
- Fingers of a newborn or infant less than 1 year old (because of the risk of hitting the bone and causing infections)
- The fifth (pinky) finger (because the tissue of this finger is considerably thinner than that of the others and there is a risk of hitting the bone)
- The thumb (because it has a pulse)
- The index (pointer) finger (because it may be more sensitive or it may be callused)
- Swollen or previously punctured sites (because accumulated fluid may contaminate the specimen and the site may be bruised, thus causing more pain if it is punctured again)
- Fingers on the side of a mastectomy (because the removal of lymph nodes during surgery may result in excessive lymph fluid on the side of the surgery; consult with the ordering physician in the case of a bilateral mastectomy)

WARMING THE SKIN PUNCTURE SITE

Although the research and clinical practices are variable, some believe that warming the skin puncture site helps facilitate phlebotomy by significantly increasing arterial blood flow to the area. Several easy-to-use methods of warming are commercially available, or the site can be warmed with a heated surgical towel or a washcloth heated with warm water to 42°C, which will not burn the skin.

CLEANSING THE SKIN PUNCTURE SITE

The skin puncture site should be cleaned with a 70% aqueous solution of isopropyl alcohol and allowed to thoroughly dry before being punctured. If alcohol pools at the site, it can cause hemolysis and contaminate testing for glucose determinations. Also, alcohol present during the puncture will sting the patient and prevent the formation of rounded drops of blood, which are best for making blood smears on microscopic slides. Povidone-iodine (Betadine) preparations are not recommended for disinfecting skin puncture sites because they can falsely elevate potassium, phosphorus, or uric acid determinations.[1]

Skin Puncture Procedure

Because skin punctures require different procedures when performed on infants, refer to Chapter 10 for information about skin puncture collections on newborn babies, blood spot testing for newborn screening, heel puncture procedures, and specimens for pediatric blood gases. However, there are some precautions that are applicable to both adult and infant skin punctures. Safety retractable puncture devices are currently available on the market. Health care workers should understand and follow the manufacturer's directions for the use of each device. Puncture devices are made to control for variable depth and length, depending on the patient's age and weight. The average depth of a skin puncture should be 2 to 2.5 mm for adults and less than 2.0 mm for small children and infants, to avoid injuring the bone. Laser devices are also available as skin puncture alternatives. They provide a smaller hole (about 250 μm wide and 1–2 mm deep).

Clinical Alert ⚠

If the bone is repeatedly punctured, it can lead to **osteomyelitis**, which is an inflammation of the bone caused by bacterial infection, or **osteochondritis**, inflammation of the bone and cartilage.

Manual, nonretractable lancets are *not recommended* for acquiring capillary specimens because they can cause more bruising and inflammation than automated retractable devices, and they are more likely to cause accidental injuries with the exposed sharp. However, unfortunately, in some facilities their use is still in practice. If a sterile lancet is used, it should be carefully removed from its packaging. (If the lancet accidentally touches clothing or brushes against the countertop, it is no longer sterile, and a new device should be opened and used.) The manufacturer's directions should be followed. The finger or heel should be held, so as to prevent sudden jerking movements during the puncture. If applicable, remove the protective shield or cap from the lancet. The puncture should be in one continuous movement, perpendicular to the skin surface, with the lancet orientation across the fingerprint grooves. As soon as the lancet has penetrated the skin, it should be quickly removed and immediately discarded into a puncture-proof biohazard sharps container.

Procedure 9-1

Basic Skin Puncture or Fingerstick Using a Retractable Device

RATIONALE

To obtain smaller amounts of blood specimens in a less invasive manner than venipuncture procedures.

EQUIPMENT

- Disposable gloves
- Automatic, retractable, sterile safety puncture devices
- Disinfectant pads (70% isopropyl alcohol)
- Sterile bandages
- Prepackaged gauze pads (2 × 2 or 3 × 3 inches)
- Glass microscope slides
- Diluting fluids for specified tests
- Plastic microcollection tubes or plastic-coated capillary tubes
- Capillary tube sealers or closures
- Laboratory request slips or labels
- A marking pen
- A puncture-proof biohazard discard container

PREPARATION

1 Be emotionally prepared and greet the patient to put him or her at ease.	**2** Ensure proper patient identification in a variety of situations.
3 Exercise standard precautions and perform hand hygiene and gloving techniques.	**4** Prepare supplies and the collection device(s).
5 Position the patient in a safe chair, comfortable bed, or reclining chair.	**6** Verify dietary conditions and that the patient does not have latex allergies.

PROCEDURE

7 Ask about hand preference; check hand dominance.

8 Choose a finger that is not cold, **cyanotic** (blue in color due to O_2 depletion), or swollen. If possible, stick the tip of the third or fourth finger of the nondominant hand (Figure 9-4 ▪).

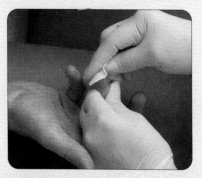

FIGURE ▪ 9-4

---

9 Gently massage the finger a few times from base to tip to aid blood flow. If the patient's hands are cold, wrap one of them in a warm towel for 3 to 5 minutes, use a commercially available warming device, or ask the patient to wash their hands in warm water before the puncture is performed.

10 Decontaminate the site with an alcohol pad (70% isopropanol) and allow it to air dry.

---

11 Remove the puncture device and/or lancet from its packaging and follow the manufacturer's instructions. Hold the patient's finger (or heel, in the case of an infant) firmly with one hand, with your thumb away from the puncture site, next to the patient's fingernail (Figure 9-5 ▪).

   With the other hand, position the puncture device on the site. Activate the release mechanism on the retractable safety puncture device and hold it perpendicular to the finger surface. Orient the cut across the fingerprints (perpendicular to the fingerprint grooves) to generate a large, round drop of blood. If the puncture is made along the lines of (i.e., parallel to) the fingerprint, a well-rounded drop will not form and the blood, tends to run down the finger). Discard the puncture device

in a puncture-proof biohazard container. (If a biohazard container is not within reach, discard the device immediately after completing the collections.)

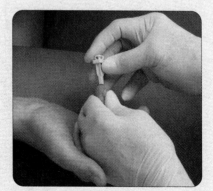

FIGURE ▪ 9-5

(continued)

12 Wipe the first drop of blood away with clean gauze (Figure 9-6 ■) unless otherwise indicated. (Some point-of-care instruments do not require this step; refer to Chapter 10.) Always follow the manufacturer's instructions.

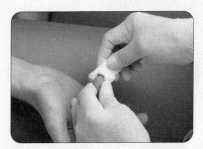

FIGURE ■ 9-6

13 Collect the second drop of blood by touching it to the tip of the microcollection device. The blood will flow into the tube by **capillary action** whereby blood flows freely into the tube on contact, without suction. If the blood becomes jammed in the collection top, a gentle tap on a hard surface will usually dislodge it so the blood can flow freely again to the bottom of the tube (Figure 9-7 ■).

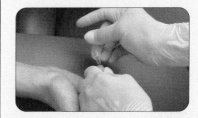

FIGURE ■ 9-7

14 Gently apply pressure to the finger and hold the puncture site in a downward position to encourage the free flow of blood, thereby getting the proper amount of blood. Do not use excessive milking/massaging of the finger or forceful scooping-up of blood, because it may result in excess tissue fluid and/or hemolysis of the specimen.

15 Each type of microcollection laboratory test has different tube and blood volume requirements. Follow the appropriate manufacturer's instructions. Gently invert containers with additives to mix the blood with the additives. Carefully and safely seal microcollection tubes with a sealant or with other commercially available devices. When filling capillary tubes, do not allow air bubbles to enter the tubes, because air bubbles can cause erroneous results in many laboratory tests. Blood flow is better and air bubbles are less likely if the puncture site is held downward and gentle pressure is applied.

16 Blood smears can also be made from subsequent drops of blood. Refer to Procedure 9-2.

17 Using a clean gauze pad, apply gentle pressure to the site until bleeding has stopped. (If collecting blood from an infant's heel, apply the gauze pad and elevate the heel until bleeding stops (Figure 9-8 ■).

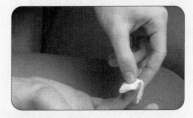

FIGURE ■ 9-8

18 Label the specimens and/or outside containers to prepare them for transport.

19 Discard all other biohazardous supplies before removing gloves.

AFTER THE PROCEDURE

20 Remove and dispose of gloves in a biohazard container and perform hand hygiene.

21 Ensure that bleeding has stopped and thank the patient before leaving with specimens and remaining supplies.

NOTES

- In health care facilities, the puncture devices used are typically small, single-use, disposable devices. However, in home settings, a patient may have a multiuse device in which only the lancet is changed after each use from that single patient. In this case, discard the lancet and clean the multiuse device according to the manufacturer's instructions if it becomes contaminated.
- A free flow of blood is essential to obtain accurate test results. Do not use excessive squeezing or massaging to obtain blood.

- If the blood drop used for the specimen is allowed to remain on the skin too long, some evaporation may occur and the drop may dry out. If this happens, wipe away this drop and use the next one; otherwise, it may result in erroneous laboratory values.
- If the sample is not adequate and blood has stopped flowing from the puncture site, use a new sterile retractable lancet to repuncture at a *different* site.

Order of Collection

The order of filling microcollection tubes with capillary blood is different than for venipuncture. If multiple laboratory tests have been ordered, the order of collection should be as follows:[1]

- EDTA specimen for hematology tests
- Other tubes with additives
- Nonadditive tubes

Blood Films for Microscopic Slides

Procedure 9-2 demonstrates the procedure for making blood smears on microscopic glass slides for performing white blood cell **differentials**, or diff, which is a hematological laboratory test to approximate percentages and determine morphology of the white blood cells.

Clinical Alert !

There are several preanalytical variables that require special attention when collecting skin puncture specimens.

- Microcollection tubes must be adequately filled and immediately capped and gently mixed. If it takes too long to fill the tube, microclots may form.
- Excessive amounts (overfilling) can cause clot formation; inadequate amounts (underfilling) can cause cells to change morphologically because of too much anticoagulant.
- Hemolysis of the capillary blood specimen is a complication that can cause erroneous laboratory results and is usually preventable if good technique is maintained. Hemolysis is caused by:[1]
    Not removing residual alcohol at the puncture site
    Excessive milking/massaging of the finger
    Patients have increased blood cell fragility and high packed cell volume (e.g., newborns and infants)
    Excessive shaking while mixing the specimen

Procedure 9-2 Blood Films for Microscopic Slides

RATIONALE

Blood films on microscopic slides are used to evaluate the morphology (form and structure) of the blood cells. The microscopic slides are prepared with a blood drop following this procedure; they are stained with special stains in the laboratory; and evaluated under a microscope. Although some facilities no longer use this manual method, it is still used in many cases for detecting cellular abnormalities, for confirmation, and/or for a back-up method.

EQUIPMENT

- Gloves
- Microscopic glass slides

- Drying rack or other clean surface

PREPARATION

1 Prepare and assemble supplies.

2 Identify the patient properly.

3 Wash or sanitize your hands with an alcohol hand rinse, then put on gloves.

PROCEDURE

④ Make blood smears from fresh drops of blood. Perform the finger puncture in the usual way, wiping the first drop of blood away. Touch the slide to the second drop at approximately 0.5–1 in. (1.3–2.5 cm) from the end of the slide (Figure 9-9 ■). Blood smears may also be made using anticoagulated (EDTA) blood from a lavender-top tube. However, it should be done where there is minimal exposure to the blood or blood spills.

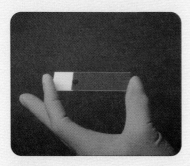

FIGURE ■ 9-9

⑤ Place the second (spreader) slide in front of the drop of blood and then pull it slowly into the drop, allowing blood to spread along the width of the slide (Figure 9-10 ■).

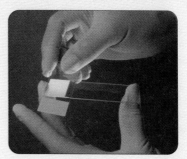

FIGURE ■ 9-10

⑥ When the blood spreads almost to the edges, quickly and evenly push the spreader slide forward at an angle of approximately 30 degrees. Do not press downward. The only downward pressure should be the weight of the spreader slide (Figure 9-11 ■).

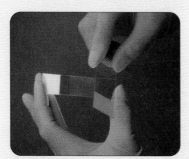

FIGURE ■ 9-11

⑦ Allow the slide to air dry; do not blow on it (Figure 9-12 ■).

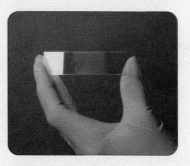

FIGURE ■ 9-12

(continued)

8. Blood films should have a **feathered edge**, as shown in the first slide. It has a visible curved edge that thins out smoothly and resembles the tip of a bird's feather, and it covers approximately half the surface of the glass slide (Figure 9-13 ■).

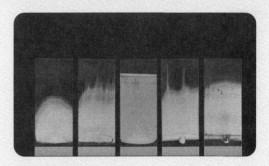

FIGURE ■ 9-13

9. No ridges, lines, or holes should be visible in the smear. Errors are often the result of too large a drop, too long a delay in making the smear, blowing on the slide, or using a chipped slide. In the figure, the last four blood films are unacceptable for analysis.

10. Label the slides and prepare them for safe transport to the laboratory.

AFTER THE PROCEDURE

11. Discard any unusable slides and all biohazardous waste in an appropriate container.

12. Wash or sanitize your hands.

13. Thank the patient for cooperating and depart with *all* specimens and *all* remaining supplies.

14. Deliver the slides immediately to the laboratory.

Lancet Disposal, Labeling the Specimen, and Completing the Interaction

Used disposable lancets should always be placed into a rigid, puncture-resistant biohazard container with a lid. All tubes must be appropriately labeled immediately after collection and mixing and the information on the labels confirmed. Several tubes may be placed together in a larger labeled container. All supplies and equipment that were brought in should be removed or discarded appropriately. Hand hygiene must be performed again after contact with *each* patient. Before leaving the patient's side, check the puncture site to make sure that the bleeding has stopped, then thank the patient for their cooperation. An adhesive bandage may be applied; however, bandages are not recommended for infants or young children because of possible irritation and the potential of swallowing or aspirating the bandage.

Self Study

Study Questions

For the following questions, select the one best answer.

1. Which of the following is the best site for a capillary puncture on an adult?

   a. middle finger
   b. pinkie finger
   c. ankle
   d. heel

2. Controlling the depth of the skin puncture prevents:

   a. puncturing a vein
   b. bacterial contamination
   c. excessive bleeding
   d. osteomyelitis

3. Skin puncture is not useful for patients who have which of the following conditions?

   a. obesity
   b. burns
   c. fragile veins
   d. healthy adults who need many laboratory tests

4. Which fingers are used most often for skin puncture?

   a. thumb
   b. second, or index, finger
   c. third or fourth finger
   d. fifth, or pinky, finger

5. What is the disinfectant of choice for a capillary puncture procedure?

   a. iodine preparation
   b. 100% ethyl alcohol
   c. 70% isopropyl alcohol
   d. 10% bleach solution

6. Which drop(s) of blood should be used for specimen collection during a fingerstick?

   a. first
   b. second
   c. twelfth
   d. blood mixed with alcohol

7. Which drop should be wiped away before beginning the capillary collection?

   a. first
   b. second
   c. twelfth
   d. blood mixed with alcohol

8. What does the *feathered edge* refer to?

   a. the point of the lancet
   b. alcohol pad
   c. edge of the blood film on a microscope slide
   d. blood drop on a microscope slide

9. Capillary blood is composed of:

   a. venous blood only
   b. arterial blood only
   c. venous, arterial, and capillary blood, and tissue fluids
   d. venous blood and tissue fluids

10. Plastic microcollection tubes should be filled with blood in which of the following ways?

   a. using a syringe to fill the tube
   b. allowing the tube to fill by itself using capillary action
   c. using suction to pull blood into the tube
   d. using the tube to scoop droplets off the skin carefully

Case Study

A health care worker was assigned to a specimen collection station in the clinic where most of the patients were having fingersticks. The first patient encountered was an 18-year-old named Sarah W., who had a fear of needles. She was shaking, her hands were cold, and she was about to cry. The second patient, Henry C., had very wrinkled, dry skin and calluses on his fingers.

Question

What should the health care worker do to make the best of these two situations and collect the blood specimens?

Self Assessment

Check Yourself

Patient Preference

Think about the last time you experienced a venipuncture or a fingerstick. Discuss your preference between the two procedures. Also, explain which finger you would prefer to have stuck and why.

Competency Checklist: Capillary Blood Collection

Each step must be successfully completed. If one step is not completed successfully, the individual/student should restudy the text and seek guidance from a supervisor or educator. He or she must try again until competency has been achieved.

(1) Completed   (2) Needs to improve

_____ 1. Patient identification and assessment are performed appropriately.

_____ 2. Prepares the appropriate supplies and puncture device.

_____ 3. Performs hand-hygiene and gloving techniques.

_____ 4. Positions the patient appropriately.

_____ 5. Selects the correct finger.

_____ 6. Decontaminates the site appropriately.

_____ 7. Uses warming devices or other methods to improve blood flow to the site.

_____ 8. Uses a self retracting puncture device to make an incision across the fingerprint. Discards puncture device.

_____ 9. Wipes away the first drop of blood.

_____10. Collects the appropriate specimen in the correct order.

_____11. Applies appropriate pressure to produce additional drops of blood.

_____12. Applies gentle pressure to stop the bleeding.

_____13. Handles the specimens appropriately (e.g., gentle mixing, etc).

_____14. Discards all waste in appropriate containers.

_____15. Labels the specimens appropriately and prepares them for transport.

_____16. Checks the patient status before leaving.

_____17. Thanks the patient for cooperating.

Competency Checklist: Making Blood Smears for Microscopic Analysis

Many phlebotomists are no longer required to make manual blood films on microscopic slides. However, it is a skill that is still required in some settings where phlebotomists are the only ones with this educational skill. Making appropriate microscopic blood films for laboratory analysis requires repeated practice. The skill should be practiced until the phlebotomist becomes proficient.

(1) Completed   (2) Needs to improve

_____ 1. Using a practice sample of blood, the phlebotomist is able to make 50 suitable blood smears.

_____ 2. Using blood from a capillary puncture on a patient, the phlebotomist wipes away the first drop of blood.

_____ 3. The glass slide is touched to the finger about 0.5 to 1 inch from the end.

_____ 4. The second slide (the spreader) is placed in front of the drop which allows the drop of blood to spread along the width of the slide.

_____ 5. The spreader is pushed evenly toward the other end of the slide causing the blood to evenly flow across the glass.

_____ 6. The blood smear is in the shape of a feathered edge.

_____ 7. The slide is allowed to air dry.

_____ 8. The slide is labeled appropriately.

Reference

1. Clinical and Laboratory Standards Institute (CLSI): _Procedures and Devices for the Collection of Diagnostic Capillary Blood Specimens_, Approved Standard, document H4-A5. Wayne, PA: CLSI, 2004.

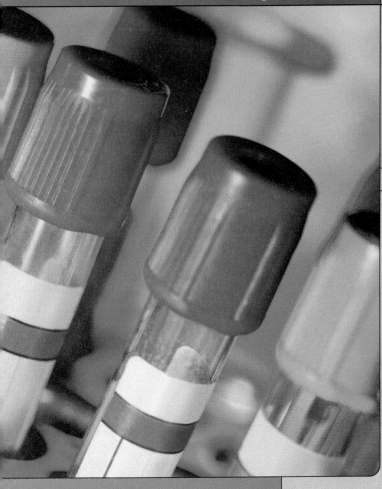

Chapter 10

Pediatric and Geriatric Procedures

KEY TERMS

blood volume

calcaneus

capillary blood gas analysis

eutectic mixture of local
   anesthetics (EMLA)

geriatric

heelstick

neonatal screening

neonates

Parkinson's disease

pediatric phlebotomy

premature infant

sucrose nipple or pacifier

Collecting blood from pediatric (baby or child) and **geriatric** (elderly) patients requires much clinical knowledge about and training for the proper techniques. Both of these age groups require extra care in blood collection.

Pediatric Patients

Children are not just little adults, and they should not be treated as such. The health care worker needs to be familiar with special types of equipment that are available, observe the various techniques as they are performed by a health care worker experienced in **pediatric phlebotomy**, and practice the techniques to develop the necessary skills. The health care worker also must learn how to talk with children of various ages to calm them for a blood collection.

Performing venipuncture or skin puncture on young patients is challenging, because children have smaller bodies and are less prepared to cope with pain and anxiety. When learning the techniques, remember to ask for help if needed and to allow adequate time to develop the necessary skills.

Preparing Child and Parent

The timing of the preparation depends on the child's age; generally, the younger the child, the closer the explanation should be to the time of the procedure.[1]

Preparing the child and the parent for the blood collection procedure involves the following steps:

1. A calm, confident approach is the first step in obtaining the cooperation of the child and parent. Introduce yourself. Be warm and friendly, establish eye contact with both the child and the parent, and show that you are concerned about the child's health and comfort. When you interact with a pediatric patient and his or her parent, provide a sense of trust and confidence.

2. Correctly identify the patient by using at least two patient identifiers.[2] The patient should have an identification bracelet with his or her name and hospital number or birth date. Verify the correct name and hospital number or birth date. A hospitalized infant usually has the identification bracelet on his or her ankle. Newborns who have not yet been named are usually identified by their last names (e.g., Baby Boy Smith and Baby Girl Jones) and identification number. If the mother is still in the hospital after delivery, the baby may wear an identification band that is cross-referenced to the mother. Keeping identifications straight is always crucial, but especially so when specimens from twin babies must be collected and labeled.

3. Find out about the child's past experience with blood collections. Ask whether the child has ever had blood collected. The child and the parent can then tell you about their experiences with past procedures and provide you with valuable information about the approaches that worked effectively for them and those that were not as successful.

4. Develop a plan. Ask the parent how cooperative his or her child will be. Parents are excellent predictors of their child's behavior and possibility for distress. Usually, the younger child with poor venous access will have more distress. A successful plan involves not only the parent's suggestions about what will be most helpful but also the health care worker's knowledge about pediatric phlebotomy techniques. If possible, allow the child to have some control by offering a choice of which arm or finger he or she prefers for blood collection.

5. Place yourself at the child's eye level to explain and demonstrate the procedure (Figure 10-1 ■).

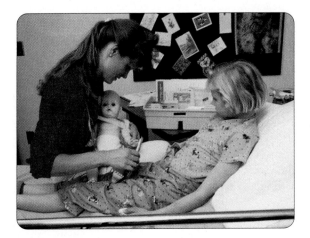

FIGURE ▪ 10-1 Talking to Child at Eye Level

When explaining what you will be doing, use words appropriate for the child's age. Use of a doll, puppet, or stuffed animal in the demonstration can help you relate to the child in a nonthreatening manner. If the child has a favorite doll, blanket, or toy, he or she should be encouraged to hug it for comfort and support.

6. Establish guidelines. Tell the child and the parent that the procedure will most likely be successful on the first attempt. If not, it will be attempted only once more by another health care worker.

7. Be honest when a child asks whether the puncture will hurt. Tell the child that if the procedure hurts too much, it can be momentarily stopped, but that the more quickly the procedure is performed the less painful it will be. Instruct the child to say when he or she feels the pain or "hurt." Tell the child that saying "ouch" or making faces is acceptable but that he or she must make an effort to keep the arm absolutely still. Reassure the child that the blood will be collected as quickly as possible so that the pain will be brief.[1]

8. Encourage parent involvement.[1] Explain how the parent can assist by holding, distracting, and soothing their child during the procedure. Some parents, however, may be reluctant to participate because they do not want to be a part of a procedure that will cause their children pain. If the parent does not wish to assist but is willing to be in the room, ask him or her to maintain eye contact with the child to reduce stress. If after discussing his or her role the parent is still reluctant to be in the room, respect his or her wishes. If the parent does not wish to participate, you may ask another health care worker to assist.

PSYCHOLOGICAL RESPONSE TO NEEDLES AND PAIN

Children especially fear needles, and an emotionally upset child has difficulty separating fear from actual pain. Children 1 to 2 years old may react extremely to painless procedures, such as taking a temperature. Children 3 to 5 years old perceive pain as a punishment for bad behavior. They may react aggressively. Children 6 to 12 years old are more likely to relate pain to past experiences. Many children perceive that a "shot," or needle, hurts more than anything else that has ever happened to them. Children 13 to 17 years old are more independent and may be embarrassed to show fear. They usually need privacy and may act hostile to

Clinical Alert ❗

It is not unusual for a sick or injured child to act younger than he or she really is. If a child who is 6 behaves like a 3 year old, use strategies appropriate for a 3 year old.[3]

The following parental behaviors and examples will have a positive effect on relieving the child's distress.[3,4]

Behaviors	Examples
Distraction	"Look at Mommy"; "Tell us about your doll"
Emotional support	Hugging, stroking hair, patting, and talking in a soothing voice
Explanation	"We need to take a tiny bit of blood from your finger"; "You will feel a little prick"; "Mommy will help you hold your arm still so that we can finish quickly"
Positive reinforcement	"You did a great job in holding your arm still!"

mask fear. With proper preparation, the child and the parent can develop coping skills to help lessen the fear and thereby diminish the "hurt."

DISTRACTION TECHNIQUES

Children older than 3 years respond well to distraction techniques to help them cope and lessen distress. Distraction helps the child refocus on a more pleasant experience. A parent or another health care worker can provide the distraction. Some examples of distraction are blowing bubbles, pinwheels, counting, reading a book or looking at a video, listening to music, singing, or talking in a gentle voice about something enjoyable. School-age children may respond to strategies such as picturing themselves in a pleasant setting or participating in the procedure.[3,4]

ROOM LOCATION

For psychological reasons, the best room location for a painful procedure is a treatment room away from the child's bed or play room. For a hospitalized child, the bed should be a safe, secure place to rest and sleep, not a place associated with pain. If the child shares a room with another child, performing the procedure at the bed side can be upsetting to the roommate as well. If the child cannot be moved to a treatment room, maintain privacy by drawing a curtain between the beds and speaking in a calm, quiet manner.

EQUIPMENT PREPARATION FOR A FRIENDLIER ENVIRONMENT

Just the sight of needles, syringes, and a person in a white laboratory coat can be frightening to a child. When working with children, wear bright, colorfully printed uniforms or smocks to create a child-friendly environment. Prepare the phlebotomy equipment and supplies before entering the child's room so that the child does not become even more anxious by watching the preparation. Use shorter needles if possible, and keep threatening-looking supplies (such as needles) covered and out of sight until you are ready to proceed with the procedure. If the hospital policy requires goggles or face shields for blood-exposure precautions, put this equipment on after greeting the child. Praise the child throughout the procedure. At the completion, reward the child with a colorful bandage, a sticker, an age-appropriate toy, or, with parental permission, a lollipop. If a parent is not present to assist in relieving the anxiety, offer a pacifier to an infant or gently stroke or talk softly to soothe a small child.

Positions for Restraining a Child

Holding the child may be required to ensure that the child does not move his or her limb (i.e., arm, finger, or foot) during blood collection. Restraining techniques should be compassionate, safe, and performed quickly. A supportive parent who has been properly instructed can assist with restraining while providing comfort to the child.

Two preferred comfort methods of restraining a child to immobilize the arm are the vertical position and the horizontal, or supine position (Figures 10-2 ■ and 10-3 ■).[3,4]

In both cases, the parent's face is close to the child's, thereby providing a comforting and secure feeling. The vertical technique, which works well for toddlers, requires the child to be held on the parent's lap. As the parent hugs and holds the child's body and the arm not being used, the health care worker can firmly hold the other arm to perform the procedure.

In the horizontal position, a baby can easily be held by a parent. However, more restraint may be needed for an older child. If the child lies supine, with the health care worker on one side of the bed and the parent on the opposite side, the parent can gently but firmly lean over the child, restraining the child's arm not being used while holding the opposite, extended arm securely for the health care worker.

Neonates and infants younger than 3 months usually do not require restraint and can be managed by the health care worker alone. Swaddling helps to control and comfort an upset newborn.

Combative Patients

At times, a child will become uncooperative even after the proper steps have been followed to gain cooperation. Children may become combative—kicking and thrashing—if force is used. Because sharps are involved in blood collection, the health care worker must be certain that the procedure can be performed safely. Using force to the point of potential physical injury is unethical and unprofessional. Therefore, if the risk of injury to the child or the health care worker is likely, discontinue the blood collection attempt and notify the nurse or the physician.

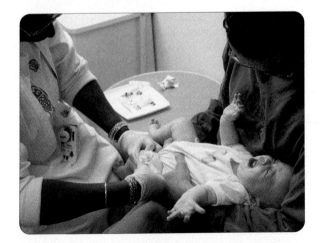

FIGURE ■ **10-2** Supine (Lying) Position for Restraining Child to Perform Blood Collection

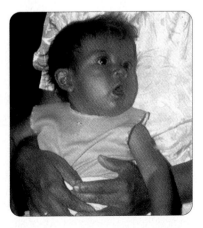

FIGURE ■ **10-3** Vertical Position for Restraining a Child to Perform Blood Collection

Decreasing the Needlestick Pain

A topical anesthetic (pain reliever), **EMLA (eutectic mixture of local anesthetics)**, can be rubbed on the skin when a needlestick is going to be used for venipuncture to a child. This local anesthetic is ideal for use before venipuncture or starting intravenous (IV) therapy because it does not require a needle. It is applied to the skin as a patch or a cream that is then covered with a transparent adhesive dressing (see Figure 10-4 ■). Optimal anesthesia occurs after 45 to 60 minutes and may last as long as 2 to 3 hours. Drawbacks to the use of EMLA are cost, the need to apply it 60 minutes before the procedure, and having to know in advance the location of the vein to be used. Two separate locations may be anesthetized if the child has difficult veins from which to obtain blood. Do not use EMLA if the child is allergic to local anesthetics.[4,5,6]

ORAL SUCROSE

Sucrose (a sugar) is effective in reducing pain and crying time during a procedure for an infant up to 6 months old. A 25% solution of sucrose can be prepared by mixing 4 teaspoons of water with 1 teaspoon of sugar. The sucrose can be carefully administered by oral syringe, dropper, nipple, or on a pacifier. A **sucrose nipple** or **pacifier** is given 2 minutes before heelsticks, and its action lasts about 5 minutes. Some studies show that infants given pacifiers or sucrose have also been shown to be more alert after the procedure, to be less fussy, and to cry for a shorter duration.[5,7]

Precautions to Protect the Child

Premature infants, newborns, and children who are chronically ill or have extensive burns are more likely to be susceptible to infections. To protect these children from potentially harmful microorganisms, some hospitals may require protective precautions. In this instance, PPE—gowns, gloves, and masks—will be worn as indicated before entering the room. After the procedure, remove the PPE according to policy and dispose of it in the appropriately marked container. Wash your hands or sanitize them according to policy. Alcohol-based waterless rubs, foams, or rinses are as effective as handwashing if the hands are not soiled.[8] Put on a clean gown and gloves before attending to the next infant or child.

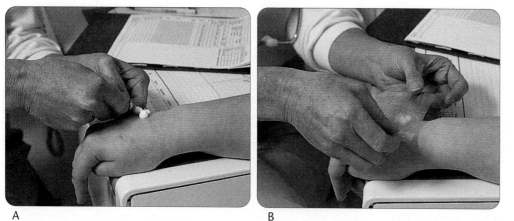

A   B

FIGURE ■ 10-4

Using EMLA. When a needlestick is planned, EMLA can be used to anesthetize the skin where the needlestick will occur. A. Apply a thick layer of the EMLA cream over intact skin (half of a 5-g tube). B. Cover the cream with a transparent adhesive dressing for 45–60 minutes

> **Clinical Alert** ❗
>
> Puncturing deep veins in children may cause cardiac arrest, hemorrhage, venous thrombosis, damage to surrounding tissues, and infection.

Pediatric Phlebotomy Procedures

Two methods are used to obtain blood from infants and children: microcapillary skin puncture and venipuncture. The previously described steps for preparing the child and the parent should be taken before either procedure is performed.

MICROCAPILLARY SKIN PUNCTURE

Skin punctures are useful for pediatric phlebotomy when only small amounts of blood are needed and can be adequately tested. It is particularly important to collect only the smallest amounts of blood necessary from neonates, infants, and children so that the effects of reductions in **blood volume** are minimal. Overcollecting during phlebotomy may require packed-blood-cell transfusion in an infant. Small infants can easily become anemic if too much blood is taken. To avoid overcollection of blood by phlebotomy, the amount of blood collected from an infant and small child must be recorded and maintained.

Each hospital treating pediatric patients should determine the amounts of blood to be drawn from patients on the basis of weight and the maximum cumulative amount of blood to be collected during a specified time period.

When performing skin punctures, collect the hematological specimens first to minimize platelet clumping, then collect for chemical and blood-bank specimens. Each laboratory has approved procedures for phlebotomy, including the volume of blood that is required for each test: always follow these procedures. Always record the amount of blood collected.

SKIN PUNCTURE SITES

The heel is the most desirable site for skin puncture on an infant or neonate. Use the most medial or most lateral section of the plantar, or bottom, surface of the heel (Figure 10-5 ■).

DO NOT use the central area of the infant's heel for blood collection. For children older than 1 year, the palmar surface of the distal phalanx (fingertip section) of the third (middle) or fourth (ring) finger is most frequently used, because the thumb has a pulse and the index finger may be more sensitive. The fifth finger is not used because the skin is too thin. The plantar surface of the great toe is NOT recommended for skin puncture. Using the proper pediatric size skin-puncture device, make an incision that is less than 2.0 mm deep (see Figure 10-6 ■). Major blood vessels lie 0.3 to 1.6 mm beneath the skin at the dermal—subcutaneous junction in newborns.[9,10] If an incision goes deeper, the **calcaneus** or heel bone may be hit, which may lead to osteomyelitis and/or osteochondritis.[11,12]

> **Clinical Alert** ❗
>
> Do not obtain blood by skin puncture from the toes or the central area of an infant's heel, because this may result in injury to nerves, tendons, and cartilage; do not use fingers of infants less than 1 year old or previously punctured sites. If an infant has compromised circulation to the extremity, as in shock, or has edema, bruises, rashes, or infection at the heel, use another site (i.e., venipuncture procedure).

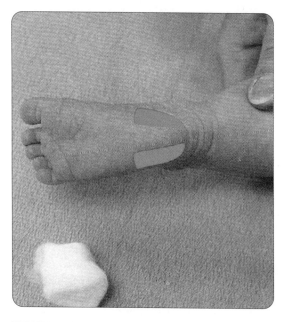

FIGURE ■ 10-5 Heel Sites for Capillary Puncture

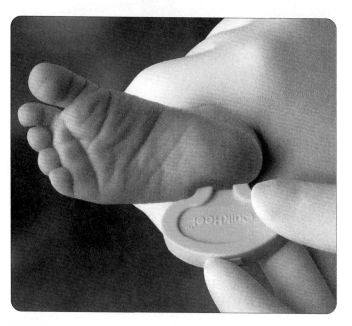

FIGURE ■ 10-6 Performing a Heelstick on an Infant

Courtesy of BD VACUTAINER Systems, Preanalytical Solutions, *Franklin Lakes, NJ.*

Procedure 10-1

Heelstick Procedure

RATIONALE

To perform a blood collection from the infant's heel.

EQUIPMENT

The following equipment is necessary for pediatric skin puncture:

- Sterile, automatic, disposable pediatric skin-puncture safety devices in different manufacturers' incision depths (0.65–0.85 mm for premature neonates, 1.0 mm for larger infants). (Please see Chapter 6, Blood Collection Equipment, for photo examples)
- 70% isopropyl alcohol swabs
- Sterile 2″ × 2″ gauze sponges
- Plastic capillary collection tubes and sealer or caps

- Microcollection containers, plastic capillary tubes, and BD Unopettes
- Glass slides for smears
- Puncture-resistant sharps container
- Disposable gloves (nonlatex if the child is allergic)
- Compress (towel or washcloth) to warm heel if necessary
- Marking pen
- Laboratory request slips or labels

(continued)

PREPARATION

(1) Prepare and assemble supplies. Remember, DO NOT place the specimen collection tray on the infant's bed or in the bassinet.

(2) Introduce yourself to the parents, explain the procedure and use appropriate comfort techniques.

(3) Identify the infant properly. Identify the infant by name, address, and identification number and/or birth date and compare with laboratory test request form. If the infant is not wearing an identification bracelet the name of the person who performs this identification procedure must be documented in the medical records and charts.

PROCEDURE

(4) Wash or sanitize your hands with an alcohol hand rub, then put on gloves. If required, don a gown and a mask.

(5) Inspect the selected area and assess it for proper warmth. If it is cool or a blood gas specimen is to be collected, prewarm the foot ▶ with a warm, wet towel or a chemical heel-warming pack, according to policy. Wipe the heel dry after removing the warm towel.

A CLOSER LOOK

▶ Heel Warming

RATIONALE

The amount of blood that can be obtained from a single **heelstick** is limited; therefore, to obtain an adequate sample, prewarming the heel may be indicated. Prewarming the heel increases blood flow and arterializes the specimen. This step is essential for collecting specimens for **capillary blood gas analysis**.

PROCEDURE

(A) Prepare and assemble supplies; warm wet towel and a plastic bag or a chemical heel-warming pack.

(B) Warm the site with a commercially available warming pack or wrap a warm, wet towel at a temperature no more than 42°C around the infant's foot. If the temperature of the towel exceeds 42°C, it may burn the infant.

(C) Encase the towel in a plastic bag to help retain heat and to keep the patient's bed dry. Use caution if the towel is heated in a microwave oven, because heating is uneven and the towel may have hot spots.

(D) Prewarm the site for 3 to 5 minutes.

(E) Depending on the institution's policy, call in advance to prewarm the infant's heel.

(6) Position the baby in a supine (lying) position with the knee at the open end of the bassinet. This position allows the foot to hang lower than the torso, improving blood flow. When the baby is in an acceptable position for this procedure, clean the incision of the heel with an antiseptic

swab. Allow the heel to air dry. Do not touch the incision site or allow the heel to come into contact with any nonsterile item or surface (Figure 10-7 ■).

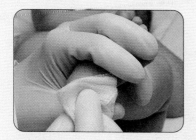

FIGURE ■ 10-7 *Courtesy of ITC, Edison, NJ.*

(7) Remove the appropriate Tenderfoot puncture device from its blister pack, taking care not to rest the blade slot end on any nonsterile surface (Figure 10-8 ■).

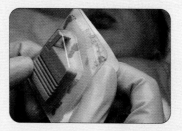

FIGURE ■ 10-8 *Courtesy of ITC, Edison, NJ.*

(8) Remove the safety clip. Note: The safety clip may be replaced if the test is momentarily delayed; however, prolonged exposure of any Tenderfoot device to uncontrolled environmental conditions before use may affect its sterility. Once the safety clip is removed, DO NOT push the trigger or touch the blade slot (Figure 10-9 ■).

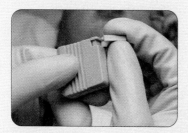

FIGURE ■ 10-9 *Courtesy of ITC, Edison, NJ.*

(9) Hold the infant's foot firmly but gently to prevent sudden movement. Holding the foot too tightly may cause bruising and restrict blood flow. Also, it can lead to erroneous laboratory tests results.

Clinical Alert !

Avoid excessive milking or squeezing, which causes hemolysis and dilutes the blood with interstitial and intracellular fluid.

(10) Raise the foot above the baby's heart level and carefully select a safe incision site (avoid any edematous area or site within 2.0 mm of a prior wound). Place the blade-slot surface of the device flush against the heel so that its center point is vertically aligned with the desired incision site (Figure 10-10 ■).

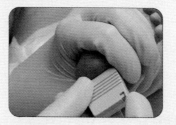

FIGURE ■ 10-10 *Courtesy of ITC, Edison, NJ.*

(continued)

11 Ensure that both ends of the device have made light contact with the skin, and depress the trigger. After triggering, immediately remove the device from the infant's heel and dispose of it in the biohazard sharps container (Figure 10-11 ■).

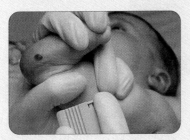

FIGURE ■ **10-11** *Courtesy of ITC, Edison, NJ.*

12 Using only a dry sterile gauze pad, gently wipe away the first droplet of blood that appears at the incision site (Figure 10-12 ■).

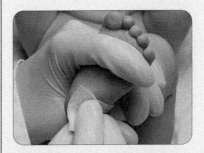
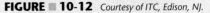

FIGURE ■ **10-12** *Courtesy of ITC, Edison, NJ.*

13 Taking care not to make direct wound contact with the collection container or capillary tube, fill to the desired specimen volume (Figure 10-13 ■).

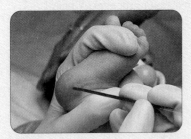

FIGURE ■ **10-13** *Courtesy of ITC, Edison, NJ.*

14 After blood collection, gently press a dry sterile gauze pad to the incision site until bleeding has ceased. This step will help prevent a hematoma from forming. (Figure 10-14 ■).

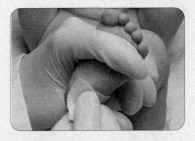

FIGURE ■ **10-14** *Courtesy of ITC, Edison, NJ.*

15 Label the specimen container and verify identification. Record the time of collection.

AFTER THE PROCEDURE: CARE OF THE HEEL

16 Elevate the heel slightly above the body and ensure that bleeding has stopped.

17 Check the infant's heel puncture site for late bleeding or inflammation.

CLEAN UP

(18) Dispose of the used skin-puncture devices in a sharps container with a biohazard label.	(19) Check the infant's bed for any equipment or trash left behind.
(20) Discard blood-soaked gauze sponges, grossly contaminated items, and gowns or gloves used in isolation rooms in biohazardous waste containers.	(21) Dispose of gowns and gloves that are not from isolation rooms in the regular trash.
(22) Wash or sanitize your hands after removing the gloves.	

Capillary Blood Gases

Arterial blood is the specimen of choice for blood gas testing (i.e., pH, oxygen [O_2] content, and carbon dioxide [CO_2] content of the blood). However, capillary (skin puncture) blood can be collected from infants and small children for blood gas analysis because this procedure is safer than an arterial puncture. Skin puncture blood is less desirable as a specimen because it contains blood from capillaries, venules and arterioles, and fluids from the surrounding tissue. In addition, common collection methods for capillary blood gas specimens use an open collection system in which the specimen is temporarily exposed to room air, which allows for a brief exchange of gases (both O_2 and CO_2) before the specimens are sealed from the air. The air exposure must be minimized to avoid falsely elevated blood oxygen levels.

NEONATAL SCREENING

In the United States, newborn babies, or neonates, are routinely screened for a variety of metabolic and genetic defects by analysis of blood collected on a special filter paper. **Neonatal screening** is important for the early detection, diagnosis, and treatment of certain genetic, metabolic, and infectious diseases. Many of these diseases can result in severe abnormalities, including mental retardation, if they are not discovered and treated early.

Blood spot testing for screening is performed before the newborn is 72 hours old. If the blood specimen is collected before the newborn is 24 hours old because of early discharge from the hospital, a second specimen for screening must be collected before 2 weeks of age.

Collection for Capillary Blood Gas Testing

RATIONALE

To perform a blood collection for capillary blood gas analysis. Blood for capillary blood gas analysis is often collected from small children and babies for whom arterial punctures can be too dangerous. Samples are collected from the same areas of the body as other capillary samples, such as the lateral posterior area of the heel or the ball of the finger.

EQUIPMENT

- Sterile, retractable, disposable pediatric skin-puncture safety devices in different manufacturers' incision depths (0.65–0.85 mm for premature neonates, 1.0 mm for larger infants)
- Heparinized safety plastic capillary tubes
- 70% isopropyl alcohol swabs
- Sterile 2″ × 2″ gauze sponges
- Plastic capillary collection tubes and sealer
- Microcollection containers, plastic capillary tubes, and BD Unopettes

- Glass slides for smears
- Puncture-resistant sharps container
- Disposable gloves (nonlatex if the child is allergic)
- Compress (towel or washcloth) to warm heel if necessary
- Marking pen
- Laboratory request slips or labels
- Ice water
- Minute metal filing
- A magnet

PREPARATION

1 Prepare and assemble supplies.	**2** Introduce yourself to the parents, explain the procedure, and use appropriate comfort techniques.
3 Identify the infant properly.	**4** Warm the site according to the institution's procedures.

PROCEDURE

5 Wash or sanitize your hands with an alcohol hand rinse, then put on gloves. If required, don a gown and a mask.	**6** Use a heparinized safety plastic capillary tube (Figure 10-15 ■) for the collection.

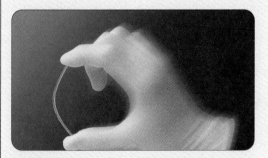

FIGURE ■ 10-15 SAFE-T-FILL Blood Gas Capillary Tube—100% Plastic for Safety

Courtesy of Ram Scientific, Inc., Needham, MA.

7 Insert a small metal filing (referred to as a "flea") into each capillary tube before collecting blood to help mix the specimen while it is entering the tube (see Figure 10-16 ■).

FIGURE ■ 10-16 Capillary Blood Gas Tube, Metal Filing (Flea), and Plastic Caps

Clinical Alert !

The specimen must be collected with no air bubbles, which can distort the values obtained from the specimen.

---

8 Perform the capillary (skin) puncture as previously mentioned and wipe away the first drop.

9 When the tube is full, seal the ends with plastic caps, and use a magnet to draw the metal filing (flea) back and forth across the length of the tube to mix the specimen completely.

---

10 Label the tube and place it in a bag surrounded by a slurry of ice water for immediate transfer to the laboratory. Notify laboratory personnel of the urgent blood gas test to be performed.

11 Press the skin puncture site with a clean gauze sponge until the bleeding stops.

AFTER THE PROCEDURE: CARE OF THE HEEL

12 Elevate the heel slightly above the body and assure that bleeding has stopped.

13 Check the infant's heel puncture site for late bleeding or inflammation.

CLEAN UP

14 Dispose of the used skin-puncture devices in a sharps container with a biohazard label.

15 Check the infant's bed for any equipment or trash left behind.

---

16 Discard blood-soaked gauze sponges, grossly contaminated items, and gowns or gloves used in isolation rooms in biohazardous waste containers.

17 Dispose of gowns and gloves that are not from isolation rooms in the regular trash.

---

18 Wash or sanitize your hands after removing the gloves.

19 Deliver the sample immediately to the laboratory. Delays of more than 15 minutes at room temperature (or more than 60 minutes at 4°C), will affect the results.

Clinical Alert ❗

Fingerstick

A fingerstick to obtain blood for routine laboratory analysis is usually preferred for children older than 1 year (Figure 10-17 ■). Also, a fingerstick may be necessary if a child has damaged veins from repeated venipuncture or if the veins are covered with bandages or casts. Do not perform a fingerstick if the finger is swollen, edematous, cyanotic, or infected.

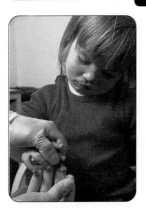

FIGURE ■ 10-17 Collecting Blood via Fingerstick from a Toddler

Procedure 10-3 — Collection of Blood for Neonatal Screening

RATIONALE

The heel of the neonate is the most frequently used site for collection of blood for screening.

Clinical Alert ❗

To prevent contamination, do not touch any part of the filter paper circles with your hands or gloves before, during, or after collection. Do not allow the filter paper to come in contact with substances such as alcohol, formula, water, powder, antiseptic solutions, or lotion.

EQUIPMENT

- Sterile, retractale, disposable pediatric skin-puncture safety devices in different manufacturers' incision depths (0.65–0.85 mm for premature neonates, 1.0 mm for larger infants)
- Appropriate collection cards
- Sterile 2″ × 2″ gauze sponges
- 70% isopropyl alcohol swabs
- Plastic capillary collection tubes and sealer

- Microcollection containers, plastic capillary tubes, and BD Unopettes
- Glass slides for smears
- Puncture-resistant sharps container
- Disposable gloves (nonlatex if the child is allergic)
- Compress (towel or washcloth) to warm heel if necessary
- Marking pen
- Laboratory request slips or labels

PREPARATION

1 Prepare and assemble supplies. Appropriate collection cards are kept in the hospital laboratory or the nursery. Circles are printed on the filter paper portion of the card.

2 Introduce yourself to the parents, explain the procedure, and use appropriate comfort techniques.

3 Identify the infant properly.

Clinical Alert !

Use a pediatric safety skin-puncture device designed for the age and size of the child. A retractable skin-puncture device controls the puncture depth, which should be less than 2.0 mm in small children. The distance from the skin surface to bone or cartilage in the middle, or third, finger is between 1.5 and 2.4 mm. Automatic puncture devices are available in sizes that incise to depths of 0.85 mm for premature infants, 1.25 mm for infants and 1.75 mm for toddlers. For a detailed description of the blood collection procedure and supplies, refer to Chapter 9, Capillary Blood Specimens.

PROCEDURE

4 Wash your hands well and put on gloves.

5 Position the baby in a supine (lying) position with the knee at the open end of the bassinet. This position allows the foot to hang lower than the torso, improving blood flow. When the baby is in an acceptable position for this procedure, clean the incision of the heel with an antiseptic swab. Allow the heel to air dry. Do not touch the incision site or allow the heel to come into contact with any nonsterile item or surface.

6 Once the puncture is made, wipe off the first drop of blood with sterile gauze. The initial drop contains tissue fluids that may dilute the sample.

7 Allow another large blood drop to form.

8 Lightly touch the printed side of the filter paper with the blood drop and fill each printed circle. Allow the blood to soak through and completely fill the circle with a single application to the large blood drop (see Figure 10-18 ■).

9 If the circle does not fill entirely, wipe the heel and express another, larger drop onto a different circle. Do not add a second drop of blood to a previously used circle.

Clinical Alert !

Use only one side of the filter paper, and the filter paper must not touch the skin puncture site.

Acceptable Specimen   Poor Quality   Poor Quality

FIGURE ■ 10-18 Collecting a Blood Sample from the Newborn for Neonatal Metabolic Screening

(continued)

Collection of Blood for Neonatal Screening (continued)

10. Dry blood spots on a clean, dry, flat nonabsorbent surface for a minimum of 4 hours.

11. Direct application of blood from the heel to the card is the technique of choice; however, blood from a heparinized capillary tube may be applied if care is taken not to scratch or dent the filter paper.

12. Correctly complete all the information on the screening card so that follow-up can be done if the results are abnormal. Place the screening card in an appropriate envelope and send it to the laboratory within 24 hours.

AFTER THE PROCEDURE: CARE OF THE HEEL

13. Elevate the heel above the body.

14. Press a sterile gauze sponge against the puncture site until the bleeding stops. This helps to prevent formation of a hematoma.

15. Monitor the infant's heel site for the first hour after the puncture for late bleeding and inflammation.

CLEAN UP

16. Dispose of the used skin-puncture devices in a sharps container with a biohazard label.

17. Check the infant's bed for any equipment or trash left behind.

18. Discard blood-soaked gauze sponges, grossly contaminated items, and gowns or gloves used in isolation rooms in biohazardous waste containers.

19. Dispose of gowns and gloves that are not from isolation rooms in the regular trash.

20. Wash or sanitize your hands after removing the gloves.

Pediatric Venipuncture

RATIONALE

Venipuncture in children is used when larger quantities of blood are needed for sampling. The veins of the antecubital fossa or the forearm (see Figure 10-19 ■) are the most accessible and are chosen for most toddlers and children. Dorsal hand veins are preferred sites for venous access in neonates and well infants (Figure 10-20 ■).[13] If a venipuncture is done on a child younger than 2 years old, limit the site to a superficial vein. Other sites used for venipuncture are the medial wrist, the dorsum of the foot, the scalp, and the medial ankle. Always check the policy at your facility before performing venipuncture on foot or ankle veins. If the neonate or child is receiving fluid or medication intravenously, avoid the distal veins for phlebotomy to preserve them for IV therapy. Venipuncture is indicated for blood sampling for routine laboratory tests, erythrocyte sedimentation rate (ESR), blood cultures, cross-matching, coagulation studies, and drug and ammonia levels. Do not use veins in an extremity or an area if there is edema or infection or if an IV line is present. Avoid deep veins in a child with hemophilia or other bleeding disorders.

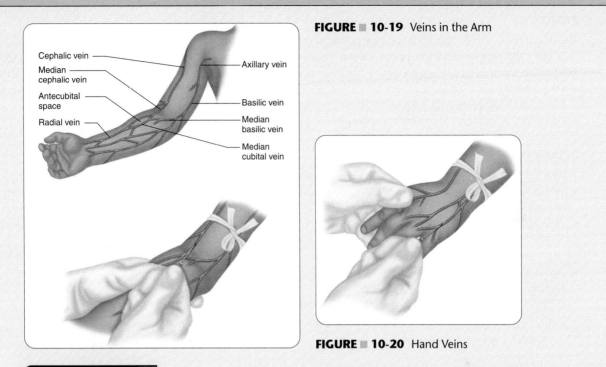

FIGURE 10-19 Veins in the Arm

Cephalic vein
Median cephalic vein
Antecubital space
Radial vein
Axillary vein
Basilic vein
Median basilic vein
Median cubital vein

FIGURE 10-20 Hand Veins

Clinical Alert !

Remove the tourniquet before withdrawing the needle. Apply pressure with a sterile gauze sponge for 3 minutes to prevent a hematoma. Do not use alcohol pads to apply pressure, because this will cause stinging and prevent hemostasis. The equipment of choice for venipuncture on a neonate is a small, winged safety (butterfly) needle. If feasible, use a winged safety needle for small children as well.

EQUIPMENT

The equipment necessary for a pediatric venipuncture includes the following:

- Winged safety infusion (butterfly) needle, 23-gauge
- Syringes slightly larger than the volume of blood needed
- Transfer device is recommended
- 70% isopropyl alcohol swab in a sterile package
- Two 2" × 2" gauze sponges
- Appropriate specimen containers
- Pediatric-size tourniquet (nonlatex if the child is allergic)
- Sterile disposable gloves (nonlatex if the child is allergic)
- For blood culture:

  a. Bottles, both aerobic and anaerobic. For smaller children, use a special pediatric bottle. The required volumes are 2–4 mL for children 2 to 12 years old and 1 mL for infants under 2 years.
  b. Iodine swabs
  c. Chlorohexidine gluconate swabs (use for infants instead of iodine)
- Paper tape and adhesive strip (for use only with older children)
- Marking pen
- Biohazardous waste container

PROCEDURE

The procedure for performing venipuncture on older children is similar to that for adults (see Chapter 8). However, special considerations may include: special preparation of the child and the parent, assistance in restraining the child, and the use of special pediatric-size needles and safety winged infusion sets. If the child's veins are difficult to locate, another option for pediatric venipuncture is the dorsal hand vein procedure.

Dorsal Hand Vein Procedure on Infant

RATIONALE

The dorsal hand vein technique is appropriate for neonates and infants who are younger than 2 years old.

Dorsal hand vein venipuncture has several advantages over skin puncture: it is less stressful for the infant and the health care worker; there is less dilution of the specimen with tissue fluids and less hemolysis; and fewer punctures are required.[14]

Although the neonate may not need restraint, an older infant can be wrapped snuggly in a receiving blanket or restrained by an assistant to minimize movement.

EQUIPMENT

- Winged safety infusion (butterfly) needle, 23-gauge
- Syringes slightly larger than the volume of blood needed
- 70% isopropyl alcohol swab in a sterile package
- 2" × 2" gauze sponges
- Appropriate specimen containers
- Sterile disposable gloves (nonlatex if the child is allergic)
- For blood culture:
  a. Bottles, both aerobic and anaerobic. For smaller children use a special pediatric bottle. The required volumes are 2–4 mL for children 2 to 12 years old and 1 mL for infants under 2 years.
  b. Iodine swabs
  c. Chlorohexidine gluconate swabs (use for infants rather than iodine)
- Paper tape and adhesive strip (for use only with older children)
- Marking pen
- Biohazardous waste container

PREPARATION

1 Positively identify the infant.	**2** Prepare and organize equipment. A 23-gauge butterfly safety needle attached to a 3- to 5-mL syringe is preferred.
3 Perform hand hygiene and put on gloves.	

PROCEDURE

4 Select the hand that has easily visible veins. No tourniquet is necessary. Warm the site if the hand is cool. **Clinical Alert !** Be careful not to bend the infant's wrist too much or the vein may collapse.	**5** Encircle the infant's wrist with your middle and forefinger and use those fingers to apply pressure to distend the dorsal veins.[a] Your finger can then be used as a "finger tourniquet." Place your thumb against the infant's fingers to flex the infant's wrist downward as the dorsum of the hand is examined.
6 Lightly palpate the back of the infant's hand to select the best vein and determine its direction. **7** Once the optimal vein has been chosen, release the finger tourniquet to allow blood to recirculate. If a vein cannot be seen or felt, do not attempt the venipuncture.	**8** Disinfect the back of the infant's hand with the 70% alcohol swab. Allow the area to air dry. **9** Select the appropriate needle according to the size of the vein.

10 Reposition the infant's wrist, apply the finger tourniquet and flex the infant's hand as described above.

11 Hold the needle with the wings of the butterfly needle folded together. Angle the needle to less than 15 degrees to the skin, bevel up and parallel to the vein. Pierce the skin 3–5 mm distal to the vein and advance slowly and carefully until the vein is punctured.

12 As soon as blood appears in the tubing of the butterfly, stop advancing and let the wings of the needle unbend. The blood may flow slowly, because venous pressure is very low. If no blood appears, it may be necessary to reposition the needle gently.

13 Pull the syringe plunger gently to fill it with the amount of blood required.

14 Release the finger tourniquet intermittently to allow the vein to refill. If the blood flow slows or stops, gently rotating the needle without advancing it may reestablish the flow.

15 Release your fingers from the infant's wrist, quickly remove the needle, and apply pressure with a dry gauze sponge placed over the puncture site.

16 Maintain direct pressure for 3 to 5 minutes or until the bleeding stops.

17 Engage the safety device on the butterfly. Disconnect the blood-filled syringe from the butterfly assembly.

18 Connect the syringe to transfer blood into the vacuum tubes with a safety blood transfer device. Let the vacuum draw the blood into the tubes according to the proper "order of draw."

Clinical Alert !

Do not use adhesive strips on neonates, because their skin is fragile.

AFTER THE PROCEDURE

19 Discard the syringe, safety blood transfer device, and needle in the sharps container.

20 Comfort the infant and offer a sucrose nipple, if permitted.

21 Discard the remaining supplies, gloves, and gown, and wash your hands.

22 Properly label the filled tubes and transport according to specimen procedural requirements.

Geriatric Patients

The elderly, or geriatric, population comprises approximately 15% of the U.S. population and uses 31% of the nation's health care services (Figure 10-21 ■). In 25 years, the geriatric population will have reached 20% of the total U.S. population.[15] Physical conditions, such as arthritis, **Parkinson's disease** (a disease causing tremors), and other debilitating diseases in elderly persons will continue to increase point-of-care testing by skin puncture because of the difficulty of obtaining blood by venipuncture. In addition, this patient population will increasingly need point-of-care testing and other health care services in their homes, nursing homes, rehabilitation centers, and other long-term-care facilities (i.e., where the length of stay is over 30 days).

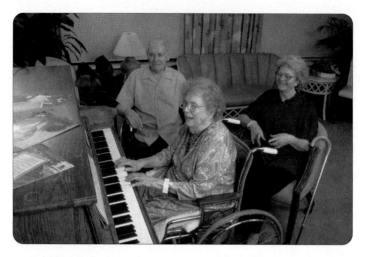

FIGURE ■ 10-21 Increasing Geriatric Population in the United States. The number of elderly citizens is rapidly increasing because of the advancing age of the Baby Boomer generation

The process of aging presents physical and emotional problems that can be challenging for health care workers. Whatever the case, treat elderly individuals with the utmost respect and dignity. Physical problems that are common in older individuals include the following:

■ Hearing loss may cause embarrassment and frustration. Repeating instructions or facing the patient to speak in the "good" ear may be necessary for the patient to truly understand a procedure.

■ Failing eyesight is common, so take care to guide the elderly individual to the appropriate seat for blood collection or to the bathroom for urine collections.

■ Loss of taste, smell, and feeling can accompany the aging process. Elderly people may lack an appetite, which may lead to malnourishment and dehydration. They may tend to drop things or not be able to make a fist because of muscle weakness. Make a note of these clues, particularly if the patient is homebound without a caregiver.

■ Memory loss can affect the patient's ability to take medications or to remember the last time he or she ate. These factors may interfere with the interpretation of laboratory results.

■ Skin tissue becomes thinner, thereby making venipuncture more difficult. Hold the skin extra taut so that the vein does not "roll." Also, do not "slap" the arm when trying to locate the vein. This causes bruising. Use of heated compresses can be helpful.

■ Muscles become smaller, so the angle of penetration of a venipuncture needle may need to be more shallow.

■ Increased susceptibility to accidental hypothermia (a subnormal drop in body temperature) can make the elderly patient feel cold. Thus, specimen collection may require warming of the site.

■ Increased sensitivities and allergies. Ask patients whether they have any allergies.

Emotional problems that are associated with aging include the possible loss of career, spouse, close friends, or relatives and can be reflected by depression or anger at life in general. Remember to address elderly persons with dignity and respect by using Mr., Mrs., Miss, and so on. Also respect the patient's privacy.

CONSIDERATIONS IN HOME CARE BLOOD COLLECTIONS

Because many elderly people have limited mobility and are unable to travel to a health care clinic, it is becoming increasingly common for health care workers to travel to homes to collect blood for diagnostic and treatment purposes. If specimens are to be collected in homes, all procedures are similar to those already covered except that health care workers should:

- Take extra supplies and equipment, including biohazard containers for disposables and a temperature-regulated specimen transport container, into the home.

- Positively identify the patient if possible. If not possible, develop and follow the procedures of the health care organization.

- Place the patient in a comfortable, preferably reclining, position in case of fainting.

- Carry a hand disinfectant with other supplies and equipment and use the disinfectant on your hands before collecting blood. Locate a bathroom for access to handwashing.

- Wait for the puncture site to stop bleeding, because many elderly patients take medications that prolong bleeding (i.e., coumadin and heparin).

- Carefully inspect the area after the procedure to ensure that all trash and used supplies have been properly discarded.

- Carefully label the specimens and place them in leakproof containers with the biohazard sign on the container. Check the appropriate temperatures for transport. Locate a bathroom for access to handwashing.

- When working in high-crime areas, take security precautions, travel with a mobile phone, and carry maps of the area to avoid getting lost on the way to or from the patient's home.

- Carefully document delays in returning specimens to the laboratory.

Chapter 8, Venipuncture Procedures, and Chapter 9, Procedures for Collecting Capillary Blood Specimens, also provide procedures that apply to the elderly patient. In these blood collections, factors to consider for older patients are the types of blood collection equipment to use. For example, using a safety butterfly needle is usually more appropriate for the elderly patient's fragile veins. Consider the physiological situation of each geriatric patient in the decision to obtain a quality blood specimen for laboratory tests.

Self Study

Study Questions

For the following questions, select the one best answer.

1. The preferred technique for preparing a child for blood collection is to:

   a. perform the blood collection when the child is asleep
   b. medicate the child for total sedation
   c. use mechanical restraint
   d. place the child in a vertical position as the parent holds him or her

2. Which of the following is an acceptable way to prepare the child for pain from venipuncture?

   a. inject pain medication in the arm that will have the venipuncture
   b. give the child oral sucrose
   c. EMLA application
   d. place an ice pack on the venipuncture site for 4 minutes before the needlestick

3. Which is the preferred site for a skin puncture for a newborn infant?

   a. dorsal side of the hand
   b. medial or lateral plantar surface of the heel
   c. central surface of the heel
   d. a previous puncture site that has healed

4. Which of the following supplies is needed to collect blood for capillary blood gases from a newborn infant?

   a. tourniquet
   b. lidocaine
   c. metal filing
   d. syringe

5. Which of the following is a debilitating disease causing tremors, particularly in elderly individuals?

   a. anemia
   b. Parkinson's disease
   c. arthritis
   d. depression

6. Which of the following supplies is needed to collect blood for a pediatric venipuncture?

   a. safety lancets
   b. plastic capillary tubes
   c. plastic capillary tube sealers
   d. safety winged infusion set

7. If a neonate or child is going to receive fluid intravenously, what veins should be avoided for blood collection?

   a. distal veins
   b. medial wrist veins
   c. scalp veins
   d. veins in the dorsum of the foot

8. If the incision made for blood collection is too deep in the infant's heel, this improper heelstick can lead to:

   a. Parkinson's disease
   b. osteochondritis
   c. genetic defects
   d. hemophilia

9. Venipuncture in an infant and/or toddler is recommended for which of the following blood tests?

   a. hematocrit
   b. blood cultures
   c. hemoglobin
   d. fasting glucose

10. For the dorsal hand vein procedure on an infant, the angle of the needle to the skin should be:

    a. 45 degrees
    b. 35 degrees
    c. 25 degrees
    d. 15 degrees

Case Study

Health care worker Maxine Berry must collect blood from a newborn infant, Baby James A. Russell. This infant is to have surgery in 2 days. The physician has requested laboratory testing for CBC, creatinine, and ABO group and Rh typing.

Question

In addition to the total blood collection process, including proper identification, what other record must be written down for possible future reference?

Self Assessment

Check Yourself

Ready to collect blood from a 5-year-old child

1. List the equipment that is needed on a blood collection tray to collect blood from a 5-year-old child.

2. After you have introduced yourself in a confident manner and then properly identified the patient (5-year-old child), describe the third through eighth steps to prepare the child and parent for a blood collection procedure.

Competency Checklist: Pediatrics and Geriatrics

This checklist can be completed as a group or individually.

(1) Completed   (2) Needs to improve

_____ 1. Lists blood collection equipment necessary for a capillary blood gas collection from a newborn infant.

_____ 2. Identifies four physical problems that are common in the elderly that can challenge blood collection efforts.

_____ 3. List three important considerations in blood collection from within an elderly patient's home.

References

1. London ML, Ladewig P, Ball J, Bindler R: *Maternal-Newborn and Child Nursing.* Upper Saddle River, NJ: Prentice Hall, 2002.

2. Clinical and Laboratory Standards Institute (CLSI): Procedures and Devices for the Collection of Diagnostic Capillary Blood Specimens, Approved Standard, document A4–A5. Wayne, PA:CLSI, 2004.

3. Markenson D: *Pediatric Prehospital Care.* Upper Saddle River, NJ: Prentice Hall, 2002.

4. Schechter N, et al.: *Reducing the Anxiety and Pain of Injections: A Guide for Managing the Pediatric Patient.* Franklin Lakes, NJ: Becton Dickinson, 1998.

5. Mitchell A, Waltman PA. Oral sucrose and pain relief for preterm infants. *Pain Manag Nurs* 2003;4(2):62–9.

6. Gradin M, et al.: Pain reduction at venipuncture in newborns: oral glucose compared with local anesthetic cream. *Pediatrics* 2002;110:1053–7.

7. Lindh V, Wiklund U, Blomquiat HK, Hakansson S: EMLA cream and oral glucose for immunization pain in 3-month-old infants. *Pain* 2003; 104(1–2):381–8.

8. Centers for Disease Control and Prevention: CDC guideline for hand hygiene in health-care hygiene in health-care settings. *MMWR Recomm Rep* 2002;RR-16:51.

9. Reiner CB, Meites S, Hayes JR: Optimal depths for skin puncture of infants and children as assessed from anatomical measurements. *Clin Chem* 1990;36(3):547–9.

10. Jain A, Rutter N: Ultrasound study of heel to calcaneum depth in neonates. *Arch Dis Child Fetal Neonatal Ed* 1999;80(3):F243–5.

11. Vertanen H, Fellman V, Brommels M, Viinikka L: An automatic incision device for obtaining blood samples from the heels of preterm infants causes less damage than a conventional manual lancet. *Arch Dis Child Fetal Neonatal Ed* 2001;84:F535.

12. Meites S, Hamlin CR, Hayes JR. A study of experimental lancets for blood collection to avoid bone infection of infants. *Clin Chem* 1992;38:908–10.

13. Johnston V: News and views: venipuncture better for newborns? *Lab Med* 1998;29(6):329.

14. Clagg ME: Venous sample collection from neonates using dorsal hand veins. *Lab Med* 1989;20(4):248–50.

15. Nixon RG: *BRADY Geriatric Prehospital Care.* Upper Saddle River, NJ: Prentice Hall, 2003.

Chapter 11

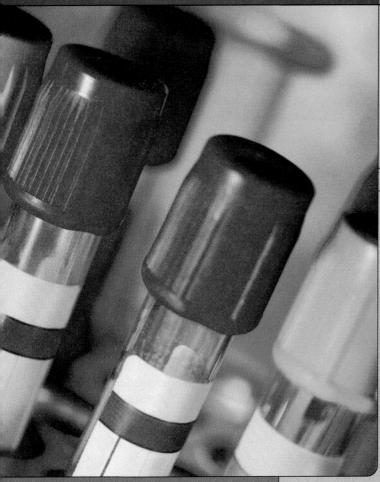

Special Collections

CHAPTER OBJECTIVES

Upon completion of Chapter 11, the learner should be able to do the following:

1. List the steps and equipment used in blood culture collections.

2. List two other terms that are synonymous with point-of-care testing.

3. Describe the most widely used applications of point-of-care testing.

4. Define quality assurance and its requirements as related to point-of-care testing.

5. Discuss the requirements for glucose testing and glucose tolerance tests.

6. Differentiate cannulas from fistulas.

7. Explain the special precautions and types of equipment needed to collect arterial blood gases.

8. List three types of urine specimen collections and differentiate the uses of the urine specimens obtained from these collections.

KEY TERMS

arterial blood gases (ABGs)

bacteremia

blood cultures

cannula

clean-catch midstream

creatinine clearance test

culture and sensitivity (C&S)

diabetes mellitus

fevers of unknown origin (FUO)

fistula

glucose tolerance test

patient-focused testing

point-of-care testing

Depending on the specific needs of individual clinical settings, health care workers may be required to perform a variety of special tests or procedures in addition to routine skin punctures and venipunctures. This chapter presents the basic techniques and precautions for various special tests and urine collections. Extensive educational skills training is required before performing these procedures because they can harm the patient if performed incorrectly.

Blood Cultures

Blood cultures are often collected from patients who have **fevers of unknown origin (FUO)**. Sometimes, during the course of a bacterial infection in one location of the body, **bacteremia** or **septicemia** (the presence of bacteria or toxins in the blood) may result and become the major clinical feature. Septicemia is a major cause of death in the United States.[1] Blood cultures aid in identifying the specific bacterial organism causing the infections.

Venipuncture is the method used for collecting blood specimens for blood cultures. However, there are important differences in a blood culture procedure that relate to the following:

- The health care worker must explain the procedure in greater detail to the patient.
- The puncture site must be decontaminated so it is sterile.
- The type of collection tubes contain media that enable bacteria to grow under laboratory conditions.

POSSIBLE INTERFERING FACTORS

- If blood culture collections are ordered with other laboratory tests, blood culture specimens must be collected first. If a vacuum blood collection tube is used before the blood culture vials or SPS evacuated tubes, the needle can become contaminated.
- When entering the needle into the venipuncture site, do not scrape the needle across the skin, because this can contaminate the needle and, thus, blood cultures.
- The anaerobic blood culture vial must be filled first in all procedures except the butterfly assembly method, because injection of air into the anaerobic bottle can cause the death of some anaerobic microorganisms and result in a false-negative culture.
- Some culture vials contain resin beads that neutralize antibiotics in the patient's blood specimen. If these vials are not gently mixed to neutralize the antibiotics in the blood, the antibiotics can inhibit bacterial growth and cause false-negative results.
- If two sets of blood cultures have been ordered, obtain the second set in the same manner as the first, performing a new venipuncture at a different site (i.e., the other arm).

After collecting the blood, remove the iodine from the patient's skin with an alcohol prep. The health care provider must initial the patient identification labels, indicate the time and date of collection on the labels, and attach a label to each vial or tube.

Disassembling or changing needles should *not* occur after collecting blood for culture, because it can lead to a needlestick injury to the health care worker. Careful skin cleansing has been shown to be the most important factor in minimizing the specimen contamination rate.

Site Preparation for Blood Culture Collection

RATIONALE

To obtain a sterile puncture site because bacteria normally located on the skin can contaminate a blood culture if it is not properly cleaned before the venipuncture.

EQUIPMENT

- Gloves (recommended sterile gloves for aseptic technique)
- 3 alcohol/acetone or alcohol preps
- 2 iodine-tincture scrub swab sticks or chlorohexidine gluconate swab sticks
- 2 blood culture vials (1 for anaerobic bacteria and 1 for aerobic bacteria)
- **Sodium polyanethole sulfonate (SPS)** evacuated tubes

- Safety needles (22- or 20-guage) or blood collection set
- Safety syringe or evacuated safety tube assembly
- Sterile gauze pads
- Nonlatex bandages
- Nonlatex tourniquet
- Patient identification labels
- Laboratory requisition slip and pen
- Biohazard waste container

PREPARATION

(1) Identify the patient properly. Briefly explain the test to the patient.

(2) Prepare and assemble supplies next to the patient.

(3) After donning gloves (nonlatex if the patient has a latex allergy), locate the vein, loosen the tourniquet, scrub the site of the venipuncture with 70% alcohol for 60 seconds to rid the site of excess dirt, then scrub with the iodine tincture (chlorohexidine gluconate for patients sensitive to iodine or for infants) for at least 30 seconds. Initially place the iodine swab at the site of needle insertion, and then move it outward in concentric circles to a diameter of approximately 4 inches, as shown in Figure 11-1 ■.

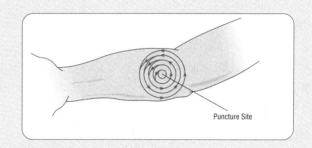

Puncture Site

FIGURE ■ 11-1 Arm Preparation for the Collection of Blood Culture Specimens

(4) Some health care facilities use a blood culture preparation kit that has a one-step application (e.g., ChloroPrep-Medi-Flex, Inc., Overland Park, KS). The application has chlorohexidine gluconate/isopropyl alcohol antiseptic combined for an effective 30-second cleansing of the venipuncture site (Figure 11-2 ■). Other blood culture preparation kits are also available commercially (Figure 11-3 ■).

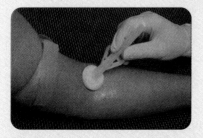

FIGURE ■ 11-2 One-Step 30-Second Application for Blood Culture Venipuncture Preparation

Medi-Flex Hospital Products, Inc., Overland Park, KS.

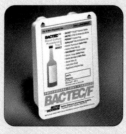

FIGURE ■ 11-3 BACTEC Blood Culture Procedural Tray

Courtesy of Becton Dickinson Microbiology Systems, Sparks, MD.

(5) Clean your gloved forefinger in the same manner.

Clinical Alert ❗

- For any of the blood collection procedures, the venipuncture site MUST NOT be repalpated after the venipuncture site is prepared for blood collection.
- Relocating the vein by repalpation after sterilization recontaminates the site.
- Make a mental note of the vein's location in relation to skin features such as a mole, crease, freckles, and so on.
- If you must repalpate, do not palpate at the actual venipuncture site.

AFTER THE PROCEDURE

(6) Collect the blood culture by syringe, vacuum tube, or safety butterfly assembly.

NOTES

- Research has shown that blood culture collection sites prepared using iodine tincture instead of iodophor (e.g., povidone) are superior in combating the contamination of sites where cultures are collected by "nonphlebotomy" personnel.[2]
- Do not go back over any area that has been prepped. Allow the area to dry for 1 minute in order for the antiseptic to be effective against skin bacteria.

- Removal of the entire metal ring on some manufacturers' bottles introduces air into the vials and can cause contamination.
- Read the maufacturer's directions about blood culture vials before using them, because they might vary in the size of blood sample needed and their preparation requirements. Place each bottle on a flat surface, and then use a marker to mark a "fill-to line."
- Treat the top of the blood culture vial as a sterile area, and take care not to contaminate it.

Procedure 11-2 — Syringe Blood Culture Collection

RATIONALE

Using a safety syringe, it is commonly recommended to do an adult collection of 20 mL and to transfer the first 10 mL to the anaerobic vial and then 10 mL to the aerobic vial.

EQUIPMENT

- Gloves (recommended sterile gloves for aseptic technique)
- 3 alcohol/acetone or alcohol preps
- 2 iodine-tincture scrub swab sticks or chlorohexidine gluconate swab sticks
- 2 blood culture vials (1 for anaerobic bacteria and 1 for aerobic bacteria)
- Safety needles (22- or 20-gauge) or blood collection set

- Safety syringe
- Sterile gauze pads
- Nonlatex bandages
- Nonlatex tourniquet
- Patient identification labels
- Laboratory requisition slip and pen
- Biohazard waste container

(continued)

PREPARATION

(1) Prepare and assemble supplies next to the patient.

(2) Identify the patient properly. Briefly explain the test to the patient.

PROCEDURE

(3) Wash or sanitize your hands with an alcohol hand rinse, then put on gloves (nonlatex if the patient has a latex allergy).

(4) Locate the vein, loosen the tourniquet, scrub the site of the venipuncture with 70% alcohol for 60 seconds to rid the site of excess dirt, and then scrub with the iodine tincture (chlorohexidine gluconate for patients sensitive to iodine or for infants) for at least 30 seconds. Initially place the iodine swab at the site of needle insertion and then move it outward in concentric circles to a diameter of approximately 4 inches.

(5) Clean your gloved forefinger in the same manner.

(6) After the collection of the blood into the syringe, activate the safety-needle cover and aseptically dispose of the needle into the sharps container without touching the needle.

(7) Then, place a blunt-tipped cannula (connector) on the syringe tip and attach the blunt-tipped connector to the direct-draw holder/adapter (Figure 11-4 ■).

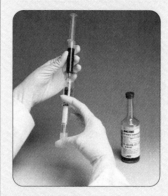

FIGURE ■ 11-4 *Courtesy of Becton Dickinson Microbiology Systems, Sparks, MD.*

(8) Starting with the vial labeled "anaerobic microbiology vial" in an upright position, place the blood-transfer device on the vial, fill to the desired amount and remove the syringe with the blood-transfer device from this vial. If anaerobic and aerobic microbiology vials are to be filled with the patient's blood, the aerobic vial is filled immediately after the anaerobic vial, and then other blood collection tubes are filled according to the "order of draw." NEVER push on the syringe plunger. Allow the vacuum in the microbiology vials to pull the blood into the vials.

(9) If the blood collector can only collect 3 mL or less, the entire amount should be placed in the aerobic vial.

(10) For infants and small children, only 1 to 5 mL of blood can usually be collected for bacterial culture. Use blood culture bottles that are designed specifically for the pediatric patient.[3]

AFTER THE PROCEDURE

(11) Discard the syringe, safety blood-transfer device, and needle in the sharps container with biohazard label. Label the specimens.

(12) Discard blood-soaked gauze sponges, grossly contaminated items, and gowns or gloves used in isolation rooms in biohazardous waste containers.

(13) Dispose of gowns and gloves that are not from isolation rooms in the regular trash.

(14) Wash or sanitize your hands.

(15) Deliver the sample immediately to the laboratory.

Safety Butterfly Assembly Blood Culture Collection

RATIONALE

To perform a blood culture collection using a safety butterfly.

EQUIPMENT

- Gloves (recommended sterile gloves for aseptic technique)
- 3 alcohol/acetone or alcohol preps
- 2 iodine-tincture scrub swab sticks or chlorohexidine gluconate swab sticks
- 2 blood culture vials (1 for anaerobic bacteria and 1 for aerobic bacteria)
- SPS evacuated tubes

- Safety needles (22- or 20-gauge) or blood collection set
- Evacuated safety tube assembly
- Sterile gauze pads
- Nonlatex bandages
- Nonlatex tourniquet
- Patient identification labels
- Laboratory requisition slip and pen
- Biohazard waste container

PREPARATION

1 Prepare and assemble supplies.

2 Identify the patient properly. Briefly explain the test to the patient.

3 Wash or sanitize your hands with an alcohol hand rinse, then put on gloves (nonlatex if the patient has a latex allergy).

PROCEDURE

4 Use a safety butterfly assembly (safety blood collection set) (Figure 6–13) for insertion of the butterfly needle into the venipuncture site after the appropriate skin preparation.

5 Place a strip of tape over the butterfly wings to keep the needle in place as the blood culture vials are filled with the blood.

6 Transfer the blood to the microbiology vials via a direct draw adapter that fits directly over the blood culture vial (Figure 11-5 ■).

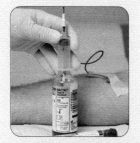

FIGURE ■ 11-5

Blood Culture Collection Using BACTEC Microbiology Vial with Blood Collection Safety Set

Courtesy of Becton Dickinson and Company, Sparks, MD.

7 Using this method, transfer the blood to the aerobic vial *first*, because the assembly tubing contains air.

Clinical Alert !

Never use the safety butterfly set without a direct draw adapter for transfer of the blood to the vials. If the needle is not covered up in this transfer of blood, the needle poses a risk of accidental needlestick as it is pushed into the microbiology vial.

Also, it is important to check with the manufacturers of blood collection safety-holder/ needle devices before attempting blood culture collections, because some of these devices do not accommodate the blood transfer to blood culture bottles. It is important to use a blood-transfer device that is compatible to the safety-holder/ needle device to avoid a needlestick injury.

(continued)

AFTER THE PROCEDURE

8 Discard the safety butterfly assembly and safety blood-transfer device in the sharps container with biohazard label.

9 Discard blood-soaked gauze sponges, grossly contaminated items, and gowns or gloves used in isolation rooms in biohazardous waste containers.

10 Dispose of gowns and gloves that are not from isolation rooms in the regular trash.

11 Wash or sanitize your hands.

12 Deliver the sample immediately to the laboratory.

Glucose Tolerance Test (GTT)

For patients who have symptoms suggesting problems in carbohydrate (i.e., sugar) metabolism, such as **diabetes mellitus**, the **glucose tolerance test** can be an effective diagnostic tool. When a glucose tolerance test is to be performed, the patient should be given complete instructions about the procedure so that his or her cooperation can be ensured (Box 11-1).

For best results, the patient should:

1. Eat normal, balanced meals for at least 3 days before the test
2. Fast for 8–12 hours before the beginning of the test
3. Drink water
4. **Do not** drink unsweetened tea, coffee, or any other beverage during fasting or during the procedure
5. **Do not** smoke, chew tobacco, or chew gum (including sugarless gum) during the fasting time or during the procedure. (NOTE: If a patient is chewing gum before or during this procedure, note this on the requisition form, because chewing gum may interfere with the test results.)

The test is performed by first obtaining a fasting blood specimen. The fasting blood specimen should be taken to the laboratory for test results. Then the patient can be given a standard load of glucose (e.g., a liquid drink called Glucola), and subsequent blood and urine samples can be obtained at intervals, usually during a 2- to 3-hour period. If the fasting specimen is abnormal, the physician must be notified before giving the load of glucose. Each specimen is then analyzed for its glucose content. In general, glucose levels should return to normal within 2 hours after ingestion of the glucose. During the test, the patient drinks a standard dose of glucose: 75 grams for adults or approximately 1 gram per kilogram of body weight for children and small adults. A dose of 50 or 75 grams is recommended for the diagnosis of gestational diabetes.[4] Gestational diabetes occurs during pregnancy, usually during the second or third trimester (See Postprandial Glucose Test). Commercial preparations of glucose are available as flavored drinks to make the glucose more palatable. The patient must start and finish the drink within 5 minutes. Water intake is encouraged throughout the procedure. If the patient should vomit at any

BOX 11-1 | **Sample Patient Information Card**

PATIENT INFORMATION CARD: GLUCOSE TOLERANCE TEST

INTRODUCTION

A glucose tolerance test (GTT) has been ordered by your physician. The purpose of a GTT is to test the efficiency of your body's insulin-releasing mechanism and glucose-disposing system.

You must prepare your body for the GTT by changing your eating and medication routines slightly for 3 days before the test. It is very important that you follow the instructions below in order for accurate results to be obtained.

Basically, you will need to follow these three guidelines to prepare for your GTT test:

1. Your carbohydrate intake must be at least 150 g per day for 3 days before the GTT.
2. Do not eat anything for 8 hours before the GTT, but do not fast for more than 12 hours before the test.
3. Do not exercise for 12 hours before the GTT.

PREPARATION: MEDICATION

Before proceeding with the GTT, you must tell your physician whether you are currently using any of the following medications, because they may interfere with test results:

- Alcohol
- Anticonvulsants (seizure medication)
- Blood-pressure medication
- Clofibrate
- Corticosteroids
- Diuretics (fluid pills)
- Estrogens (birth control pills or estrogen replacement pills)
- Salicylates (aspirin, pain killers)—only if taken in high doses, such as for rheumatoid arthritis

PREPARATION: DIET AND EXERCISE

Remember that for 3 days before your test, your diet must contain at least 150 g of carbohydrates per day. The following is a list of high-carbohydrate foods:

- **Milk and milk products**—12 g of carbohydrates per serving. One serving is equal to 8 oz. of milk (whole, skim, or buttermilk), 4 oz. of evaporated milk, or 1 cup of plain yogurt.
- **Vegetables**—5 g of carbohydrates per serving. One serving is equal to 1/2 cup of any vegetable, excluding starches (e.g., potatoes, corn, or peas).
- **Fruits and fruit juices**—10 g of carbohydrates per serving. One serving is equal to 1/2 cup of juice, 1 small piece of fresh fruit, or 1/2 cup of unsweetened canned fruit, with the following exceptions:

Apple juice	1/3 cup
Grape juice	1/4 cup
Raisins	2 Tbsp.
Watermelon	1 cup
Prunes	2 medium
Banana	1/2 small
Dates	2

(continued)

Sample Patient Information Card *(continued)*

Cantaloupe	1/4 6-inch melon
Honeydew melon	1/8 7-inch melon

- **Breads and starches**—15 g of carbohydrates per serving. One serving is equal to 1 slice of bread or 1 small roll. Other one-serving sizes are:

Bagel/English muffin	1/2
Tortilla	1
Cooked cereal	1/2 cup
Dry cereal	3/4 cup
Cooked rice, noodles, and pasta	1/2 cup
White potatoes, dried beans, and peas	1/2 cup
Yams	1/4 cup
Corn	1/3 cup
Crackers	5–6

- **Meats, cheeses, and fats**—These foods contain few or no carbohydrates.
- **Miscellaneous**

Ice cream	1/2 cup	15 g of carbohydrates
Sherbet	1/2 cup	30 g of carbohydrates
Gelatin	1/2 cup	30 g of carbohydrates
Jams and jellies	1 Tbsp.	15 g of carbohydrates
Sugar	1 tsp.	4 g of carbohydrates
Carbonated beverage	6 oz.	20 g of carbohydrates
Hard candy	2 pieces	10 g of carbohydrates
Fruit pie	1/6 pie	60 g of carbohydrates
Cream pie	1/6 pie	50 g of carbohydrates
Plain cake	1/10 cake	30 g of carbohydrates
Frosted cake	1/10 cake	38 g of carbohydrates

PREPARATION: GENERAL HEALTH

The following physical conditions should be reported to your doctor because they too may affect the results of your test:

Acute pancreatitis

Adrenal insufficiency

Diabetes mellitus

Hyperinsulinemia (excess insulin secretion, resulting in hypoglycemia)

Hyperthyroidism

Hypopituitarism (decreased function of pituitary gland)

Pregnancy

Stress

If you have any difficulty making the necessary alterations in your diet or medication schedule, please inform your doctor. For accurate test results, the instructions on this card must be followed.

Courtesy of Division of Laboratory Medicine, University of Texas M. D. Anderson Cancer Center, Houston, TX.

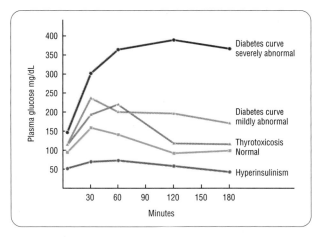

FIGURE ▦11-6 Graph of Glucose Tolerance Test Results

point in the procedure, the physician should be notified immediately to decide whether the test should be continued or stopped.[5]

When the patient finishes drinking the solution, the time is noted, and 30-, 60-, 120-, and 180-minute blood specimens are obtained.

Examples of timed blood collections for GTT are as follows:

- Fasting specimen obtained and sent to the laboratory (lab result, okay to proceed with GTT)
- Glucose load given (i.e., Glucola) at 7:00 A.M.
- 1/2-hour specimen at 7:30 A.M.
- 1-hour specimen at 8:00 A.M.
- 2-hour specimen at 9:00 A.M.

The tubes should be labeled with the time (Figure 11-6 ▦) as well as "30 minutes," "1st hour," and so on. Upon collection, each specimen should be sent to the laboratory for immediate testing. Venous blood is the preferred specimen for glucose tolerance tests, because normal glucose values are determined using venous blood. If serum samples are collected, the serum separator tube should be used. The grey-topped tubes have a preservative and can also be used for this procedure.

POSSIBLE INTERFERING FACTOR

The health care worker must be prepared to handle a situation when the patient becomes ill from drinking the glucose. Nausea and vomiting may occur early during the GTT, and it is a good idea to have towels and a basin nearby. If the patient vomits within the first 30 minutes, the test should be discontinued and will probably need to be rescheduled for another day. If the patient vomits or becomes faint later in the test, have him or her lie down and complete the testing. You do not want the patient in a position (i.e., sitting in a regular chair) where he or she may faint and fall and be injured.

Postprandial Glucose Test

The 2-hour **postprandial** (after a meal) **glucose test** can be used to screen patients for diabetes, (including gestational diabetes), because glucose levels in serum specimens collected 2 hours after a meal are rarely elevated in normal patients. In contrast, diabetic patients usually have increased values 2 hours after a meal.

For this test, the patient should be placed on a high-carbohydrate diet for 2 to 3 days before the test. The day of the test, the patient should eat a breakfast of orange juice, cereal with sugar, toast, and milk to provide an approximate equivalent of 100 g of glucose. A blood specimen is taken 2 hours after the patient finishes eating breakfast. The glucose level of this specimen is then determined, and the physician can decide whether further carbohydrate metabolism tests (such as a GTT) are needed.

Glucose Monitoring

With the increasing health care requirements of the growing U.S. elderly population, nurses, laboratorians, and other health care providers will increasingly perform on-site laboratory testing to obtain various types of laboratory test results. The demand for **point-of-care testing** is increasing because rapid turnaround of laboratory test results is necessary for prompt medical decision making.

The other terms used for these direct laboratory services include:

- Decentralized laboratory testing
- On-site testing
- Bedside testing
- Near-patient testing
- **Patient-focused testing**

During the past decade, small glucose-monitoring instruments, such as the one shown in Figure 11-7 ■ and described in Table 11-1 ■, became commonplace in the home, in the nursing home, and at the hospital bedside.[7] These "rapid" methods (Figure 11-8) require whole blood samples collected by skin puncture from the finger, heel (for infants), or a flushed heparin line. As for any blood collection procedure, appropriate safety protocols must be followed (e.g., wearing gloves), and disposal of potentially contaminated waste must be part of the quality control and safety guidelines (see Chapter 4). These bedside procedures are handy for quick screening in a hospital or outpatient setting.

To perform the blood glucose determinations, health care providers need to gather the appropriate supplies (Procedure 11–4) and must be aware of the total quality assurance procedures that are required to obtain accurate and precise results.[8,9] The timing of the reaction is critical, and most of these instruments call the time to the attention of the

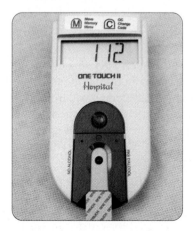

FIGURE ■ **11-7** Blood Glucose Monitor. Many types of glucose meters are available today

Instrument (Manufacturer)	Features	Test Time	Volume	TABLE ■ 11-1
Accu-Chek Active (Roche Diagnostics Corp.)	Photo-reflectance assay; 200 tests	5 seconds	1 μL	**Blood Glucose Monitors**
Medisense Soft-Tact (Abbott Laboratories)	Electrochemical assay; 450 tests	20 seconds	3 μL	
Ascensia Glucometer DEX2 (Bayer Diagnostics)	Electrochemical assay; 100 tests	30 seconds	3–4 μL	
One Touch Ultra (Life Scan)	Electrochemical assay; 150 tests	5 seconds	1 μL	
FreeStyle (TheraSense)	Electrochemical assay; 250 tests	15 seconds	0.3 μL	

operator by buzzing, sounding an alarm, or digitally displaying the glucose result. Also, the health care provider needs to know what type of blood—blood from a fingerstick and/or blood from venipuncture—can be used to perform glucose determinations with the point-of-care instrument and the patient age group for whom the blood instrument can be used.

As an example, the HemoCue β-Glucose Analyzer (Figure 11-8 ■) is an instrument that can obtain test results from capillary, venous, or arterial whole blood. It uses a microcuvette rather than a test strip and does not require blotting. Also, it can be used to monitor blood glucose in neonates as well as adults and children.

QUALITY IN POINT-OF-CARE TESTING (POCT)

Some glucose-monitoring instruments should be calibrated with glucose standards (calibrators). The glucose values must be monitored daily with **quality control material** and whenever a battery is changed or the meter is cleaned. This control material should be similar to the patient's specimen in order to determine whether the analytic system is working properly. For example, the glucose control material should be based on the use of whole blood, because this type of body fluid is used for measurements with point-of-care glucose-monitoring instruments.

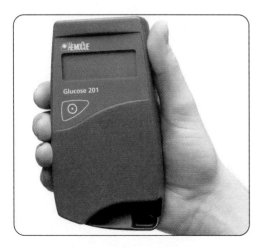

FIGURE ■ **11-8** HemoCue β-Glucose Analyzer

Courtesy of HemoCue, Inc., Lake Forest, CA.

Obtaining Blood Specimen for Glucose Testing (Skin Puncture)

RATIONALE

One of the most widely used applications of point-of-care testing is blood glucose monitoring, in which commercially available instruments, such as the one shown in this procedure, are used to determine blood glucose levels. Such determinations allow the physician to choose appropriate treatment regimens for patients with diabetes mellitus.[6]

EQUIPMENT

- Gloves (recommended sterile gloves for aseptic technique)
- Safety automatic lancet
- Antiseptic
- 3 alcohol/acetone or alcohol preps
- Sterile gauze pads
- Hemocue® blood glucose monitor

PREPARATION

1 Gather equipment: safety automatic lancet.	**2** Identify the patient properly. Briefly explain the test to the patient.
3 Clean your hands.	**4** Don gloves.

PROCEDURE

5 Select the site and cleanse with antiseptic (especially the side of a finger) (Figure 11-9A ■).	**6** Cleanse skin with alcohol wipe (Figure 11-9B ■) and allow skin to dry.
7 Gently massage the finger five or six times from base to tip to aid blood flow (Figure 11-9C ■).	**8** Decide which side of the finger to make the incision (Figure 11-9D ■).
9 Remove the safety lancet from the protective paper without touching the tip and, as you hold the patient's finger firmly with one hand, make a swift, deep puncture with the retractable safety puncture device (Figure 11-9E ■).	**10** Wipe the first three drops of blood away with clean gauze (Figure 11-9F ■).
11 Gently massage the finger from base to tip to obtain the needed drop of blood. Do not squeeze the fingertip, because this can cause hemolysis of the blood sample (Figure 11-9G ■).	**12** Apply the Hemocue® microcuvette to the drop of blood. The correct volume is drawn into the cuvette by capillary action (capillary, venous, or arterial blood can be used) (Figure 11-9H ■).
13 Wipe off any excess blood from the sides of the cuvette (Figure 11-9I ■).	**14** Place the microcuvette into the cuvette holder and insert it into the photometer (Figure 11-9J ■).

The laboratory test result is displayed automatically (Figure 11-9K ■).

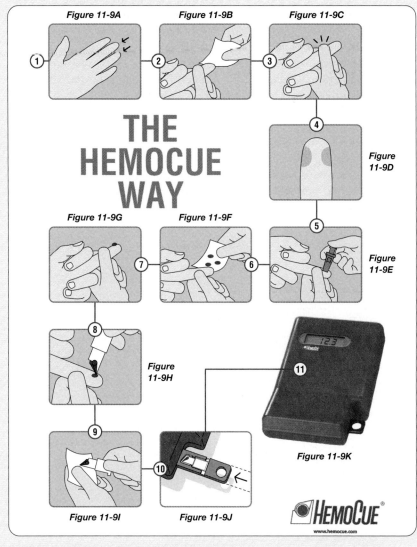

FIGURE ■ 11-9

Courtesy of HemoCue, Inc., Lake Forest, CA.

AFTER THE PROCEDURE

16 Discard the safety automatic lancet in the sharps container with biohazard label.

17 Discard the gauze, alcohol wipes, and gloves in biohazardous waste containers.

18 Wash or sanitize your hands.

In addition, some instruments have automatic control, or "electronic quality control" (EQC). The purpose of EQC is to test the electronics: the internal and analyte circuits of the instrument. Both the liquid and electronic QC should be performed.

For each day the glucose assay or other point-of-care test is performed on patients' blood specimens, control material should be analyzed so that the mean and standard deviation can be calculated. The calculations usually occur on 20 to 30 control values.[10] The control value obtained each day is plotted on a chart under the appropriate date, and the daily plots are joined with a straight line (Figure 11-10 ■). Interpretation of this chart is based on the fact that, for a normal distribution, 95% of the values about the mean, or average ($\bar{x}$), should be within plus or minus 2 standard deviations (SD) of the mean (average), and the fact that, for a normal distribution, 99% of the values are within plus or minus 3 SD of the mean. Tolerance limits are determined by pooling the data obtained during a 30-day test period and referring to the mean plus or minus 2 SD. If a daily control value exceeds the tolerance limits, corrective action must occur according to the manufacturer's directions and be documented for future reference.

Another quality control measure that can be taken when point-of-care monitoring instruments are used is purchasing the reagent strips and controls in quantities that enable health care workers to use constant pools of the same lot number. This leads to reproducibility of the results. Required preventive maintenance of each point-of-care instrument is critical for accurate results.

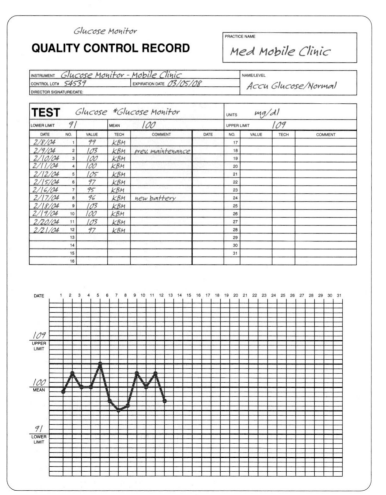

FIGURE ■ **11-10** Quality Control Record.

Specimen is inappropriately stored.

Contamination of the blood with alcohol. (After alcohol is used to cleanse the skin puncture site, the skin must dry completely before the site is punctured.)

Wrong volume of specimen is collected.

Instrument blotting/wiping technique is not performed according to manufacturer's directions.

Instrument is not clean.

Reagents are outdated.

Timing of the analytic procedure is incorrect.

Reagents are not stored at the proper temperature, leading to deterioration.

Patient has not dieted properly for the procedure.

Patient's result, time, date, or other information is mislabeled.

Recording of the result is incorrect.

Battery for the instrument is weak or dead.

Calibrators and/or controls are not properly used and/or recorded.

Results are not sent to appropriate individuals in timely manner.

Air bubbles in cuvette cause falsely abnormal low results.

Some point-of-care testing instruments can store and download calibrators, controls, and patients' results and can, thus, provide a complete instrument log for quality assurance interpretation. Table 11-2 ■ provides a list that will help lead to quality results through avoidance of these problems.

Blood Coagulation Monitoring

Similar to glucose monitoring, monitoring blood coagulation through point-of-care testing provides immediate results that can be used in monitoring bleeding or clotting disorders in patients. A blood coagulation instrument, such as the CoaguChek System from Roche Diagnostics Corp., is a handheld instrument that can measure prothrombin time (PT) from an unmeasured drop of whole blood, providing results in 2 minutes (Figure 11-11 ■).

The CoaguChek System can be used by home health care providers or other outpatient clinic providers to monitor long-term anticoagulation therapy in patients. The immediate test results allow rapid dose adjustments. Again, the health care provider using these instruments must be trained appropriately in the preventive maintenance and quality control parameters to obtain accurate results. Also, reading the manufacturer's directions is essential. For example, the CoaguChek System is calibrated to use the first drop of blood in skin puncture. The ProTime device by International Technidyne Corp. measures PT using one or two drops from a finger stick. The blood is collected directly into the disposable cuvette.

Other point-of-care coagulation systems are the Actalyke Activated Clotting Time Test (ACT) System (Figure 11-12 ■), the Hemochron Jr. Instrument, the Rapidpoint Coag analyzer, and the INRatio Meter (Figure 11-13 ■). These instruments are designed for use at the patient's point of care (i.e., home, intensive care unit, and physician's office) to monitor anticoagulation therapy such as heparin or warfarin sodium (Coumadin).

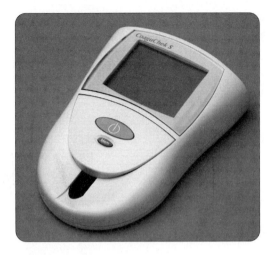

FIGURE ■ 11-11 CoaguChek System

Courtesy of Roche Diagnostics Corp. Indianapolis, IN.

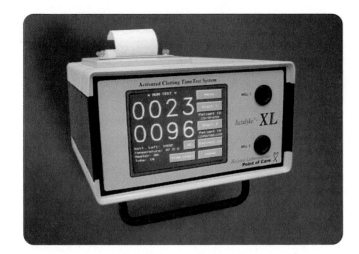

FIGURE ■ 11-12 Actalyke Activated Clotting Time Test (ACT) System

Courtesy of Helena Laboratories Point of Care, Beaumont, TX.

Hematocrit, Hemoglobin, and Other Hematology Parameters

The hematocrit (Hct, packed cell volume [PCV], or Crit) represents the volume of circulating blood that is occupied by red blood cells (RBCs). It is expressed as a percentage; thus, a hematocrit value of 38% indicates that 38 mL of each 100 mL of peripheral blood is composed of RBCs. Hematocrit values are obtained to aid in the diagnosis and evaluation of anemia, a less-than-normal number of erythrocytes. Blood collection usually occurs by skin puncture, as described in Chapter 9. For accurate test results, remember not to squeeze the tissue to obtain capillary blood, because doing so will dilute the sample with tissue fluid. It is very important to follow the healthcare facility's procedures. Plastic microcapillary tubes must be used to avoid the possibility of bloodborne pathogen exposure from a broken tube.

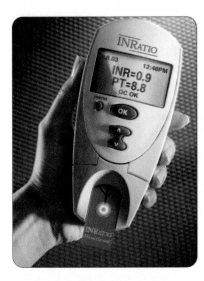

FIGURE ■ 11-13 INRatio Meter

Courtesy of HemoSense, Milpitas, CA.

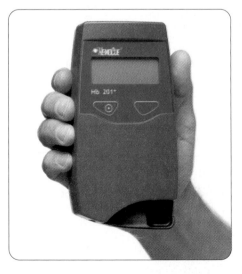

FIGURE ■ 11-14 HemoCue β-Hemoglobin Analyzer

Courtesy of HemoCue, Inc., Lake Forest, CA.

Determining a patient's hemoglobin level is another test to aid in the diagnosis and evaluation of anemia and other blood abnormalities. The hemoglobin test has been determined by the American Medical Association (AMA) to be more accurate than the hematocrit test in diagnosis and treatment. Also, the hemoglobin procedure is a safer method for the detection of anemia. A point-of-care analyzer that can be used to measure hemoglobin is the HemoCue β-Hemoglobin System (Figure 11-14 ■). A patient's venous, capillary, or arterial whole blood sample placed in the microcuvette and inserted into this instrument provides the patient's hemoglobin value.

Cannulas and Fistulas

A **cannula** is a tubular instrument that is used in patients with kidney disease to gain access to venous blood for dialysis or blood collection. Blood should be collected from the cannula of these patients only by specially trained personnel, because the procedure requires special techniques and experience.

A **fistula** is an artificial shunt in which the vein and artery have been fused through surgery. It is a permanent connection tube located in the arm of the patients undergoing kidney dialysis. Only specialized personnel can collect blood from a fistula. The health care worker should use extreme caution when collecting a blood specimen from these patients and avoid using the arm with the fistula as the site for venipuncture. If no other location can be found for the venipuncture site, the patient's arm must be cleaned thoroughly before blood collection. If the venipuncture site in this arm becomes infected, the inflammation in the blood vessels of the arm may shut down all the veins, requiring surgery to place a new shunt in the patient.

Donor Room Collections

Properly trained health care providers may be employed in a regional blood center or a hospital blood donor center to screen and collect blood from donors. This section summarizes the procedure outlined by the American Association of Blood Banks (AABB).[11] Only an experienced, properly trained health care worker or technologist should be considered for this function, because a physical, emotional, or traumatic experience may keep a donor from volunteering in the future.

DONOR INTERVIEW AND SELECTION

Not everyone who wants to donate blood is eligible, so the interviewer must determine the eligibility of each potential donor. Carefully determining donor eligibility not only helps prevent the spread of disease to blood product recipients but also prevents untoward effects on the potential donor. During this eligibility process, the health care worker needs to be in a private area for obtaining confidential donor information, and the questioning should occur in a very pleasant manner for the donor wanting to donate his or her blood.

The following confidential information on every donor should be kept on file indefinitely and is initially obtained from every prospective donor, regardless of the acceptability of his or her donation:

1. Date and time of donation
2. Last name, first name, and middle initial
3. Address
4. Telephone number
5. Gender

6. Age and birth date (Donors should be at least 17 years of age; however, minors may be accepted if written consent is obtained in accordance with applicable state law. Elderly prospective donors may be accepted at the discretion of the blood bank physician.)

7. Written consent form signed by the donor (1) allowing the donor to defer from being a donor if he or she has risk factors for HIV, the causative agent of acquired immunodeficiency syndrome (AIDS), or (2) authorizing the blood bank to take and use his or her blood

8. A record of reasons for deferrals, if any

9. Social security number or driver's license number (May be used for additional identification but is not mandatory; these data are needed for information to be retrieved in some computerized data systems.)

10. Name of patient or group to be credited, if a credit system is used

11. Race (not mandatory, but this information can be useful in screening patients for a specific phenotype [chromosomal makeup])

12. Unique characteristics about a donor's blood (Donated blood that is negative for cytomegalovirus or that is Rh-negative group-O blood is used for neonatal [infant] patients.)

To help minimize the incidence of dizziness, fainting, or other reactions to blood loss, donors are encouraged to eat within 4 to 6 hours of donating blood. Eating a light snack just before the phlebotomy may help prevent these reactions, but a donor should not be required to eat if he or she does not want to do so.

Blood bank records must link each component of a donor unit (red blood cells [RBCs], white blood cells [WBCs], platelets, etc.) to its disposition. If the donation is a "replacement for credit" for a particular patient, the donor must supply the patient's name or the group name that is to be credited.

A brief physical examination is required to determine whether the donor is in generally good condition on the day when he or she is to donate blood. The physical examination is actually a few simple procedures that are performed by the health care worker:

1. Weight. Donors must weigh at least 110 lb (50 kg); if the weight is less, the volume of blood donated must be carefully monitored and care taken that not too much blood is collected. Also, the anticoagulant in the bag must be modified for the lesser donation. Most blood banks will not routinely accept donors who weigh less than 110 lb.

2. Temperature. The donor's oral temperature must not exceed 37.5°C (99.5°F). Lower than normal temperatures are usually of no significance in healthy individuals; however, they should be repeated to verify the lower temperature.

3. Pulse. The donor's pulse should be regular and strong, between 50 and 100 beats per minute. The pulse should be taken for at least 15 seconds.

4. Blood pressure. The systolic blood pressure should measure no higher than 180 mm Hg, and the diastolic blood pressure should be no higher than 100 mm Hg. People with blood pressure outside these limits should be deferred as donors and referred to their physicians for evaluation of a possible health problem.

5. Skin lesions. Both arms should be examined for signs of drug abuse, such as needle marks or sclerotic veins. The presence of mild skin disorders, such as a poison ivy rash, does not necessarily prohibit an individual from donating unless the lesions are in the antecubital area or the rash is particularly extensive. The skin at the site of the venipuncture must be free of lesions.

6. General appearance. If the donor looks ill, excessively nervous, or under the influence of alcohol or drugs, he or she should be deferred.

7. Hematocrit or hemoglobin values. The hematocrit value must be no less than 38% for donors. The hemoglobin value must be no less than 12.5 g/dL. A fingerstick is commonly used to draw blood for such determinations. The health care worker may either collect blood in a plastic hematocrit tube for centrifuging and reading, measure hemoglobin spectrophotometrically, or use the copper sulfate method, in which the hemoglobin is qualitatively determined. (For further details on the copper sulfate method, please refer to the AABB technical manual.)

8. An extensive medical history must be taken for all potential donors, regardless of the number of previous donations on record. Most blood bank donor rooms have a simple card listing all the questions to be asked and "yes" or "no" columns that are used to indicate the donor's responses. The health care provider should refer to the protocol of the donor room at the institution's blood bank or the AABB technical manual, which sets guidelines for donor screening and acceptance.

COLLECTION OF DONOR'S BLOOD

The health care worker in a donor room must operate under the supervision of a qualified, licensed physician. Blood should be collected by using aseptic technique; a sterile, closed system; and a single venipuncture. If a second venipuncture is needed, an entirely new, sterile donor set is necessary; the first is discarded according to the biohazard disposal requirements of the institution.

A donor should never be left alone either during or immediately after blood collection. The health care worker should be well versed in donor reactions, equipment safety precautions, first-aid techniques, and the location of first-aid equipment in case it is needed during the course of donation.

Sometimes a patient must have the intentional removal of blood for treatment of a disorder. When a patient is obviously ill, his or her physician or the medical director of the blood bank should be present during this therapeutic phlebotomy. Generally, the patient should be bled more slowly than a healthy donor, and the resting period should be lengthened.

The blood obtained through therapeutic bleeding may be used for homologous transfusion if the unit is deemed to be suitable by the director of the blood bank. If it is to be used, the recipient's physician must agree to use the blood from his or her patient, and a record of the agreement should be kept. The unit is then labeled and processed in the usual manner. The label must indicate that the blood is the result of a therapeutic bleed and must include the patient's diagnosis. If the unit is unsuitable for transfusion, the entire unit is disposed of in the usual manner for contaminated wastes.

COLLECTION OF RECIPIENT'S (PATIENT'S) BLOOD FOR TRANSFUSION

A new patient safety initiative referred to as "the red armband" has been implemented at Memorial Hermann Hospital in Houston and is affecting the health care worker's blood collection responsibilities. It is designed to increase awareness about the high-risk blood transfusion process and to build in safety measures to prevent patients from receiving the wrong blood. The "red armband rules" include:

- Red armband required on all potential transfusion recipients
- Patient must have a hospital identification armband
- Two patient identifiers must be used at all times
- Specimen must be labeled at bedside

- A third unique red armband identifier must be used at all times
- Red armband must not be removed.

Arterial Blood Gases

Arterial blood gases (ABGs) provide useful information about the respiratory status and the acid-base balance of patients with pulmonary (lung) disease or disorders. In addition, critically ill patients with other diseases, such as diabetes mellitus, benefit from ABG measurement, which is used to help manage their electrolyte and acid-base balance. Arterial blood is used rather than venous blood, because arterial blood has the same composition throughout the body tissues, whereas venous blood has various compositions relative to metabolic activities in body tissues.

Arterial puncture to obtain arterial blood for blood gas evaluation requires skill and knowledge about the technique. A health care provider must undergo extensive training on arterial punctures, including demonstration of the procedure, observation, and, under the supervision of a qualified instructor, several performances on patients.

RADIAL ARTERY PUNCTURE SITE

When an ABG analysis is ordered, the experienced health care worker should palpate the areas of the forearm where the artery is typically close to the surface. The radial artery, located on the thumb side of the wrist (Figure 11-15 ■) is the artery most frequently used for blood collection for ABG analysis.

Using your index and middle fingers, the pulses from the radial artery should be palpated about 1 inch above the wrist (see Figure 11-15). This artery has widespread collateral flow, which means that the hand area is supplied with blood from more than one artery. Arterial blood flows into the hand from both the radial and the ulnar arteries. In addition, the radial artery lies over ligaments and bones of the wrist and can be easily compressed to lessen the chance of a hematoma during the procedure. A drawback to using the radial artery is its small size.

BRACHIAL AND FEMORAL ARTERY PUNCTURE SITES

The brachial artery is an alternative site for blood collection for ABG analysis. The brachial artery is in the cubital fossa of the arm, as shown in Figure 11-16 ■.

> **Clinical Alert** !
>
> The pulse of the brachial artery may be felt at the fold of the elbow on the little finger side of the arm. Puncture of the vein is a possibility, because the brachial artery is close to the veins. The brachial artery lies close to the median nerve, which can be accidentally punctured.

FIGURE ■ 11-15 Locating the Radial Artery

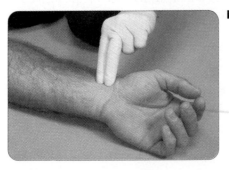

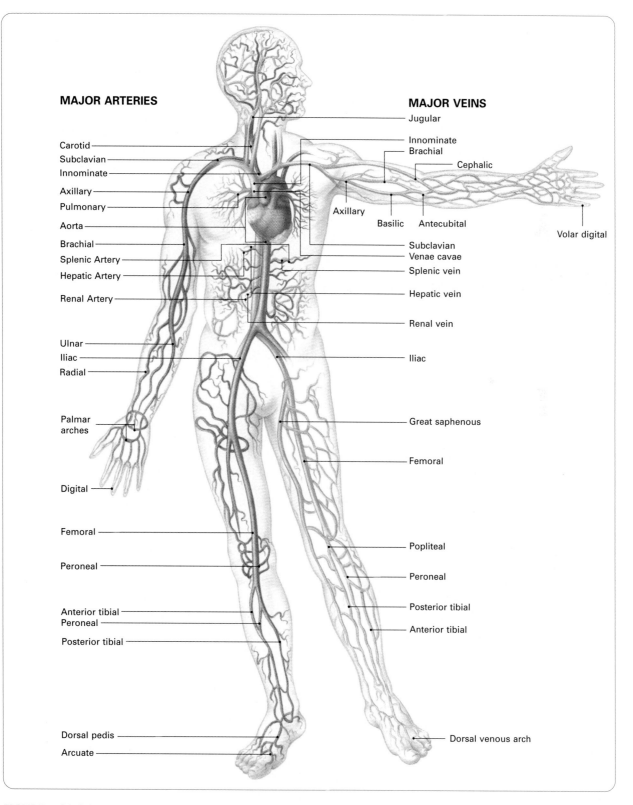

MAJOR ARTERIES

Carotid
Subclavian
Innominate
Axillary
Pulmonary
Aorta
Brachial
Splenic Artery
Hepatic Artery
Renal Artery
Ulnar
Iliac
Radial
Palmar arches
Digital
Femoral
Peroneal
Anterior tibial
Peroneal
Posterior tibial
Dorsal pedis
Arcuate

MAJOR VEINS

Jugular
Innominate
Brachial
Cephalic
Axillary
Basilic
Antecubital
Volar digital
Subclavian
Venae cavae
Splenic vein
Hepatic vein
Renal vein
Iliac
Great saphenous
Femoral
Popliteal
Peroneal
Posterior tibial
Anterior tibial
Dorsal venous arch

FIGURE ■ 11-16 Arteries in the Arm and Leg for Puncture Sites

Another choice, the femoral artery, is the largest artery used in ABG collections. It is located in the groin area of the leg, lateral to the femur bone, as shown in Figure 11-16. Even though the brachial and femoral arteries are larger than the radial artery, they are used less frequently because they lack collateral circulation. A 4-year study of blood collections from the brachial artery has demonstrated that brachial artery puncture is an acceptably safe procedure and a very reasonable alternative to radial artery puncture. The femoral artery is a site sometimes used on patients with cardiovascular disorders. The possibility of releasing plaque from the inner wall of the artery in geriatric patients, however, is a definite disadvantage of using the femoral artery as a puncture site. Usually, the femoral artery is the last choice for an arterial puncture site, and the health care provider must have expertise in obtaining blood from this artery.

Procedure 11-5 | Radial ABG Procedure

RATIONALE

To perform a blood collection for arterial blood gas analysis using the radial artery.

EQUIPMENT

- Tincture of iodine solution or chlorohexidine gluconate
- 0.5%–1% lidocaine to numb site
- Prefilled heparinized safety syringe, 1–5 mL (especially designed plastic syringe for collections for ABG analysis)
- Safety needles (20- to 22-gauge, for collections for ABG analysis)
- Needles (25- to 26-gauge, for lidocaine administration)
- Safety syringe for lidocaine administration (1- or 2-mL plastic syringe)
- Gauze squares to be held on site after puncture
- Plastic bag or cup with crushed ice and water

- Patient identification label
- Laboratory requisition slip
- Waterproof ink pen
- Alcohol pad
- Adhesive bandage strip
- Oxygen-measuring device to record on laboratory requisition slip the oxygen concentration on patient receiving oxygen
- Thermometer to record patient's temperature on laboratory requisition slip
- Mask
- Gloves (nonlatex if the patient has a latex allergy)
- Protective laboratory coat or smock
- Biohazardous waste containers for sharps

PREPARATION

1 Gather and organize the necessary equipment and supplies for a successful arterial puncture.	**2** Properly identify and inform the patient of the arterial puncture procedure.
3 Determine that the patient has been in a stable state for at least the previous 30 minutes (i.e., no respiratory changes).	**4** Attempt to calm the patient before collecting the specimen if the patient appears anxious. The anxiety can lead to hyperventilation, which will falsely alter the ABG levels.

5 Before proceeding, determine whether the patient is receiving anticoagulant therapy or is allergic to iodine or lidocaine, and record the patient's temperature, oxygen concentration from the respirator (if applicable), and respiratory rate.

PROCEDURE

6 Wash your hands, put on gloves, a facial mask, and a protective laboratory coat, and then palpate the radial artery in the forearm. The radial artery in the patient's nondominant hand is usually the best choice.

7 With the forefinger or first two fingers, press at these sites to find the artery (see Figure 11-15). Never use the thumb for palpating, because there is a pulse in the thumb that may be confused with the patient's pulse. Avoid any site that has a hematoma or that was previously used for an arterial puncture.

8 Position the patient's arm with the wrist slightly extended and rotated. Check for adequate collateral circulation using the modified Allen test. ▶

A CLOSER LOOK

▶ **Modified Allen Test**

RATIONALE

To use the radial artery for blood collection for ABG analysis, the health care provider must first perform the modified Allen test to make certain that the ulnar and radial arteries are providing collateral circulation (Figure 11-17 ■).[12]

FIGURE ■ 11-17

Modified Allen Test
A. Using the index and middle fingers, the health care worker compresses the patient's ulnar and radial arteries. The patient tightly clenches his or her fist. B. The patient opens their hand and the health care worker releases the pressure. C. If the patient's hand refills with blood (i.e., color returns) within 5 to 10 seconds, the test is positive; if not, the test is negative.

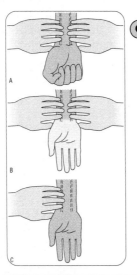

PROCEDURE

A Compress both arteries with your index and middle fingers, and ask the patient to tightly clench his or her fist.

B Ask the patient to open their hand, and release the pressure on the ulnar artery.

C The hand should fill with blood within 5 to 10 seconds; if so, the Allen test is positive. If color does not return to the hand after 5 to 10 seconds, the Allen test is negative. A negative Allen test indicates the inability of the ulnar artery to supply blood to the hand adequately and shows a lack of collateral circulation. Thus, the radial artery should *not be used* in a negative Allen test, because this artery might be accidentally damaged during puncture, resulting in a total lack of blood flow to the hand.

(continued)

9 Once the radial artery site is chosen, clean the area well with tincture of iodine.

10 If a local anesthetic is desired by the patient, fill a 1-mL syringe with lidocaine and inject the lidocaine with the 25- to 26-gauge needle subcutaneously around the anticipated puncture site.

11 No tourniquet is required, because the artery has its own strong blood pressure. Use a prefilled heparinized safety syringe (1–5 mL) with a needle to withdraw the sample.

12 Hold the syringe or collection device in one hand as one would hold a dart, pull the skin taut with a finger of the other hand over the artery and pierce the pulsating artery at a high angle, usually an angle of 30 to 45 degrees against the blood stream (Figure 11-18 ▪). Little or no suction is needed, because the blood pulsates and flows quickly into the syringe under its own pressure.

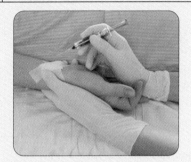

FIGURE ▪ 11-18 Completing Arterial Blood Gas Collection

Courtesy of Radiometer America, Inc.

13 When approximately 1 mL of blood is collected, withdraw the needle carefully to avoid introducing bubbles into the syringe and apply gauze and direct manual pressure on the site for at least 5 minutes.

14 Engage the safety syringe cover to cover the needle exposure, gently mix the blood in the syringe with the heparin, and label the syringe and immediately place it in ice water in an effort to prevent blood gases from escaping into the atmosphere.

15 Before leaving the patient, clean the puncture site with an alcohol pad to remove the excess iodine solution; leave a pressure bandage on.

16 If bleeding from the site persists, apply more manual pressure and ring for assistance from the patient's primary nurse. Never leave a patient who is bleeding, particularly after an arterial puncture.

AFTER THE PROCEDURE

17 Notify the primary nurse after an arterial puncture is performed so that the area may be checked frequently for deep or superficial bleeding.

18 Ideally, the specimen should be analyzed within 10 minutes of collection. Therefore, transport the specimen immediately to the laboratory.

19 Discard the syringe and needle in the sharps container with biohazard label.

20 Discard blood-soaked gauze, grossly contaminated items, and gowns or gloves used in isolation rooms in biohazardous waste containers.

21 Dispose of gowns and gloves that are not from isolation rooms in the regular trash.

22 Wash or sanitize your hands.

Arterial blood results for some analytes (e.g., ammonia, glucose, lactic acid, and alcohol) may differ from venous blood results because of metabolic activities. Therefore, arterial blood samples should be collected for the blood gas measurements only when specifically requested by the attending physician. In such situations, the request slip must indicate that arterial blood was collected for the analytes.

Urine Collections

In addition to collecting and transporting blood specimens, health care workers usually are involved in the collection and/or transportation of urine and other body-fluid specimens. The health care worker should be careful when transporting body fluids because they are difficult to obtain and because the quality of the clinical laboratory test result is only as good as the specimen that is collected and transported to the testing site. Also, because such specimens may be biohazardous, the health care worker must adhere to standard precautions (see Chapter 4, Safety and Infection Control) during the collection and transportation of these specimens. Just as for blood collections, the laboratory request slip must accompany the specimen, which must be properly labeled with the patient's name, the patient's identification number, the date, the time of collection, the type of specimen, and the attending physician's name. The label should be affixed on the container, NOT the lid, as shown in Figure 11-19 ■.

If different patients' urine specimens are in the same location for testing and the labeled lids are taken off the unlabeled containers for testing each urine specimen, it is highly likely that mismatching of the tests' results to the patients will occur.

Routine urinalysis (UA) is one of the most frequently requested laboratory procedures, because it can provide a useful indication of body health. It can be performed on a "first morning" or "random" urine specimen. Some of the more common types of urine specimen collections and their uses are provided in Table 11-3 ■. The routine UA includes a physical, chemical, and sometimes microscopic analysis of the urine sample. The physical properties include the following: color, transparency vs. cloudiness, odor, and concentration as detected through a specific gravity measurement.

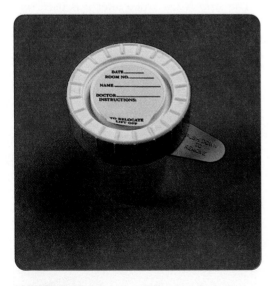

FIGURE ■ 11-19 Urine Collection Container. The label with necessary patient's information should be affixed to the container, NOT the lid

TABLE ■ 11-3

Types of Urine Specimen Collections and Their Uses

Specimen Type	Reason for Collection	Use
Random	This type of specimen is most convenient to obtain.	Routine UA Quantitative and qualitative
First urine of the morning	This urine excretion is the most concentrated.	Protein, nitrate, microscopic analysis Routine urinalysis (UA)
Fasting	Metabolic abnormalities are suspected	Glucose level determinations for diabetes mellitus testing
Clean-catch midstream	The specimen is free of contamination.	Culture for bacteria and/or microscopic analysis
Timed (e.g., 2 hour, 4 hour, or 24 hour)	The excretion rate of the analyte can be determined.	Creatinine clearance test, urobilinogen determinations, hormone studies
Tolerance test	Timed blood and urine specimens are obtained to detect metabolic abnormalities.	GTT and other tolerance tests

The chemical analysis for abnormal constituents is determined by using plastic reagent strips impregnated with color-reacting substances that test for the presence of glucose, protein, blood (red blood cells [RBCs] and hemoglobin), white blood cells (WBCs), ketones, bacteria, bilirubin, and other constituents (Figure 11-20 ■). The plastic reagent strip, which has a separate reagent pad for each chemical test, is dipped into the urine briefly (Figure 11-21 ■). The color of each reagent pad is compared to a color chart usually shown on the outer label of the reagent strip container. The results are reported according to the reagent label specifications (e.g., trace, 1+, 2+, and so on for a positive result or negative when no reaction occurs). The strip is discarded after it is used one time. As for all types of point-of-care testing, quality control monitoring must be used to ensure accurate results. Other tests that can be performed on urine specimens are the pregnancy, myoglobin, and porphyrin tests. Urine is also the specimen of choice for drug abuse testing.

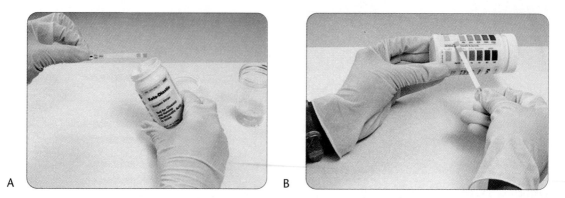

A   B

FIGURE ■ 11-20 Keto-Diastix Strip. A. The Keto-Diastix strip is used to check urine for ketone bodies. B. The Keto-Diastix strip is checked against the chart found on the bottle after dipping the strip in the urine

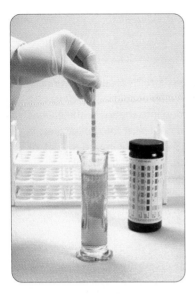

FIGURE ▪ 11-21 Dipping the Plastic Urinalysis Strip into the Urine for Chemical Analysis

SINGLE-SPECIMEN COLLECTION

The preferred urine specimen for most analyses is the first voided urine of the morning (Figure 11-22 ▪), when urine is the most concentrated. The urine collection containers must be clean and dry before the collection process. For routine UA procedures, appropriate containers include plastic disposable cups or bags (for infants) with a capacity of 50 mL. The containers must be properly labeled (label on container, not the lid), free of interfering chemicals, able to be tightly capped, and leak proof (Figure 11-23 ▪).

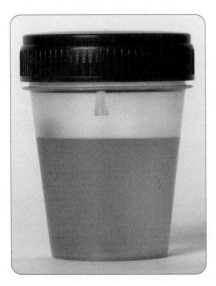

FIGURE ▪ 11-22 Single Specimen Collection. Urine is most concentrated in the morning

Source: Dorling Kindersley Media Library.

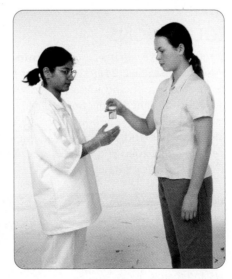

FIGURE ▪ 11-23 Patient's Labeled Urine Specimen Given to Health Care Worker

Source: Dorling Kindersley Media Library.

BOX 11-2 **Clean-Catch Midstream Urine Collection Instructions for Women**

1. After washing her hands, the woman should separate the skin folds around the urinary opening and clean this area with mild antiseptic soap and water or special towelettes.
2. Holding the skin folds apart with one hand and after urinating into the toilet, the patient should urinate into a sterile container. The container should not touch the genital area. It must be covered with the lid provided after urination. It is extremely important not to touch the inside or lip of the container with the hands or other parts of the body.
3. The health care worker or, sometimes, the patient will label the container with her name and the time of collection and deliver it to the requested location.
4. Health care personnel should refrigerate the urine specimen immediately.

The specimen should be transported to the UA section promptly for analysis within 30 minutes after the patient voids. If transportation or analysis cannot occur within this time period, the urine should be refrigerated.

Another type of single-specimen urine test is the urine **culture and sensitivity (C&S)** test. This specimen requires a clean-catch midstream urine collection. The patient is instructed to void approximately one half of the urine into the toilet, collect a portion in a readily available sterile container, and allow the rest to pass into the toilet.[13]

If asked, "What is a clean-catch urine specimen?" the procedure should be described, stating that this type of specimen is used to detect the presence or absence of infecting organisms. The specimen must be free of contaminating matter that may be present on the external genital areas. Thus, the steps in Box 11-2 should be explained to a female patient who is to obtain a clean-catch midstream urine specimen. For a male patient, the procedure in Box 11-3 should be adhered to for obtaining a clean-catch midstream urine specimen.

The urine specimen must be transported to the microbiology section promptly. If it cannot be taken to the area for microbiological culturing within 1 hour of collection, the specimen should be refrigerated to prevent an overgrowth of contaminate bacteria.

TIMED COLLECTIONS

For some laboratory assays, such as the **creatinine clearance test**, urobilinogen determinations, and hormone studies, 24-hour (or other timed period) urine specimens must be obtained. Incorrect collection and improper preservation of this type of specimen are two frequent errors affecting timed collections. Thus, the health care worker should be aware of the protocol for collecting a 24-hour urine specimen so that he or she can assist other health care professionals and the patient in preventing collection errors. The steps in Procedure 11-6 should be followed for a 24-hour urine collection.[14]

BOX 11-3 **Clean-Catch Midstream Urine Collection Instructions for Men**

1. The man should wash his hands and the end of his penis with soapy water or special towelettes and then let it dry.
2. After allowing some urine to pass into the toilet, the patient should collect the urine in the sterile container. The container should not touch the penis. Steps 3 and 4 are the same as those for a woman (Box 11-2).

Collecting a 24-Hour Urine Specimen

RATIONALE

To collect a 24-hour urine specimen for a creatinine clearance test, urobilinogen determinations or hormone studies.

EQUIPMENT

- Wide-mouthed, 3- to 4-liter container with lid
- Preservative, if required
- Label for specimen
- Requisition slip
- Container with ice, if required

Clinical Alert !

To obtain accurate test results, the laboratory needs the ENTIRE 24-hour urine specimen.

PREPARATION

1 Explain the whole procedure to the patient and also provide written directions. Provide instructions in the patient's native language. Explain the importance of handwashing for the urine collection.

2 Give the patient the container and lid. Add any required preservatives to the container before giving it to the patient. Write the preservative and any precautions on the collection container label. Place the label on the container, not on the lid. Include the following information on the label:

- Patient's name
- Patient's identification number
- Starting collection date and time
- Ending collection date and time
- Name of the requested laboratory test

Other information may be required by the facility.

PROCEDURE

3 Instruct the patient verbally and give them written instructions that the collection of the 24-hour urine specimen begins with emptying the bladder and discarding the first urine passed. This first step in the collection process should start between 6 and 8 A.M., and the exact time should be written on the container label.

4 Except for the first urine discarded, all urine should be collected during the next 24-hour period. Remind the patient to urinate at the end of the collection period and to include this urine in the 24-hour collection. Tell the patient to urinate before having a bowel movement, because fecal material in the urine specimen will make the specimen unacceptable for collection.

5 Instruct the patient to refrigerate the entire specimen after adding each collection during the 24-hour period.

6 Some preservatives for 24-hour urine collection are corrosive if accidentally spilled or if the patient comes into contact with them during collection. Thus, warn the patient of any preservatives in the container.

(continued)

Collecting a 24-Hour Urine Specimen *(continued)*

(7) Inform the patient not to add anything except urine to the container and not to discard any urine during the collection period.

(8) A normal intake of fluids during the collection period is desirable unless otherwise indicated by the physician.

(9) Some laboratory assays require special dietary restrictions; give these instructions to the patient.

(10) If possible, discontinue medications for 48 to 72 hours preceding the urine collection as a precaution against interference in the laboratory assays.

(11) Transport the 24-hour urine specimen to the clinical laboratory as soon as possible. Place the specimen in an insulated bag or a portable cooler to maintain their cool temperature.

Self Study

Study Questions

For the following questions, select the one best answer.

1. What is a fistula?

   a. the fusion of a vein and an artery
   b. a good source of arterial blood
   c. a tubular instrument used to gain access to venous blood
   d. an artificial shunt that provides access to arterial blood

2. What is the first step to obtain blood for glucose monitoring?

   a. choose and wash patient's fingertip
   b. use an alcohol pad to cleanse the skin on the fingertip
   c. check the patient's ID according to the health care facility's protocol
   d. squeeze the patient's finger to make a big first drop of blood for the monitor

3. Which of the following tests is measured through blood coagulation monitoring by point-of-care testing?

   a. glucose
   b. pO_2
   c. PTP
   d. pH

4. Which of the following supplies is not needed to test with the CoaguChek System?

   a. tourniquet
   b. safety lancet
   c. alcohol swab
   d. gloves

5. What is the reason for collecting a 24-hour urine specimen from a patient?

   a. to test for creatinine clearance
   b. to determine whether the patient can follow the collection instructions
   c. to test for the possibility of a hematoma
   d. to test for the hemoglobin level

6. Which of the following evacuated tubes is preferred for the collection of a blood culture specimen?

   a. yellow-topped evacuated tube
   b. green-topped evacuated tube
   c. light blue–topped evacuated tube
   d. red-topped evacuated tube

7. During a glucose tolerance test, which procedure is acceptable?

   a. a fasting blood collection is performed and then a standard amount of glucose drink is given to the patient
   b. the patient should be encouraged to drink tea, water, or coffee throughout the procedure
   c. the patient is allowed to chew sugarless gum
   d. all of the patient's specimens are timed from the fasting collection

8. The ABG analysis uses which of the following for the preferred blood collection site to obtain accurate results?

   a. heelstick
   b. femoral artery
   c. ulnar artery
   d. radial artery

9. When arterial blood is collected for an ABG determination, the needle should be inserted at an angle of no less than

   a. 15 degrees
   b. 30 degrees
   c. 45 degrees
   d. 65 degrees

10. If blood culture collection is requested on a patient that is allergic to iodine, what alternative cleansing solution should be used?

    a. chlorophenol
    b. chlorohexidine gluconate
    c. formaldehyde
    d. 1% phenol

Case Study

As a health care worker, you provide point-of-care testing for patients in the ambulatory care center. Today, Mrs. Hamilton came to the ambulatory care center and had a physician request slip for her PT to be tested. To provide the test, you collected the blood by fingerstick and applied the drop of whole blood from the patient's finger to the analyzer blood collection site for the instrument to provide the result. You waited the required number of minutes for the test result to appear on the instrument's screen, and the screen image printed out "Error in testing." Provide four possible problems that could have led to this error message.

Self Assessment

Check Yourself: Providing Proper Instructions to a Patient for a 24-Hour Urine Specimen Collection

1. Write out the instructions that you would give to a patient for a proper 24-hour urine specimen collection. Also, include the types of collection containers that are used by the health care facility for this type of collection.

2. Practice giving the instruction to a friend or coworker. Practice your communication techniques by double checking that they are completely understood; ask them to give a constructive critique of your instructions.

Competency Checklist: Special Collections

This checklist can be completed as a group or individually.

(1) Completed (2) Needs to improve

_____ 1. List the dietary instructions that should be given to a patient who is going to have a GTT performed in the next few days.

_____ 2. List five essential pieces of information that must be kept on file from a blood donor.

References

1. Ruge D, Sandin R, Siegelski S, Greene J, Johnson N: Reduction in blood culture contamination rates by establishment of policy for central intravenous catheters. *Lab Med* 2002;33(10):797–800.

2. Schifman R, Pindur A: The effect of skin disinfection material on reducing blood culture contamination. *Am J Clin Pathol* 1993;99:536–8.

3. Forbes B, Sahm D, Weissfeld A: *Bailey & Scott's Diagnostic Microbiology.* 11th ed. St. Louis, MO: Mosby Publishers, 2002.

4. American Diabetes Association: Gestational diabetes mellitus—position statement. *Diabetes Care* 2000;23(Suppl.1):1–6. http://journal.diabetes .org.

5. Report of the Expert Committee on the Diagnosis and Classification of Diabetes Mellitus. *Diabetes Care* 2000;23(Suppl. 1). http://journal.diabetes.org.

6. Clinical and Laboratory Standards Institute (CLSI): *Point-of-Care Blood Glucose Testing in Acute and Chronic Care Facilities.* Approved Guideline, 2nd ed. Wayne, PA: CLSI, 2002.

7. Clinical and Laboratory Standards Institute (CLSI): *Glucose Monitoring in Settings Without Laboratory Support.* Approved Guideline, 2nd ed. Wayne, PA: CLSI, 2005.

8. US Food and Drug Administration: *Center for Devices and Radiological Health, Current Lab Safety Tips.* http://www.fda.gov/cdrh/oivd/laboratory. html5/21/2003.

9. Jacobs E: Point-of-care (near-patient) testing, In *Clinical Chemistry: Theory, Analysis, Correlation,* edited by LA Kaplan, AJ Pesce, S Dazmierczak. St. Louis: Mosby Publishers, 2003.

10. Westgard J, Klee G: Quality management. In *Tietz Textbook of Clinical Chemistry and Molecular Diagnostics,* edited by C Burtis, E Ashwood, D Bruns. St Louis: Elsevier/Saunders Publishers, 2006.

11. Brecher M (ed): *Technical Manual of the AABB,* 15th ed. Bethesda, MD: AABB, 2005.

12. Clinical and Laboratory Standards Institute (CLSI). *Procedures for the Collection of Arterial Blood Specimens.* Approved Standard, 4th ed. Wayne, PA: CLSI, 2004.

13. Garza D: Urine collection and preservation. In *Textbook of Urinalysis and Body Fluids,* edited by DL Ross, AE Neely. New York: Appleton-Century-Crofts, 1983:61.

14. Clinical and Laboratory Standards Institute (CLSI). *Urinalysis and Collection, Transportation, and Preservation of Urine Specimens.* Approved Guideline, 2nd ed. Wayne, PA: CLSI, 2001.

Appendix Contents

Finding a Job

Finding a job that is a good fit for both the applicant and the employer is a time-consuming, often challenging process. However, the time and effort spent researching and applying for a position can have a wonderful payoff in terms of job satisfaction, salary, benefits, environment, and personal gratification. The keys to finding the right job are to spend time searching, be prepared with documentation and with questions during the interview, and keep an open mind. Here are some essential factors to think about. This list can be used as a checklist for your application process.

Places to Seek Employment	Newspaper, professional journals, and Internet
	Health care organizations
	Friends and relatives
	School faculty and advisors
	Bulletin boards
	Employment agencies
Contacting an Employer	Check employer's Web site
	Call for an appointment
	Send a cover letter (see example on page 260)
	Send a resume (see example on page 261)
	Complete a job application (provided by employer)
Cover Letter	Be neat and use correct spelling
	State where you heard about the job
	State the specific job for which you are applying
	State why you are qualified for this position
	Give a brief summary of your education, experience, and qualifications
	Refer to your resume
	Request an interview
	Give your name, address, and phone number
Resume	List name, address, phone number(s), and e-mail address
	Career plans (1 to 3 statements about your short-term and long-term career goals)
	Education (high school and beyond)
	Work experience (part-time or full-time, dates, duration of employment)

Volunteer activities (community service, religious activities, etc.)

Interests (sports, music, art, hobbies)

Special skills and abilities (computer skills with particular software, telephone expertise, use of special equipment, etc.)

Reference names and contact information (always ask permission of those you use as references before listing them)

Interview	Be well groomed and do not chew gum
	Dress neatly and professionally
	Be on time or a few minutes early
	Greet the interviewer with your name and a smile
	Shake hands firmly
	Stand until you are asked to sit
	Answer questions truthfully and sincerely
	Prepare a few questions about the job
	Avoid discussing personal problems
	Be enthusiastic and maintain eye contact
	Do not criticize former employers or teachers
	Thank the interviewer for his or her time and leave promptly

After the Interview	Send a thank-you letter to the interviewer

SAMPLE COVER LETTER FOR JOB INQUIRY

Jane Doe
8200 West Jersey Avenue
Lubbock, Texas 79452
511-799-9990
jdoe@nnn.com

July 20, 2007

Ms. A. D. Jones
Director, Laboratory Services
Muncy Hospital
P.O. Box 22333
San Antonio, Texas 78277

Dear Ms. Jones,
I am responding to an advertisement in the *San Antonio Press* on July 5, 2007, for an entry-level phlebotomy technician. I graduated from Lamar High School in 2004. Since then, I have worked part time and been a part-time student at Hilltop Community College. I recently completed a phlebotomy training program, and my goal is to utilize my skills while pursuing additional studies in laboratory sciences.

I have enclosed my resume, which includes a list of skills and experience. I feel that I am well qualified for this position because of my work with adults and children coupled with my organizational skills. I hope to arrange an interview as soon as is convenient for you. Please feel free to contact me at 511-799-9990 to schedule an interview or for additional information. Thank you.

Sincerely,
Jane Doe

SAMPLE RESUME

Jane Doe
8200 West Jersey Avenue
Lubbock, Texas 79452
511-799-9990
jdoe@nnn.com

Career Plans	To become an experienced phlebotomist while continuing my education in laboratory sciences
Experience	2004–present Community college phlebotomy student and part-time library assistant; responsibilities include clerical duties (filing, answering multiple telephone lines, word processing), greeting customers, and providing assistance in locating reference materials.
	2002–2004 Part-time caretaker for 3 children; responsibilities included carpooling, providing after-school snacks, assistance with homework, monitoring activities.
	2001–2002 Part-time employee at ABC Grocery; responsibilities included assisting customers in locating products, restocking groceries, checking out grocery items at cash register, assisting with inventory.
Education	2004 Graduated from Lamar High School
Skills/Strengths	Excellent verbal and written communication skills in both English and Spanish
	Computer skills include proficiency with both MAC and PC, word processing, Internet research, Excel, and PowerPoint
Interests	Reading, camping, art, church youth group, Girl Scouts
References	Available on request

Appendix 2

Units of Measurement and Symbols

The Joint Commission has updated the 2007 National Patient Safety Goals that includes a list of "do not use" abbreviations, acronyms, and symbols. This recommendation is to prevent confusion among caregivers when communicating test orders and results. In addition, the Institute for Safe Medication Practices (ISMP) has published a "List of Error-Prone Abbreviations, Symbols, and Dose Designations" with additional abbreviations to avoid. The aim is to eliminate misinterpretations of written information. Using both lists, selected recommendations of terms that may apply to phlebotomy practice have been incorporated into this appendix. However, this list is not exhaustive. For more comprehensive information, consult the organizations' Web sites: www.jointcommission.org and www.ismp.org respectively.

a	alpha	h	hecto- (10^2)
Å	angstrom	hpf	high-power field on microscope
amp	ampere (unit of electric current)	international unit	formerly written as IU, it should now be spelled out, *not* abbreviated
and	formerly written as symbol &, should now be spelled out		
at	formerly written as symbol @, should now be spelled out	k	kilo- (10^3)
		˚K	degrees Kelvin (thermodynamic temperature)
c	centi- (10^{-2})		
˚C	degrees centigrade or Celsius (unit of temperature)	kg	kilogram (1000 g, or 2.2 lb)
		l	liter (1000 ml, unit of volume)
cubic centimeter	(same as ml) formerly written as cc, it should now be spelled out, *not* abbreviated	less (greater) than	formerly written as symbols, should now be spelled out
		lpf	low-power field on microscope
cd	candela (unit of luminous intensity)	mcg	microgram (1/1000 mg)
		m	meter (unit of length)
cm	Centimeter	m	milli- (10^{-3})
cu mm	cubic millimeter	mCi	millicurie
d	deci- (10^{-1})	mEq or meq	milliequivalent
discharge	formerly written as D/C, it should now be spelled out, *not* abbreviated	mg	milligram (1/1000 g)
		mg%	milligrams in 100 ml (same as dl)
discontinue	formerly written as D/C, it should now be spelled out, *not* abbreviated	min	minutes
		mL	milliliter (1/1000 L, same as a cubic centimeter)
dl	deciliter (1/10 of a liter)		
˚F	degrees Fahrenheit (unit of temperature)	mm	millimeter (1/10 cm)
		mm³	cubic millimeter
g or gm	gram (1/1000 of a kilogram, unit of mass)	mm Hg	millimeters of mercury
		mmole	millimole
G%	grams in 100 mL	mol, M	mole (unit of substance)

mOsm	milliosmol	TPN	total parenteral nutrition
N	normality	TPR	temperature, pulse, respirations
n	nano- (10^{-9})	Unit	formerly written as U, it should now be spelled out, *not* abbreviated
ng	nanogram (1/1000 mg)		
p	pico- (10^{-12})		
pg	picogram (1/1000 ng)	WNL	within normal limits
QNS	quantity not sufficient	WNR	within normal range
sec or s	second (unit of time)	wt	weight
sp g	specific gravity	w/v	weight/volume

Clinical Alert !

Trailing Zeros, Decimal Points, Periods, Spacing, and Latin Abbreviations

Be particularly mindful when you are handwriting data or reading handwritten information. The following symbols are often misread and can lead to errors in patient care. If you read symbols that are unclear, you should ask for clarification before proceeding with any type of phlebotomy procedure.

Trailing zeros: Do not use a zero alone *after* a decimal point because the reader may not notice the decimal point (e.g., 3.0 ml might be mistaken for 30 ml; instead write 3 ml).

Decimal point: Always use a zero before a decimal point when the measurement is less than a whole unit so the reader notices the decimal point (e.g., .5 ml might be mistaken for 5 ml; instead write 0.5 ml).

Periods: Do not use a terminal period after a symbol for a unit of measurement because it may be interpreted as another symbol (e.g., 7 ml. might be mistaken for 7 ml1, which is meaningless; instead write 7 ml).

Spacing: Use adequate space between numbers and letter symbols so that they will not run together (e.g., 8ml might be mistaken as 8001 if the *m* is mistaken for zeros; instead write 8 ml).

Latin abbreviations: Use the exact meaning of words rather than Latin abbreviations (e.g., instead of the terms *q.i.d.*, *q.o.d.*, and *t.i.d.*, write or say *once daily*, *every other day*, and *three times per day* respectively).

Military Time (24-Hour Clock)

Military time uses a 24-hour time clock (Figure A3-1) and eliminates the need for the A.M. and P.M. designations that are used in civilian or Greenwich time (12-hour time clock). The 24-hour clock is particularly useful in health care settings so that confusion is eliminated when documenting time for treatment procedures, specimen collections, tests, drug administration, surgical procedures, and so on. It is important that all health care workers understand and use it correctly.

Military time is expressed by four numerals; the first pair is *hours* (00 to 24), and the second pair is *minutes* (00 to 59). Each day begins at midnight, 0000, and ends at 2359.

The first 12 hours are equivalent in Greenwich and military time; that is, 3:00 A.M. is equivalent to 0300 in military time, but conversion of afternoon and evening times from a 12-hour clock to military time requires adding 12 to each hour (2:00 P.M. is 1400 in military time). The following examples illustrate:

1:00 A.M. = 0100	1:00 P.M. = 1300
5:00 A.M. = 0500	4:00 P.M. = 1600
10:00 A.M. = 1000	9:00 P.M. = 2100
11:00 A.M. = 1100	10:00 P.M. = 2200
12:00 noon = 1200	12:00 midnight = 2400/0000

Military time is usually stated in terms of hundreds (e.g., 1500 is stated as "fifteen hundred hours"; 0300 is stated as "zero three hundred").

Reference

Badasch, SA, and Chesebro, DS: *Introduction to Health Occupations, Today's Health Care Worker*, 5th ed. Upper Saddle River, NJ: Prentice Hall Health, 2000.

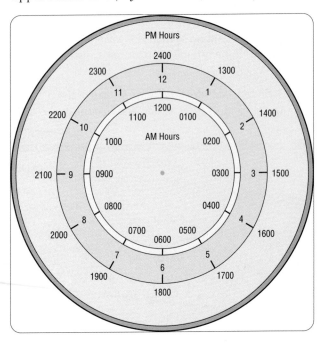

FIGURE ▓ A3-1

24-Hour Clock
(Military time is indicated in the light green areas)

Guide for Maximum Amounts of Blood to Be Drawn from Patients Younger than 14 Years

Patient's Weight		Maximum amount to be drawn at any one time (ml)	Maximim amount of blood (cumulative) to be drawn during a given hospital stay (1 month or less) (ml)
Pounds	Kilograms		
6–8	2.7–3.6	2.5	23
8–10	3.6–4.5	3.5	30
10–15	4.5–6.8	5	40
16–20	7.3–9.1	10	60
21–25	9.5–11.4	10	70
26–30	11.8–13.6	10	80
31–35	14.1–15.9	10	100
36–40	16.4–18.2	10	130
41–45	18.6–20.5	20	140
46–50	20.9–22.7	20	160
51–55	23.2–25.0	20	180
56–60	25.5–27.3	20	200
61–65	27.7–29.5	25	220
66–70	30.0–31.8	30	240
71–75	32.3–34.1	30	250
76–80	34.5–36.4	30	270
81–85	36.8–38.6	30	290
86–90	39.1–40.9	30	310
91–95	41.4–43.2	30	330
96–100	43.6–45.5	30	350

Courtesy of Memorial Hermann Hospital Laboratory, with permission.

Appendix 5

Basic Spanish for Specimen Collection Procedures

The following translations present the health care worker with a very basic means of communicating with patients who speak Spanish. Before speaking with patients, the health care worker should practice using these phrases with someone who knows the correct pronunciation. Otherwise, the patient may become even more confused. Remember that in Spanish, the letter *h* is always silent. Also, if a word ends in *a*, it is usually feminine gender; if it ends in *o*, it is masculine. Another alternative is to have the key phrases printed on cards that the health care worker may point to or use as a reference when he or she is communicating with the patient. Also, use your hands when speaking; pantomime, point, or use facial expressions to assist in communicating your verbal or written message.

English	Spanish
one	uno
two	dos
three	tres
four	cuatro
five	cinco
six	seis
seven	siete
eight	ocho
nine	nueve
ten	diez
twenty	veinte
thirty	treinta
forty	cuarenta
fifty	cincuenta
sixty	sesenta
seventy	setenta
eighty	ochenta
ninety	noventa
one hundred	ciento/cien
Hello.	Hola.
Good day.	Buenos dias/Buendia.
Good morning.	Buenos dias.
Good afternoon.	Buenas tardes.
Good evening.	Buenas noches.
mother	madre/mama
father	padre/papa
sister	hermana

brother	hermano
son	hijo
daughter	hija
husband	esposo/marido
wife	esposa/marida
infant/baby	niño/niña
grandfather	abuelo
grandmother	abuela
friend	amigo/amiga
Mister	Señor
Mrs.	Señora
Miss	Señorita
doctor	doctor/medico
technician	técnico
nurse	enfermera
alcohol	alcohol
fasting	enayunas
gloves	guantes
needle	aguja
sterile	estéril
syringe	jeringa
tourniquet	torniquete
pathology	patología
procedure	procedimiento
hematology	hematología
complete blood count (CBC)	biometría hemática complete
blood bank	banco de sangre
coagulated	coagulado
reports	reportes
specimen	muestra
tubes	tubos
My name is . . .	Me llamo . . . /Mi nombre es . . .
I work in the laboratory.	Trabajo en el laboratorio.
I speak . . .	Hablo . . .
We are going to analyze	Vamos analizar
. . . your blood.	. . . su sangre.
. . . your urine.	. . . su orina.
. . . your sputum.	. . . su esputo.
Do you understand?	¿Entiende usted (ud.)?
I do not understand.	No entiendo.
Please (pls.)	Por favor (p.f.)
Thank you.	Gracias.

You are welcome.	De nada.
Speak slower, pls.	Hable mas despacio, p.f.
Repeat, pls.	Haga me el favor de repetir, p.f.
Can you hear me?	¿Puede oírme?
Can you speak?	¿Puede hablar?
Relax.	Relajese.
What is your name?	¿Como se llama?
What is your address?	¿Que es su domicillo?
What is your birth date?	¿En que fecha nacio?
How old are you?	¿Cuantos años tiene ud.?
Have you been here before?	¿Ha estado ud. aquí antes?
Who is your doctor?	¿Quien es su doctor?
Your doctor wrote the order.	El doctor/la doctora escribio la orden.
Here is the bathroom.	Aquí esta el baño.
Here is the call light.	Aquí esta la luz de emergencia.
You may not eat/drink anything except water.	No debe de comer/beber nada solamente agua.
You may not smoke.	No puede fumar.
Have you had breakfast?	¿Ya tomo el desayuno?
We need a blood/urine/stool sample.	Necesitamos una muestra de su sangre/orina/del excremento.
Please stay in bed.	Por favor, quédese en la cama.
Please do not eat after midnight.	Por favor, no coma después de medianoche.
Please	Haga me el favor de
. . . make a fist.	. . . cerrar el puño.
. . . bend your arm.	. . . doblar el brazo.
. . . roll up your sleeve.	. . . levantarse la manga.
. . . open your hand.	. . . abrir la mano.
. . . sit down here.	. . . sientese aquí.
. . . change your position.	. . . cambiarse de posición.
. . . turn over.	. . . voltearse.
. . . change to the left.	. . . cambiarse a la izquierda.
. . . change to the right.	. . . cambiarse a la derecha.
I am going to lift your sleeve.	Voy levantar la manga.
I need to	Necesito
. . . take a blood sample.	. . . sacar una muestra de sangre.
. . . stick/prick your finger.	. . . picarle su dedo.
. . . two tubes of blood.	. . . dos tubos de sangre.
Open your hand.	Abra la mano.
It will hurt a little.	Le va a doler un poquito.
Please do not move.	No se mueva, por favor.
This is done quickly.	Esto se hace rapido.
The needle will stay in your arm while I am collecting the blood sample.	La aguja se quedara en su brazo durante el tiempo necessario para obtener la muestra.

I am finished. Thank you.	Ya termine. Gracias.
Press this gauze on your arm/finger until I can make sure that the bleeding has stopped.	Comprese esta banda en su brazo/su dedo hasta que pare la sangre.
I am going to put a bandage on you.	Voy a ponerle una cinta adhesiva/un curita/un bandaid.
Are you lightheaded?	¿Esta usted mareado/mareada?
Do you feel as if you are going to faint?	¿Se siente como si se va a desmayar?
Do you feel all right?	¿Se siente bien?
You must lie down.	Necesita acostarse.
Collect the midstream portion of the urine in the container or bottle.	Coleccione la porción del medio de la orina en el vaso.
Void a little, then put urine in this cup.	Orine un poco, luego ponga la orina en esta taza.

Source: Joyce, EV, Villanueva, ME: *Say It in Spanish, A Guide for Health Care Professionals*, 2nd ed. Philadelphia: W. B. Saunders Co, 2000.

NAACLS Phlebotomy Competencies and Matrix

This table describes competencies from the National Association for Accreditation of Clinical Laboratory Sciences (NAACLS) for accredited programs in Phlebotomy. It cross-references the competencies with chapters in two textbooks where the topic or related topics are covered. It also provides a brief overview of the depth of coverage (beginning, intermediate, or advanced) in the context of a curriculum for phlebotomists. While some of the text discussions are not exhaustive, this matrix provides an overview of where material can be obtained and a basis on which students and instructors can seek out further information.

Depth of Coverage: B = Beginning   I = Intermediate   A = Advanced

NAACLS Competencies	*Phlebotomy Simplified*	Chapter(s) where related topics are found	*Phlebotomy Handbook: Blood Collection Essentials, 7e*	Chapter(s) where related topics are found
1.1 Identify the health care providers in hospitals and clinics and the phlebotomist's role as a member of this health care team.	B	1	I	1
1.2 Describe the various hospital departments and their major functions in which the phlebotomist may interact in his or her role.	B	1	I	1
1.3 Describe the organizational structure of the clinical laboratory department.	B	1	I	1
1.4 Discuss the roles of the clinical laboratory personnel and their qualifications for these professional positions.	B	1	B	1
1.5 List the types of laboratory procedures performed in the various sections of the clinical laboratory department.	B	3	I-A	3, 4, Appendix
1.6 Describe how laboratory testing is used to assess body functions and disease.	B	3	I-A	3, 4
1.7 Define medical terminology commonly used in the laboratory.	B	3, Glossary	I-A	3, 9, 10, Glossary
2.1 Identify policies and procedures for maintaining laboratory safety.	B	4	A	6
2.2 Demonstrate accepted practices for infection control, isolation techniques, aseptic techniques, and methods for disease prevention.	B	4	B	5
2.2.1 Identify and discuss the modes of transmission of infection and methods for prevention.	B	4	I-A	5, 6
2.2.2 Identify and properly label biohazardous specimens.	B	5, 8	I-A	5, 7, 9
2.2.3 Discuss in detail and perform proper infection control techniques, such as handwashing, gowning, gloving, masking, and double-bagging.	B	4, 8	I	5, 9
2.2.4 Define and discuss the term *nosocomial infection*.	B	4	I	5

2.3 Comply with federal, state, and local regulations regarding safety practices.	B	4, 8	I-A	5, 6
2.3.1 Use the OSHA Standard Precautions.	B	4, 8	I-A	5, 6, 9
2.3.2 Use prescribed procedures to handle electrical, radiation, biological, and fire hazards.	B	4	I	6
2.3.3 Use appropriate practices, as outlined in the OSHA Hazard Communication Standard, including the correct use of the Material Safety Data Sheet as directed.	B	4	I	6
2.4 Describe measures used to insure patient safety in various patient settings, e.g., inpatient, outpatient, pediatrics.	B	4	I-A	6, 12, 14
3.0 Demonstrate basic understanding of the anatomy and physiology of body systems and anatomic terminology in order to relate major areas of the clinical laboratory to general pathologic conditions associated with the body systems.	B	3	I-A	3, 4
3.1 Describe the basic functions of each of the main body systems, and demonstrate basic knowledge of the circulatory, urinary, and other body systems necessary to perform assigned specimen collection tasks.	B	3	I-A	3, 4
3.2 Identify the veins of the arms, hands, legs, and feet on which phlebotomy is performed.	B	3, 8, 10	I-A	3, 4, 9, 12
3.3 Explain the functions of the major constituents of blood, and differentiate between whole blood, serum, and plasma.	B	3	A	4
3.4 Define hemostasis, and explain the basic process of coagulation and fibrinolysis.	B	3	I-A	4
3.5 Discuss the properties of arterial blood, venous blood, and capillary blood.	B	3	A	4, 9, 10
4.0 Demonstrate understanding of the importance of specimen collection and specimen integrity in the delivery of patient care.	B-I	5	A	7, 9, 10
4.1 Describe the legal and ethical importance of proper patient and sample identification.	B-I	2, 8	I	2
4.2 Describe the types of patient specimens that are analyzed in the clinical laboratory.	B	3, 11	A	3, 4, 9, 10, 15, Appendix
4.3 Define the phlebotomist's role in collecting and/or transporting these specimens to the laboratory.	B	5, 11	A	7, 9, 10, 15
4.4 List the general criteria for suitability of a specimen for analysis and reasons for specimen rejection or recollection.	B	5, 11	A	7, 9, 13, 15
4.5 Explain the importance of timed, fasting, and stat specimens as related to specimen integrity and patient care.	B	5, 8, 11	A	9, 13, 14, 15
5.0 Demonstrate knowledge of collection equipment, various types of additives used, special precautions necessary, and substances that can interfere in clinical analysis of blood constituents.	B	6, 8, 11	A	8, 9, 10, 11,13, 14, 15
5.1 Identify the various types of additives used in blood collection, and explain the reasons for their use.	B-I	6	A	8

NAACLS Competencies		*Phlebotomy Simplified*	Chapter(s) where related topics are found	*Phlebotomy Handbook: Blood Collection Essentials,* 7e	Chapter(s) where related topics are found
5.2	Identify the evacuated tube color codes associated with the additives.	B	6	A	8
5.3	Describe substances that can interfere in clinical analysis of blood constituents and ways in which the phlebotomist can help to avoid these occurrences.	B	5, 7	A	7, 8, 9, 11
5.4	List and select the types of equipment needed to collect blood by venipuncture, capillary, and arterial puncture.	B	6, 8	A	7, 8, 9, 13
5.5	Identify special precautions necessary during blood collections by venipuncture, capillary, and arterial puncture.	B	8, 9, 10, 11	I-A	8, 9, 13
6.0	Follow standard operating procedures to collect specimens.	B	8	A	9
6.1	Identify potential sites for venipuncture, capillary, and arterial punctures.	B	8, 9, 10	A	9, 10, 12, 13
6.2	Differentiate between sterile and antiseptic techniques.	B	4	A	5, 9
6.3	Describe and demonstrate the steps in the preparation of a puncture site.	B	8, 9, 11	A	9, 10, 13
6.4	List the effect of tourniquet, hand squeezing, and heating pads on capillary puncture and venipuncture.	B	8, 9, 10	A	9, 10, 12
6.5	Recognize proper needle insertion and withdrawal techniques, including direction, angle, depth, and aspiration, for arterial puncture and venipuncture.	B	8, 10, 11	A	9, 12, 13
6.6	Describe and perform correct procedure for capillary collection methods on infants and adults.	B	9, 10	A	10, 12
6.7	Identify alternate collection sites for arterial, capillary, and venipuncture. Describe the limitations and precautions of each.	B	3, 8, 9, 11	A	9, 10, 12, 13
6.8	Name and explain frequent causes of phlebotomy complications. Describe signs and symptoms of physical problems that may occur during blood collection.	B	7, 8	A	9, 10, 11, 12
6.9	List the steps necessary to perform an arterial, venipuncture and/or capillary puncture in chronological order.	B	8, 9, 11	A	9, 10, 12, 13
6.10	Follow standard operating procedures to perform a competent, effective venipuncture on a patient.	B	8	A	9
6.11	Follow standard operating procedures to perform a competent, effective capillary puncture on a patient.	B	9, 10	A	10, 12
7.0	Demonstrate understanding of requisitioning, specimen transport, and specimen processing.	B	5	A	7, 9
7.1	Describe the standard operating procedure for a physician requesting a laboratory analysis for a patient. Discuss laboratory responsibility in responding to physician requests.	B	1	I-A	1, 7
7.2	Instruct patients in the proper collection and preservation for various samples, including blood, sputum, and stools.	B	5	I-A	15, 16

7.3	Explain methods for transporting and processing specimens for routine and special testing.	B	5, 11	I-A	7, 9, 15
7.4	Explain methods for processing and transporting blood specimens for testing at reference laboratories.	B	5	I-A	7
7.5	Describe the potential clerical and technical errors that may occur during specimen processing.	B	5	A	1, 7, 11
7.6	Identify and report potential preanalytical errors that may occur during specimen collection, labeling, transporting, and processing.	B	5, 7	A	7, 11
7.7	Describe and follow the criteria for specimens and test results that will be used as legal evidence, e.g., paternity testing, chain of custody, blood alcohol levels.	B	2	I	2, 16
8.0	Demonstrate understanding of quality assurance and quality control in phlebotomy.	B	1, 11	I	1, 14
8.1	Describe the system for monitoring quality assurance in the collection of blood specimens.	B	1	I	1
8.2	Identify policies and procedures used in the clinical laboratory to assure quality in the obtaining of blood specimens.	B	1, 8, 9	I	1, 9, 10
8.2.1	Perform quality control procedures.	B	11	I	5, 6, 8, 14
8.2.2	Record quality control results.	B	11	I	5, 6, 8, 14
8.2.3	Identify and report control results that do not meet predetermined criteria.	B	11	I	5, 6, 8, 14
9.0	Communicate (verbally and nonverbally) effectively and appropriately in the workplace	I	1	A	1, 9
9.1	Maintain confidentiality of privileged information on individuals.	I	1, 2	A	1, 2
9.2	Value diversity in the workplace.	B	1	I	1
9.3	Interact appropriately and professionally with other individuals.	B	1	I	1
9.4	Discuss the major points of the American Hospital Association's Patient's Bill of Rights or the Patient's Bill of Rights from the institution.	B	2	I	1, 2
9.5	Model professional appearance and appropriate behavior.	B	1	I	1
9.6	Model professional appearance and appropriate behavior.	B	1	I	1
9.7	Define the different terms used in the medicolegal aspect for phlebotomy, and discuss policies and protocol designed to avoid medicolegal problems.	B	2	I	2
9.8	List the causes of stress in the work environment, and discuss the coping skills used to deal with stress in the work environment.	B	1	I	1
9.9	Demonstrate ability to use computer information systems necessary to accomplish job functions.	B	5	I	7

Answers to Study Questions, Case Studies, and Competency Checklists

CHAPTER 1

Study Questions

1. a, b, d
2. a, b, c
3. a, b, c
4. d
5. a, b, d
6. b
7. c
8. b
9. a
10. a

Case Study Answers

1. There are several tips that might help to communicate with Mrs. Gonzales:
   - Remain calm, professional, respectful, and courteous
   - Make sure she is comfortable and approach her more slowly
   - Check to see if she would prefer to speak a language other than English; if so, seek out a translator or written instructions in her language of choice
   - Ask if she has family members who might support her during the procedure
   - Double-check for understanding of your instructions

2. Factors that might contribute to her anger or anxiety are:
   - Fear of the procedure or pain
   - Inability to communicate effectively due to language barriers
   - Possible deafness or vision loss

3. Cultural issues that may affect communication with Mrs. Gonzales include the following:
   - Cultural values, such as the presence or absence of her family
   - Language preferences
   - Beliefs, such as about health care, religion, or medical staff
   - Customs and traditions

Competency Checklist: Communication

Refer to pages 10–20

Competency Checklist: Quality Basics

Refer to pages 24–30

CHAPTER 2

Study Questions

1. c	5. a	8. c
2. c	6. c	9. b
3. b	7. b	10. c
4. a		

Case Study Answers

1. Mr. Riley needs to apply pressure to the venipuncture site for additional minutes and then check to see if continuous bleeding is occurring under the skin. If the hematoma continues to enlarge, even with the pressure applied for additional minutes, the health care worker must call his or her supervisor or a nurse.

2. After the patient is provided communication to calm her, Mr. Riley and the supervisor must have the patient evaluated by the attending physician to make certain that she has not had any damage to her median nerve by the needle stick. If she is still complaining of pain, the physician can send her for diagnostic procedures to determine if there was nerve injury.

3. The health care worker must provide a written detail of everything that occurred when he attempted the blood collection from Ms Dickinson, including her jumping as he entered the vein with the needle. This written report will be the incident report that will be filed. If the patient files a malpractice lawsuit, the incident report will provide needed documentation of the venipuncture attempt. If any witnesses, such as other health care workers, or a supervisor, were in the outpatient clinic at the time of this incident and saw the event, they need to provide a written report also.

Competency Checklist: Ethical, Legal, and Regulatory Issues

1. Refer to pages 39, 42
2. Refer to pages 36, 41–42

CHAPTER 3

Study Questions

1. b	5. a	8. c
2. c	6. a	9. c
3. c	7. b	10. d
4. d		

Case Study Answers

1. The health care worker can briefly explain to the patient, "Basically, veins are thin-walled blood vessels that carry deoxygenated blood from the tissues to the heart. Venous blood is dark red, and the veins appear bluish in color. Arteries carry oxygenated blood from the heart and lungs to the tissues so arterial blood appears brighter red in color. However, if you would like a more detailed explanation, please ask your doctor. Would you like to get more information from your doctor before I continue with the blood collection procedure, or may I continue with the procedure?" It is important to provide the patient with information; however, it must be truthful and accurate. It is better not to provide any information than to make up information. Remember that the patient must agree to have the procedure done prior to the venipuncture, so it is best to assure that his or her concerns have been addressed before proceeding. If necessary, the doctor or nurse in charge of the patient can be contacted to answer further questions.

Competency Checklist: Prefixes

1. without, lack of
2. away from
3. toward
4. both
5. without, lack of
6. up
7. before
8. against
9. self
10. two, double
11. short
12. slow
13. bad
14. down
15. a hundred
16. around
17. against
18. ten
19. through
20. double
21. two
22. bad, difficult
23. within
24. upon, above
25. good, normal
26. out, away from
27. outside, beyond
28. half
29. different
30. similar, same
31. water
32. above, excessive
33. below, deficient
34. below
35. between
36. within
37. bad
38. large, great
39. middle
40. small
41. one-thousandth
42. many, much
43. none
44. scanty, little
45. all
46. beside
47. around
48. many
49. first
50. false
51. four
52. five
53. backward
54. half
55. below, under
56. above, beyond
57. together
58. together
59. four
60. three
61. one

Competency Checklist: Root Words

1. vessel
2. to choke
3. artery
4. artery
5. fatty substance, porridge
6. hair-like
7. heart
8. heart
9. heart
10. elbow, forearm
11. cell
12. skin
13. electricity
14. to cast, to throw
15. work
16. red
17. blood
18. necrosis of an area
19. fat
20. study
21. thin
22. muscle
23. vein
24. vein
25. lung
26. rhythm
27. hardening
28. serum
29. pulse
30. chest
31. tension
32. clot
33. vessel
34. vein

Competency Checklist: Suffixes

1. pain
2. immature cell, germ cell
3. hernia, tumor, swelling
4. surgical puncture
5. cell
6. binding
7. pain
8. surgical excision
9. vomiting
10. a weight, mark, record
11. to write, record
12. one who specializes, agent
13. inflammation
14. study of
15. destruction, separation
16. enlargement, large
17. measure
18. resemble
19. tumor
20. to view
21. condition of
22. disease
23. deficiency
24. surgical fixation
25. to eat
26. to speak
27. attraction
28. fear
29. to obstruct
30. growth
31. formation, produce
32. surgical repair
33. paralysis, stroke
34. breathing
35. formation
36. drooping
37. spitting

38. bursting forth	42. rupture	46. new opening	50. nourishment, development
39. bursting forth	43. instrument	47. treatment	
40. suture	44. to view	48. instrument to cut	51. urine
41. flow, discharge	45. control, stopping	49. incision	

Competency Checklist: Identifying Medical Terms

1. coagulate	4. hyperglycemia	7. pathology	9. leukopenia
2. anticoagulant	5. leukocyte	8. antecubital	10. arteriosclerosis
3. hematology	6. erythrocyte		

Competency Checklist: Spelling

1. immunology	4. hematocrit	7. hematology	9. thrombus
2. phlebotomy	5. leukemia	8. embolus	10. millimeter
3. hemorrhage	6. erythrocyte		

Competency Checklist: Cardiovascular System

1. H	5. N	9. J	13. E	17. D
2. I	6. L or M	10. Q	14. F	18. A
3. K	7. P	11. R	15. G	19. S
4. M or L	8. O	12. T	16. C	20. B

CHAPTER 4

Study Questions

1. c	5. b	8. a
2. a	6. b	9. a
3. c	7. c	10. c
4. b		

Case Study Answers

1. In this case, Clara has exposed herself to definite harm by having an open wound that could have been contaminated by the patient's blood. She must immediately cleanse the area with isopropyl alcohol and apply an adhesive bandage.

2. Even though Clara knows she made a drastic error in not taking the gloves with her for the blood collections, she must notify her supervisor, fill out the necessary incident and medical forms, and undergo the appropriate laboratory tests. In addition, Clara will need to be counseled and evaluated for HIV and hepatitis C infection at periodic intervals.

Check Yourself: Infection Control Procedures and Safety

1. Handwashing is essential in the performance of any phlebotomy procedure on any patient. Remember, even though you are using a different set of gloves for each patient's blood collection procedure, handwashing has to occur before another set of gloves is placed on your hands.

2. Health care workers, as well as patients, can become allergic to latex products. Many of the gloves used in health care facilities are made of latex. Also, some tourniquets, syringes, adhesive tape, and blood pressure cuffs contain latex that could lead to an allergic reaction in the patient and/or health care worker.

3. The recommendations are to:

Wear gloves; use 1:10 bleach solution or commercially prepared solution; first clean the area with visible blood and then disinfect the entire area of possible contamination; and keep the bleach in contact with the contaminated area for at least 20 minutes to ensure complete disinfection. If it had been a "large" spill, a spill kit should have been used for the clean-up process.

Competency Checklist: Infection Control and Safety

1. Type ABC extinguishers contain a dry chemical and are used on fires of wood, cloth, paper, oil, grease, and gasoline. They are multipurpose in combating fires and are located in fire stations throughout health care facilities.

2. Always unplug before maintenance performance on the centrifuge or any other electrical equipment.

3. Examples: gloves, facial masks, respirators, gowns, shields

4. Isopropyl alcohol   It is an antiseptic for skin.
   Iodine   It is an antiseptic for skin.
   Chloramine   It is a disinfectant for wounds.

CHAPTER 5

Study Questions

1. a	5. c	8. b
2. b	6. b	9. c
3. b	7. a	10. c
4. a		

Case Study Answers

1. The most likely cause of the hemolysis in so many specimens is that the phlebotomist probably shook the blood specimens too vigorously when trying to mix the anticoagulant with the specimen. Another possibility is that the specimens were not properly situated in the pneumatic tube carrier case and may have been excessively agitated during the tube transportation to the laboratory. If this had been the case, the specimen tubes may have broken or cracked and leaked, causing a serious biohazard.

2. Communication with the phlebotomist who collected the specimens should be open, and she should be asked about her technique for mixing specimens and her methods of positioning the specimen tubes for transport in the pneumatic tube. Appropriate counseling and retraining should occur. The situation should be documented for all patient specimens concerned, the physicians should be notified, and recollections should be initiated.

Competency Checklist: Specimen Transportation

Refer to pages 100–108

CHAPTER 6

Study Questions

1. c	5. c	8. a
2. a	6. b	9. b
3. a	7. a	10. c
4. c		

Case Study Answers

1. Gray-topped vacuum tubes contain an additive to maintain the glucose level in the blood until it is tested for a result. The additive is usually potassium oxalate and sodium fluoride.

2. Because the sodium fluoride in the gray-topped tube destroys many enzymes (e.g., AST, CK, ALP, ALT), in the blood, it should not be used for enzyme collections.

Self Assessment: Identifying the Proper Equipment for Blood Collection

1. Refer to pages 113–117
2. Refer to pages 118–126
3. Refer to pages 126–131

CHAPTER 7

Study Questions

1. a	5. c	8. b
2. d	6. b	9. c
3. c	7. c	10. d
4. c		

Case Study Answer

The normal fasting blood glucose values are based on fasting blood specimens collected some time between 8 and 12 hours after eating food. If the patient has not eaten for 14 hours, as Mrs. Gonzalez indicated, her blood glucose value could be erroneous because it is not based within the time period allotted for fasting specimens.

However, Dorothy should proceed with the blood collection and document as required by written or computer entry that the patient had fasted for 14 hours rather than the normal 8 to 12 hour time limit. The physician will have to decide whether to use that blood glucose result in his or her diagnosis and treatment or to request another fasting specimen.

Competency Checklist: Preanalytical Complications in Blood Collection

1. Refer to pages 136–138
2. Refer to page 143

CHAPTER 8

Study Questions

1. b	5. d	8. a
2. a, b, c, d	6. d	9. c
3. b	7. b	10. b
4. d		

Case Study Answers

Case Study 1

There are several key issues that are important for the health care worker in this confusing situation:

confirming the patient's identity;

dealing with a comatose patient; and

collecting blood from a patient with an IV.

Procedurally, the health care worker should ask the patient her name even though the patient may appear asleep or comatose. If the patient does not respond, which would be likely in this case, the health care worker should seek confirmation of the identity from an authorized nurse or family member. If the patient's armband confirms the identity on the laboratory requisitions, (e.g., Ann Beaumont), then the health care worker may proceed with the specimen collection process. However, the health care worker should notify the nurse or supervisor about the incorrect sign on the patient's bed. *Never* rely on a bed sign for identity confirmation.

Regarding the comatose condition, the health care worker should ask the nurse to assist her in positioning the patient's arm in a secure manner so that if the patient flinches during the needle puncture, it will not cause injury or disrupt the specimen collection process. And, in consideration of the IV in one arm, the health care worker should use the other arm for the venipuncture. If there are no palpable veins in the non-IV arm, the health care worker may select a dorsal hand vein on this arm or on the IV arm *below* the IV site. Remember, that venous blood is flowing from the tips of the fingers toward the heart, so IV fluid contamination into the blood specimen would be *less* likely below the IV site (on the side closest to the fingers) rather than above the IV site (on the side closest to the heart). If the specimen is collected from the dorsal side of the hand below the IV site, a notation should be made to indicate this situation. Generally speaking, the health care worker should always "go the extra mile" to confirm identity and collect an accurate specimen with the least amount of discomfort to the patient. If there is any question about identity, venipuncture site, or patient condition, seek clarification from a supervisor *before* beginning the procedure.

Case Study 2

Since the patient had a mastectomy on her *left* side, it would be best to draw the blood from the *right* arm in the antecubital area. If there are no suitable veins in this area, the second area to search for a good vein would be the dorsal side of the right hand.

The correct order of draw would be as follows:

Blood cultures (yellow)—Keep in mind that blood cultures require sterile preparation of the site

PT & PTT (light blue)—Coagulation tests

electrolytes (red)—Chemistry test

HGB & HCT, cell counts (lavender)—Hematology tests

Competency Checklist: Patient Identification

Refer to pages 151–153

Competency Checklist: Preparing for the Patient Encounter

Refer to pages 154–156

Competency Checklist: Use of a Tourniquet and Site Selection

Refer to pages 163–165

Competency Checklist: Decontamination of the Puncture Site

Refer to pages 165–166

Competency Checklist: Performing a Venipuncture

Refer to pages 166–171

Competency Checklist: Order of Draw

Refer to pages 174–175

Competency Checklist: Leaving the Patient

Refer to pages 178–179

CHAPTER 9

Study Questions

1. a
2. d
3. d
4. c
5. c
6. b
7. a
8. c
9. c
10. b

Case Study Answers

In the case of Sarah W., who was obviously fearful of the specimen collection procedure and whose hands were cold, the health care worker can take several positive steps to help the situation. First, a polite, sympathetic, and professional conversation with Sarah about the procedural steps could help Sarah understand that a fingerstick is not as invasive as a venipuncture procedure. Allow Sarah to see the equipment and ask questions about it. Second, ask Sarah to hold a warming device in her hands, and/or to dangle her arm low, or to run warm water over her hand to increase the blood flow to the area. Let her know that warming her hands will facilitate the fingerstick process and help the blood flow quickly into the collection tubes. Inform her that the volume of blood needed for the procedure is very small, so it will be over quickly. Ask her if she has ever fainted during or after a blood collection procedure. If possible, place her in a reclining collection chair for comfort and safety or in a secure blood collection chair with adjustable arm rests.

As for Henry C., his skin condition may indicate that he is dehydrated. He may benefit from drinking a glass of water and coming back after a short period of time. Check the fingers of both hands, and ask him which is his dominant hand. Seek a finger site on the nondominant hand because it may be less likely to have calluses. Use of a warming device or warm water on his hand may help increase blood flow to the area. If none of these methods increases the blood flow to the hand, or the fingers appear too calloused to prick, it may be best to consult a supervisor. However, if one of the fingers appears suitable, continue with the puncture procedure. Try to focus on the fleshy side, (i.e., the thick section), of the third or fourth finger tip of the nondominant hand.

Competency Checklist: Capillary Blood Collection

Refer to pages 193–196

Competency Checklist: Making Blood Smears for Microscopic Analysis

Refer to pages 189–193

CHAPTER 10

Study Questions

1. d
2. c
3. b
4. c
5. b
6. d

7. d   9. b   10. d

8. b

Case Study Answers

1. The skin puncture performed on this infant will require that the hematology specimen (i.e., CBC, hemoglobin) will be collected first, followed by the chemistry specimen (i.e., creatinine) and then the blood-bank specimen (i.e., ABO group and Rh typing).

2. The phlebotomist must *always* record the amount of blood collected from the infant. Overcollecting blood during numerous blood collections may lead to a blood transfusion in an infant. Thus, the cumulative amount of blood collected from an infant or child during a hospital stay must be continuously checked so that too much blood is not collected, leading to anemia in the infant or child.

Self Assessment: Check Yourself

1. Refer to page 212

2. Refer to page 220

3. Refer to page 221

CHAPTER 11

Study Questions

1. a   5. a   8. d
2. c   6. a   9. c
3. c   7. a   10. b
4. a

Case Study Answer

Problems That Could Have Led to Point-of-Care Testing Error

Contamination of the blood with alcohol. (After alcohol is used to cleanse the skin puncture site, the skin must completely dry before puncturing the site.)

Wrong volume of specimen is collected.

Instrument blotting/wiping technique is not performed according to manufacturer's directions.

Instrument is not clean.

Reagents are outdated.

Timing of the analytic procedure is incorrect.

Reagents are not stored at the proper temperature, leading them to deterioration.

Battery for instrument is weak or dead.

In addition to this list of possible problems, the instrument will have troubleshooting guidelines to help identify the problem so that the correct result can be obtained.

Competency Checklist: Special Collections

1. Refer to page 231–232

2. Refer to page 241–243

Glossary

The terms in this glossary are defined as they would most likely be used by clinical laboratory personnel—more specifically, by phlebotomists. The definitions are not exhaustive or elaborate.

acid-citrate-dextrose (ACD) an additive commonly used in specimen collection for blood donations to prevent clotting. It ensures that the RBCs maintain their oxygen-carrying capacity.

active listening a set of skills that enables an individual to become a more effective listener. The skills include concentrating on the speaker, getting ready to listen by clearing one's mind of distracting thoughts, use of silent pauses when appropriate, providing reassuring feedback, verifying the conversation that took place, keeping personal judgments to oneself, paying attention to body language of the person speaking, and maintaining eye contact.

additives substances (gels, clotting activators, or anticoagulants) that are added in small amounts to specimen collection tubes to alter the specimen so as to make it appropriate for laboratory analysis or handling.

age-specific care considerations providing services that are age-appropriate and considerate (e.g., special considerations are needed for different ages of children (toddler versus teen) and also for geriatric patients). Factors typically relate to age-related fears/concerns, communication styles, procedures for comforting the patient, and safety.

alcohol colorless liquid that can be used as an antiseptic.

Allen test a procedure used prior to drawing specimens (for ABGs) from the radial artery. It assures that the ulnar and radial arteries are providing collateral circulation to the hand area. Basically, it entails compressing the arteries to the hand and emptying the hand of arterial blood, then releasing the compression to see if the circulation is immediately restored. A negative test would indicate that collateral circulation is not sufficient and an alternative artery (brachial or femoral) should be used for ABG collections.

aliquot a portion of a blood sample that has been removed/separated from the primary specimen tube.

ambulatory care health care services that are delivered in an out-patient or nonhospital setting. It implies that the patients are able to ambulate, or walk, to the clinic to receive their services.

American Society for Clinical Laboratory Scientists (ASCLS) professional organization for laboratory personnel that provides continuing education, conference activities, and certification examinations for specified groups.

American Society for Clinical Pathology (ASCP) professional organization that certifies many types of laboratory personnel based on their passing a certification examination. ASCP offers clinical and research conferences, many types of continuing education activities, and ongoing certification programs.

analytic phase refers to the phase in laboratory testing whereby the specimen is actually assessed or evaluated, and results are confirmed and reported.

anatomic pathology major area of laboratory services whereby autopsies are performed and surgical biopsy tissues are analyzed.

anemia medical condition where by there is a reduction in hemoglobin thus lowering the O_2 carrying capacity of blood cells.

antecubital area of the forearm (around the crease of the elbow) most commonly used for venipuncture.

anterior surface region of the body characterized by the front (or ventral) area and including the thoracic, abdominal, and pelvic cavities.

anticoagulant substance introduced into the blood or a blood specimen to keep it from clotting.

antimicrobial chemical or therapeutic agent that destroys microorganisms such as bacteria, viruses, and fungi.

antiseptic hand rub applying/rubbing a waterless antiseptic product onto all surfaces of the hands to reduce the number of microorganisms present; the hands are rubbed until the product has dried.

antiseptic hand wash washing hands with soap and water or other detergents containing an antiseptic agent.

antiseptics chemicals (e.g., 70 percent isopropyl alcohol, iodine, chlorohexidine, chlorine, hexachlorophene, chlorooxylenol, quarternary ammonium compounds, and triclosan) used to clean human skin by inhibiting the growth of microorganisms.

arterial blood gases (ABGs) analytical test that measures oxygen and carbon dioxide in the blood. Provides useful information about respiratory status and the acid–base balance of patients with pulmonary disorders.

arteries highly oxygenated blood vessels that carry blood away from the heart.

arterioles smaller branches of arteries.

aseptic a degree of cleanliness that prevents infection and the growth of microorganisms. The technique to achieve this condition includes frequent handwashing, use of barrier garments and personal protective equipment (PPE), waste management of contaminated materials, use of proper cleaning solutions, following standard precautions, and using sterile procedures when necessary.

assault a legal term referring to the unjustifiable attempt to touch another person or the threat to do so in circumstances that cause the other person to believe that it will be carried out, or to cause fear. An assault may be permissible if proper consent has been given (e.g., consent to obtain a blood specimen).

assessments a measurement term referring to factors that affect both the analytic (quantitative) and nonanalytic (qualitative) components of health care. Competency assessments are used to measure an individual's ability to perform specified job tasks.

automated skin-puncture device a single-use apparatus that pierces the skin with a lancet that automatically retracts into a protective casing.

bacteremia presence of bacteria in the blood; an infection of the blood.

bar codes series of light and dark bands of varying widths that relate to alphanumeric symbols. They can correspond to the patient's name and/or identification numbers.

basal state for phlebotomy procedures, this refers to the patient's condition in the early morning, approximately 12 hours after the last ingestion of food. In hospitals, most laboratory tests are analyzed on basal state specimens.

basilic vein vessel of the forearm that is acceptable for venipuncture.

battery a complex legal term referring to the intentional touching of another person without consent, and/or beating or carrying out threatened physical harm. Battery always includes an assault and is therefore commonly used with the term in *assault and battery*.

beta-carotene a photosensitive analyte.

bevel slanted surface at the end point of a needle.

bilirubin a photosensitive analyte.

blood circulating fluid and cells in the cardiovascular system.

blood cells components of blood, the three main types of circulating blood cells are erythrocytes, leukocytes, and thrombocytes.

bloodborne pathogens (BBPs) pathogenic microorganisms, including hepatitis B virus and human immunodeficiency virus, that are present in human blood and can cause disease in humans.

blood cultures tests that aid in identifying the specific bacterial organism causing infections in the blood. In the case of a patient that is experiencing fever spikes, it is recommended that the blood culture specimens be collected before and after the fever spike, when bacteria are most likely present in the peripheral circulation. Care must be taken by the phlebotomist not to contaminate the specimen, so special sterile preparation of the collection site is required.

blood-drawing chair a chair specifically designed to hold a patient comfortably and safely in a proper position during and after a blood collection procedure. The design typically includes a moveable armrest on both sides of the chair.

blood gas analysis refer to *arterial blood gases*.

blood urea nitrogen (BUN) analytic testing procedure to determine the amount of urea in the blood.

blood vessels key component of the circulatory system, these vessels transport blood throughout the body.

blood volume the total amount of blood in an individual's body. This is particularly important in pediatric phlebotomies because withdrawing blood can cause a significant decrease in the total blood volume of a small infant, thus resulting in anemia. Blood volume is based on weight and can be calculated for any size person.

body planes imaginary dividing lines of the body that serve as reference points for describing distance from or proximity to the body. Body planes include the sagittal, frontal, transverse, and medial planes.

brachial artery an artery located in the cubital fossa of the arm and used as an alternative site for ABG collections. Phlebotomists must be specially trained to perform collections from this site.

breach of duty a legal term referring to an infraction, violation, or failure to perform.

buffy coat in blood specimens that contain anticoagulants, the WBCs and platelets form a thin white layer above the RBCs called the *buffy coat*.

butterfly system also called a winged infusion system or scalp needle set, the system can be used for difficult venipunctures due to small or fragile veins. The needle is typically smaller, and has a thin tubing with a Luer adapter at the end so that it can be used on a syringe or an evacuated tube system during venipuncture. Most models have needle safety devices such as retractable needles and/or needle coverings/sheaths.

calcaneus heel bone.

cannula a tube that can be inserted into a cavity or blood vessel and used as a channel for transporting fluids. The term is most commonly used in dialysis for patients with kidney disease. The cannula is used to gain access to venous blood for dialysis or for blood collections. Specialized training and experience are required to draw blood from a cannula.

capillaries microscopic blood vessels that carry blood and link arterioles to venules.

capillary action a term used when referring to micro-collection procedures that indicates the free flowing movement of blood into the capillary tube without the use of suction.

capillary blood a specimen from a skin puncture that contains a blend of blood from venules, arterioles, and tissue fluid.

capillary blood gas analysis using microcollection methods on infants (usually the heel site) to collect specimens for blood gas analyses; these analytical tests measure oxygen and carbon dioxide in the blood. Provides useful information about respiratory status and the acid–base balance of patients with pulmonary disorders.

capillary tubes disposable narrow-bore pipettes that are used for pediatric blood collections and/or micro-hematocrit measures. The tubes may be coated with anticoagulant such as heparin, and for safety reasons are usually made of plastic.

cardiopulmonary resuscitation (CPR) the method used to revive the heart and/or breathing of a patient whose heart or respiration has stopped. It is advisable for health care workers to be appropriately trained in the use of CPR.

cardiovascular system body system that provides for rapid transport of water, nutrients, electrolytes, hormones, enzymes, antibodies, cells, and gases to all cells of the body.

cause-and-effect diagrams (Ishikawa) a quality improvement tool that uses diagrams to identify interactions between equipment, methods, people, supplies, and reagents.

Centers for Disease Control and Prevention (CDC) federal agency responsible for monitoring morbidity (disease) and mortality (death) throughout the country.

centrifugation the process of separating cellular elements from the liquid portion of a blood specimen. It is done by spinning the specimen in a specially designed centrifuge.

centrifugation phase period of time when a blood specimen is inside the centrifuge.

cephalic vein a vein of the forearm that is acceptable for venipuncture.

cerebrospinal fluid (CSF) fluid that surrounds the brain and meninges within the spinal column.

chain of infection the process by which infections are transmitted; components include the source of the infection (nonsterile items, contaminated equipment or supplies, etc.), the mode of transmission (direct contact, airborne, medical instruments, etc.), and the susceptible host (patient).

circulatory system body system referring to the heart, blood vessels, and blood; responsible for transporting oxygen and nutrients to cells and transports carbon dioxide and wastes until they are eliminated; transports hormones, regulates body temperature, and helps defend against diseases.

citrate type of anticoagulant additive for blood collection tubes; prevents the blood clotting sequence by removing calcium and forming calcium salts.

civil law different from criminal law; in civil law, the plaintiff sues for monetary damages.

clean-catch midstream a urine specimen that is used for detecting bacteria and/or for microscopic analysis. Normally, the specimen should be free of contamination because the patient should be instructed to clean and decontaminate themselves prior to urination. The urine specimen should be collected into a sterile container. Urine should be voided and the specimen should be collected mid-urination.

clinical laboratory a workplace where analytic procedures are performed on blood and body fluids for the detection, monitoring, and treatment of disease.

Clinical Laboratory Improvement Amendments (CLIA) federal guidelines that regulate all clinical laboratories across the United States. Regulations apply to any site that tests human specimens, including small POLs, or screening tests done at the patient's bedside.

Clinical and Laboratory Standards Institute (CLSI) nonprofit organization that recommends quality standards and guidelines for clinical laboratory procedures, formerly National Committee for Clinical Laboratory Standards (NCCLS).

clinical pathology major area of laboratory services where blood and other types of body fluids and tissues are analyzed.

clinical record see *medical records*.

coagulation a phase in the blood-clotting sequence in which many factors are released and interact to form a fibrin meshwork, or blood clot.

competency statements performance expectations that include entry-level skills, tasks, and roles performed by the designated health care worker.

confidentiality the protected right and duty of health care workers not to disclose any information acquired about a patient to those who are not directly involved with the care of the patient.

constituents chemical or cellular elements that make up blood.

contaminated sharps used objects that can penetrate the skin, including needles, scalpels, broken glass, broken capillary tubes, and exposed wires.

contamination presence of blood or potentially infectious substances on an item or surface.

continuous quality improvement (CQI) a theoretical framework and management strategy to improve health care structures, processes, outcomes, and customer satisfaction. It is ongoing and involves all levels of the administrative structure of an organization.

creatinine clearance test analytic procedure to determine whether or not the kidneys are able to remove creatinine from the blood.

criminal actions legal recourse for acts against the public welfare; these actions can lead to imprisonment of the offender.

critical test result a term that should be defined by each health care organization and typically includes test results that are abnormal, STAT test results, or other results that require an immediate response.

critical value a laboratory result that indicates a pathophysiologic state at such variance with normal as to be life threatening; these values should be defined and reported to the patient's physician as soon as possible.

culture a system of values (importance of education), beliefs (spiritual, family bonding), and practices (food, music, traditions) that stem from an individual's concept of reality. Culture influences decisions and behaviors in many aspects of life.

culture and sensitivity (C&S) microbiologic test to determine the growth of infectious microorganisms in bodily specimens (e.g., urine), and to determine which antibiotics are most effective on the microorganism.

cyanotic bluish in color due to oxygen deficiency.

date of birth (DOB) personal information, i.e., birthday, included in a patient's medical record and on laboratory test requests.

decontaminate use physical or chemical means to remove or destroy bloodborne pathogens on a surface (including skin) or item so that pathogens are no longer able to transmit disease. Prior to venipuncture, decontamination involves cleaning with a sterile swab or sponge to prevent microbiological contamination of either the patient or the specimen. This is usually accomplished with a sterile swab containing 70 percent isopropyl alcohol (or isopropanol).

defendant individual (e.g., a health care worker), against whom a legal action (civil or criminal) or lawsuit is filed.

dehydration loss of body water.

diabetes mellitus metabolic disease in which carbohydrate utilization is reduced due to a deficiency in insulin and characterized by hyperglycemia, glycosuria, water and electrolyte loss, ketoacidosis, and in serious conditions, coma. In milder forms of noninsulin-dependent diabetes mellitus, dietary regulation may keep the disorder under control.

diagnostic test results the results from all tests performed on the patient: laboratory, radiology, and so on.

diastolic pressure the second measure reported in a blood pressure measurement.

differentials a laboratory test that categorizes blood cells and any abnormalities present.

digestive system body system referring to organs in the gastrointestinal (GI) tract that break down food chemically and physically into nutrients that can be absorbed by the body's cells and allow the elimination of waste products of digestion.

disinfectants chemical compounds used to remove or kill pathogenic microorganisms; typically used on medical instruments or countertops.

disposable sterile lancet sterile sharp device, preferably retractable, used in skin puncture collections to penetrate the skin at specified depths (e.g., no more than 2.0 mm for infant heelsticks).

distal distant or away from point of attachment (e.g., the birthmark was *distal* to the wrist).

diurnal rhythms opposite of nocturnal (nighttime) rhythms, "diurnal" rhythms are variations in the body's functions or fluids that occur during daylight hours or every 24 hours (e.g., some hormone levels decrease in the afternoon). Also referred to as circadian rhythms.

dizziness lightheadedness, unsteadiness, loss of balance.

dorsal surface region of the body characterized by the back (or posterior) area and including the cranial and spinal cavities.

double bagging practice of using two trash bags for disposing of waste from patient's rooms, particularly those in isolation.

edematous condition in which tissues contain excessive fluid and it often results in localized swelling.

electronic medical record (EMR) computerized version of a medical/clinical record.

e-mail electronic mail often used in health care facilities. Guidelines for using e-mail, including a patient's

consent to use e-mail, are now required of health care facilities.

engineering controls refer to devices that isolate or remove bloodborne pathogen hazards from the workplace (e.g., needleless devices, shielded needle devices, plastic capillary tubes). "Work practice" controls are activities that reduce the risk of exposure (e.g., "no-hands" procedures for discarding sharps).

Environmental Protection Agency (EPA) federal agency that, among its other responsibilities, regulates the disposal of hazardous substances and monitors and regulates disinfectant products.

ethics a branch of philosophy that deals with distinguishing right from wrong and with moral consequences of human actions.

ethylenediamine tetra-acetic acid (EDTA) anticoagulant additive used to prevent the blood-clotting sequence by removing calcium and forming calcium salts. EDTA prevents platelet aggregation and is useful for platelet counts and platelet function tests. Fresh EDTA samples are also useful for making blood films or microscopic slides, because there is minimal distortion of platelets and WBCs.

eutectic mixture of local anesthetics (EMLA) a topical anesthetic (pain reliever) that is an emulsion of lidocaine and prilocaine and can be applied to intact skin.

evacuated tube system method of blood collection using double-sided needles whereby the needle is attached to a holder/adapter and allows for multiple specimen tube fills and changes without blood leakage.

expiration date the date after which products or supplies should not be used.

exposure control plan a document required in health facilities that details the process for medical treatment, prophylaxis, and/or follow-up after an employee has been exposed to potentially harmful or infectious substances (e.g., in the case of a percutaneous needlestick injury).

extrinsic factors substances involved in the clotting process that are stimulated when tissue damage occurs.

fainting see *syncope*.

fasting refers to no food or drinks (except water).

fasting blood tests tests performed on blood taken from a patient who has abstained from eating and drinking (except water) for a particular period of time.

feathered edge a term used to describe blood smears on microscopic slides; it is a visible curved edge that thins out smoothly and resembles the tip of a bird's feather.

femoral artery located in the groin area of the leg and lateral to the femur bone, it is the largest artery used as an alternative site for ABG collections. Phlebotomists must be specially trained to perform collections from this site.

fibrin substance that forms a blood clot.

fibrinolysis the final phase of the hemostatic process whereby repair and regeneration of the injured blood vessel occurs and the clot slowly begins to dissolve or break up (lyse).

fistula an artificial shunt or passage, commonly used in the arm of a patient undergoing kidney dialysis; the vein and artery are fused through a surgical procedure. Only specially trained personnel can collect blood from a fistula.

fomites inanimate objects that can harbor infectious agents and transmit infections (e.g., toilets, sinks, linens, door knobs, glasses, phlebotomy supplies).

frontal plane imaginary line running lengthwise on the body from side to side, dividing the body into anterior and posterior sections.

gauge number refers to the size (diameter) of the internal bore of a needle. The larger the number, the smaller the bore size, and vice versa.

gauze loosely woven material used for bandages that are sterile or chemically clean.

geriatric refers to an elderly patient.

gestational diabetes diabetes that begins during pregnancy (often the second or third trimester). It occurs in 1–4% of pregnancies and usually subsides after delivery.

glucose tolerance test (GTT) diagnostic test for detecting diabetes. The test is performed by obtaining blood and urine specimens at timed intervals after fasting, then after ingesting glucose. Each specimen is analyzed for its glucose content to determine if the glucose level returns to normal within 2 hours after ingestion.

granulocytes (basophils, neutrophils, eosinophils) mature leukocytes (WBCs) in the circulating blood; when stained and viewed microscopically, granules are present.

hand hygiene term that applies to handwashing (with non-antimicrobial soap and water), antiseptic handwashing, antiseptic hand rub (with waterless antiseptic), or surgical hand antisepsis.

health care–acquired (nosocomial) infections infections acquired after admission into a health facility.

Health Insurance Portability and Accountability Act (HIPAA) federal law (1996) expanded in 2000 to protect security, privacy, and confidentiality of personal health information.

heart a key component of the cardiovascular system, it is the pump that forces blood throughout the body.

heelstick pediatric phlebotomy procedure that requires puncturing one of specified areas of an infant's heel.

hematocrit a commonly ordered laboratory test to assess the circulatory system; it describes the concentration of RBCs and therefore provides an indirect measure of the oxygen-carrying capacity of the blood.

hematology the study of blood.

hematoma a localized leakage of blood into the tissues or into an organ. In phlebotomy, it can occur as a result of blood leakage during the vein puncture, thereby causing a bruise.

hematopoiesis the process of blood cell formation that occurs in the bone marrow.

hemoconcentration increased localized blood concentration of large molecules such as proteins, cells, and coagulation factors. This can be caused by excessive application of a tourniquet.

hemoglobin the molecules that carry oxygen and carbon dioxide in the RBCs.

hemolysis rupture or lysis of the blood cells.

hemostasis maintenance of circulating blood in the liquid state and retention of blood in the vascular system by prevention of blood loss.

heparin an anticoagulant that prevents blood clotting by inactivating thrombin and thromboplastin, the blood-clotting chemicals in the body.

histograms bar graphs often used as quality improvement tools.

holder (adapter) plastic apparatus needed in specimen collecting using the evacuated tube method. The adapter/holder secures the double-pointed needle: one end of the needle goes into the patient's vein, and on the other end of the needle is placed an evacuated tube.

home health care services provision of health care services in a patient's home under the direction of a physician.

homeostasis means literally "remaining the same"; also referred to as a steady-state condition, it is a normal state that allows the body to stay in a healthy balance by continually compensating with necessary changes.

human immunodeficiency virus (HIV) a virus spread by sexual contact or exposure to infected blood.

hypoxia a condition in which body tissues are not receiving enough oxygen.

iatrogenic anemia a type of induced blood-loss resulting in anemia when too much blood is withdrawn in a short period of time, a patient may require a blood transfusion.

immunology the study of diseases of the immune system.

incision a cut into the skin. The term is used to describe the puncture made by an automatic skin puncture device.

infection control programs guidelines designed to address surveillance, reporting, isolation procedures, education, and management of community-acquired and health-care-associated infections.

informed consent a complex legal term; basically, it refers to voluntary permission by a patient to allow touching, examination, and/or treatment by health care workers after they have been given information about the procedures and potential risks and consequences. It allows patients to decide what may be performed on or to their bodies.

inpatients hospitalized patients.

insulin a chemical produced by the pancreas that is released into the bloodstream to facilitate glucose absorption from the blood into the tissues where it is used for energy. When insulin is not produced (as in diabetes mellitus), blood glucose levels increase because it cannot be absorbed into the tissues.

integumentary system body system referring to skin, hair, sweat and oil glands, teeth, and fingernails; involved in protective and regulatory functions.

interstitial space between tissues and/or organs.

interstitial (tissue) fluid minute amounts of liquid forming between gaps/layers of tissue; a natural component of capillary blood.

intravenous (IV) catheter vascular access device inserted into a blood vessel for administration of medications and nutrients and for blood collection.

intrinsic system part of the coagulation process that involves the clotting factors contained in the blood.

invasion of privacy a legal term referring to objectionable or personal intrusion upon an individual such that it is offensive (e.g., the publishing of confidential information).

iodine used to make tincture of iodine (2% solution) which is used as a skin disinfectant. Some patients are allergic to iodine.

isolation procedures methods used to protect individuals (health care workers) from patients with infectious diseases. Formally divided into two types (category-specific and disease-specific), newer guidelines combine isolation practices for moist and potentially infectious body substances, to be used for all patients. The new categories of isolation are based on the mode of transmission and include airborne, droplet, and contact precautions.

The Joint Commission independent, nonprofit organization that sets quality standards for healthcare.

judicial law legal processes designed to resolve disputes.

lancet/lancing device a sharp apparatus (similar to a needle) used to puncture skin to acquire a capillary blood specimen.

lateral directional term meaning towards the sides of the body.

latex allergy reaction to certain proteins in latex rubber, a natural ingredient in some varieties of gloves. Allergic reactions range from skin redness, rash, hives, or itching to respiratory symptoms and, in rare instances, shock.

law societal rules or regulations designed to protect society and resolve conflicts; laws are rules that must be observed.

liable a legal term that refers to a legal obligation when damages are concerned.

light sensitive refers to laboratory specimens; some chemical constituents (bilirubin, vitamin B_{12}, carotene, folate, urine porphyrins) decompose if exposed to light and therefore should be protected/covered during transportation and handling.

lipemic when referring to serum, it is a cloudy or milky appearance, usually due to a temporarily elevated lipid level after the ingestion of fatty foods.

lithium iodoacetate antiglycolytic agent and anticoagulant; not to be used for hematology testing or enzymatic determinations.

litigation process a legal action to determine a decision in court. Many malpractice cases are negotiated and settled out of court.

lymphatic system body system responsible for maintaining fluid balance, providing a defense against disease, and absorption of fats and other substances from the blood stream.

lymphocytes type of white blood cell that is nongranular in appearance; plays a role in immunity and in the production of antibodies.

lymphostasis obstruction and/or lack of flow of the lymph fluid.

malice a legal term referring to a reckless disregard for the truth (e.g., knowing that a statement is false).

malpractice a legal term referring to improper or unskillful care of a patient by a member of the health care team, or any professional misconduct, unreasonable lack of skill, or infidelity in professional or judiciary duties; often described as "professional negligence."

mastectomy removal of a breast.

medial directional term meaning toward the midline of the body.

median cubital vein forearm vein that is most commonly used for venipuncture.

Medicaid a shared federal- and state-funded program designed to provide health insurance for individuals with low incomes.

medical records definitive documents, paper or electronic medical records (EMR), that contain a chronological log of a patient's care. It must include any information that is clinically significant or relevant to the patient's care.

Medicare federal program designed to provide health insurance for the elderly and members of special groups.

melanin pigment in the skin that provides color and protects underlying tissues from absorbing ultraviolet rays.

metabolism an important bodily function that allows the formation or breakdown of substances (e.g., proteins) for the purpose of using energy.

microbiology the study of microbes.

microcollection process by which small amounts of blood are collected in small containers or tubes using specially designed devices.

microcontainers specialized collection devices designed for small quantities of blood; some containing anticoagulants. These devices are typically used for pediatric or geriatric patients with fragile or inaccessible veins, and/or for finger sticks.

microorganisms living organisms that are too small to see with the naked eye such as bacteria, viruses, and fungi.

misdemeanor a legal term referring to many types of criminal offenses that are not serious enough to be classified as felonies.

mode of transmission refers to the method by which pathogenic agents are transmitted (e.g., direct contact, air, medical instruments, other objects, and other vectors).

monocytes type of white blood cell that is nongranular and also plays a role in defense.

multiple-sample needles used with the evacuated tube method of blood collection, these needles are attached to a holder/adapter and allow for multiple specimen tube fills and changes without blood leakage.

muscular system body system referring to all muscles of the body.

National Fire Protection Association (NFPA) developed the labeling system for hazardous chemicals that is used in healthcare facilities.

National Phlebotomy Association (NPA) professional organization for phlebotomists that offers continuing educational activities and a certification examination for phlebotomists.

needleless system a device that does not use needles for procedures that are normally associated with needle use. This includes collection of bodily fluids or withdrawal of body fluids after initial venous or arterial access is performed. It includes any procedure that has the potential for occupational exposure to bloodborne pathogens from contaminated sharp objects.

needlestick skin puncture using a needle.

negligence a legal term referring to the failure to act or perform duties according to the standards of the profession.

neonatal screening typically refers to mandatory (required by law) laboratory testing of infants for specified disorders such as PKU and hypothyroidism. There is wide variability in what tests are required by each state.

neonate a newborn infant; term used during the first 28 days after birth.

nervous system body system that includes organs that provide communication in the body, sensations, thoughts, emotions, and memories.

obesity an unhealthy abundance of body fat.

occluded veins closed or constricted veins.

occult blood analysis that detects hidden (occult) blood in the stool.

occupational exposure contact via skin, eye, mucous membranes, or parenteral with potentially infectious materials as a result of an individual's work duties.

Occupational Safety and Health Administration (OSHA) an agency of the U.S. Department of Labor requiring employers to provide a safe work environment including measures to protect workers exposed to biological and occupational hazards.

osteochondritis inflammation of the bone and its cartilage.

osteomyelitis inflammation of the bone due to bacterial infection.

osteoporosis a condition of the bone whereby the mineral density is reduced, making the bone more fragile.

outcomes used as a quality improvement term to refer to what is accomplished for the patient (e.g., healing, return to wellness, or return to normal functions). Poor patient outcomes have been described as the "5 Ds": death, disease, disability, discomfort, and dissatisfaction.

oxalates anticoagulants that prevent blood-clotting sequence by removing calcium and forming calcium salts.

panic value see *critical value*.

parental involvement during pediatric phlebotomy procedures, a parent's support and presence during the procedure is often helpful in reducing stress/anxiety for the patient. On the other hand, some parents are reluctant to be involved, so the phlebotomist must assess each situation to determine the level of parental involvement that would optimize the phlebotomy encounter.

Parkinson's disease a neurological disease characterized by muscular tremors and rigidity of movement.

pathogenesis the origin of a disease.

pathogenic agents disease-causing bacteria, fungi, viruses, or parasites that are transmitted by direct contact, air, medical instruments, other objects, or vectors.

pathology the study of all aspects of disease and abnormal conditions of the body.

patient confidentiality see *confidentiality*.

patient-focused testing laboratory services usually designed around a team concept and focused on convenience to the patient.

patient–physician relationship the professional communication linkage that a patient has with his or her doctor.

Patient's Bill of Rights a statement developed to affirm the rights of patients. Key elements involve the right to respectful and considerate care; accurate information about diagnoses, treatment, and prognoses; informed consent; refusal of treatment; privacy; confidentiality; advance directives; reviewing records about own treatment; knowing identity and role of personnel involved in care; information about research procedures; billing information; and knowing business relationships of those providing care.

peak a term used for therapeutic drug monitoring to describe the blood sample that is taken when the drug is at its highest concentration in the patient's serum (e.g., "the *peak* level").

pediatric phlebotomy procedures performed on infants and children and require specialized training and management. Often done by skin puncture, pediatric phlebotomies also entail matching the procedure with the specimen requirements for testing, the patient's age and emotional condition, and possible parental involvement.

percutaneous through the skin.

peripheral circulation near the surface of the body.

personal protective equipment (PPE) equipment designed to protect the health care worker from hazards in the workplace (e.g., goggles, gloves, gowns).

petechiae minute, pinpoint hemorrhagic spots in the skin that may be indicative of a coagulation abnormality. For phlebotomists, it should be a warning sign that the patient may bleed excessively.

phenylketonuria (PKU) a congenital disorder, usually diagnosed at birth, that can cause brain damage resulting in severe retardation, often with seizures and other neurologic abnormalities.

phlebotomist individual who practices phlebotomy (i.e., a blood collector); *phlebo* is related to "vein," and *tomy* relates to "cutting."

phlebotomy a cut or incision into the vein.

photosensitive sensitive to light.

physician–patient relationship the association between the patient and the physician providing clinical and consultative services; the communication between them is private and confidential.

physician's office laboratories (POLs) nonhospital laboratories usually based in a physician's office/clinic at the private practice.

plasma liquid portion (unclotted or anticoagulated) of the blood in which blood cells are suspended.

platelets (thrombocytes) blood cells that aid in blood clot formation.

pleural fluid fluid from the lung cavity.

pneumatic tube systems transportation system used in many health care facilities for specimens and paper-based documentation. Considerations for use of these systems involves evaluation of speed, distance, control mechanisms, shock absorbency, sizes of carriers, and breakage/spillage rates.

point-of-care (POC) testing refers to tests and procedures that are actually performed at the patient's bedside or at the "point of care." The tests are not sent to a laboratory in a remote location; rather, they are rapid methods designed to produce quick results.

porphyrins a type of photosensitive analyte.

postcentrifugation phase period of time after a specimen has been centrifuged but before serum or plasma has been removed for testing.

posterior surface region of the body characterized by the back (or dorsal) area and including the cranial and spinal cavities.

postprandial glucose test a glucose test performed after ingestion of a meal; useful for screening patients for diabetes, because glucose levels in serum specimens drawn 2 hours after a meal are rarely elevated in normal patients. In contrast, diabetic patients have elevated glucose values 2 hours after a meal.

preanalytical phase laboratory testing phase in which tests are ordered and specimens are collected and prepared for testing. Preanalytical variables include patient variables (fasting versus nonfasting, stress, availability, etc.), transportation variables (specimen leakage, tube breakage, excessive shaking, etc.), specimen processing variables (centrifugation, delays, contamination of the specimen, exposure to heat or light), and specimen variables (hemolysis, inadequate volume, inadequate mixing of the tube, etc.).

precentrifugation phase period of time after a specimen has been collected but before centrifugation.

premature infant an infant born before 37 weeks of gestation (normal gestation is 40 weeks).

primary care health care services that are provided to maintain and monitor normal health and provide preventive services.

primary tube tube containing the patient's blood sample.

privacy the patient's right to respectful consideration of the confidential nature of his or her health information.

proficiency testing (PT) testing that is part of the quality management of laboratory services and involves subscribing to an outside source to provide "unknown" or "blind" specimens to see how one laboratory's results compare with other laboratories' results. Performance reviews on proficiency tests are part of the accrediting process for most laboratories.

protective (reverse) isolation precautionary measures and procedures designed to protect patients who are particularly susceptible or at increased risk of acquiring infections (e.g., patients with low WBC counts (neutropenic or leukopenic), patients with burns, and/or immunosuppressed patients).

proximal near the point of attachment (e.g., the leg broke on the *proximal* side of the knee).

pulmonary circuit the circulatory pathway when blood leaves the heart and enters the right and left pulmonary arteries.

puncture proof a surface that can withstand punctures from sharp objects such as needles.

qualitative test pertains to the presence or absence (positive or negative) of a substance in the specimen.

quality refers to a specimen that is correctly identified, collected, and transported.

quality control material daily controls that are used in analytic testing to determine acceptable ranges of test results (i.e., tolerance limits).

quantitative test pertains to the exact measurement or quantity of substance in the specimen.

radial artery located on the thumb side of the wrist, this artery is most commonly used to collect blood specimens for arterial blood gases. Phlebotomists must be specially trained to perform collections from this site.

radio frequency identification (RFID) a newer form of identification for specimens with the following characteristics: tiny silicon chips that transmit data to a wireless receiver, does not require line-of-sight reading with a scanner, can be detected at various distances, identifies and/or tracks many items simultaneously, and can be used in combination with a bar code for multiple purposes.

random urine sample urine sample taken at random time(s).

red blood cells (RBCs or erythrocytes) blood cells that function to transport oxygen and carbon dioxide in the body.

reference ranges when referring to laboratory values, these are laboratory test value ranges that are considered within "normal" limits.

reproductive system body system referring to organs involved in sperm production, secretion of hormones (e.g., testosterone, estrogens, and progesterone), ovulation, fertilization, menstruation, pregnancy, labor, and lactation.

requisition form paper-based method for requesting laboratory tests.

respiratory system body system referring to parts that assist in respiration or breathing (e.g., nose, pharynx, larynx, trachea, bronchi, and lungs).

sagittal plane imaginary line running lengthwise on the body from front to back, dividing the body into right and left halves.

sclerosed veins veins that have become hardened.

secondary tube tube containing removed plasma/serum (an aliquot) *after* specimen centrifugation of a primary tube containing the patient's blood sample.

separated plasma/serum serum or plasma that has been removed or separated from contact with blood cells. It is referred to as an *aliquot*. It can be removed from the primary tube after centrifugation using a pipette, or separated from cellular contact with a chemical or physical barrier.

septicemia formally called "blood poisoning," the term now means the presence of toxins or multiplying bacteria in the blood.

serum when blood is allowed to clot, sera separates from the blood cells, which are meshed in a fibrin clot. Serum contains the same constituents as plasma except that the clotting factors are contained within the clot.

sharps any devices or tools that can potentially cut, puncture, or cause injury.

single-sample needle used for collecting a blood sample from a syringe.

skeletal system body system referring to all bones and joints.

skin puncture a cut into the skin (e.g., of the finger or heel) with a retractable puncture device or a nonretractable lancet.

sodium fluoride an additive (antiglycolytic agent) present in specific blood collection tubes that is used for glycolytic inhibition tests.

sodium polyanethole sulfonate (SPS) an additive typically used in blood culture bottles to prevent clotting.

source the origin of an infection (e.g., human hands, lab coats or other clothing, contaminated medical instruments).

specimen collection manual electronic or paper-based document required by accrediting agencies that includes instructions for patient preparation, type of collection containers, amounts of specimen required for specified tests, timing requirements, preservatives or anticoagulants needed, special handling instructions, proper labeling requirements, and other test-specific or situation-specific requirements for specimens.

specimen integrity high quality blood sample that can be adversely affected or compromised by the method of transport, timing delays, temperature, agitation, exposure to light, and centrifugation methods.

specimen rejection relates to the suitability of a specimen for testing or when it may *not* be used for laboratory analyses.

stakeholders individuals, groups, organizations, and/or communities that have an interest in or are influenced by health care services. Stakeholders can be internal to the organization or external (i.e., outside the organization).

standard of care the practices or guidelines that a reasonably prudent person would follow in any particular circumstance. Many agencies, licensing boards, certifying boards, and accrediting organizations write standards of care or standards of practice to guide health care workers in their duties.

standard operating procedures (SOP) instructions to achieve uniform or consistent performance of a function.

Standard Precautions a set of safeguards designed to reduce the risk of transmission of microorganisms; guidelines apply to *all patients and all body fluids, nonintact skin, and mucous membranes and include the use of barrier protection (protective equipment such as gloves, gowns, etc.), hand hygiene, and proper use and disposal of needles and other sharps.* Policies must comply with OSHA Standards are available from the U.S. Centers for Disease Control and Prevention.

STAT an emergency situation that requires immediate action; in the case of blood collection and analysis, tests that are ordered "STAT" should be given the highest priority for collection, delivery to the laboratory, analysis, and reporting.

steady state also referred to as homeostasis, it is a condition that allows the normal body to stay in balance by continually compensating with necessary changes, thereby remaining in a healthy condition.

sterile gauze pads typically used in blood collection procedures either during the decontamination process and/or after blood collection to aid in stopping the bleeding; it is a sterile cotton mesh pad that is packaged in individual units.

sterile technique use of procedures that produce an aseptic condition (i.e., free from all living microorganisms and their spores).

sucrose nipple or pacifier a sucking device for infants and toddlers that is used to pacify or comfort the child.

superficial near the surface of the body (e.g., *superficial* veins show up easily on the skin).

superior vena cava one of the two large veins that brings oxygen-poor blood to the heart from the head, neck, arms, and chest region.

supine reclining position.

susceptible host a component in the chain of infection; the degree to which an individual is at risk for acquiring an infection. Factors affecting susceptibility are age, drug use, degree and nature of the patient's illness, and status of the patient's immune system.

syncope the transient (and frequently sudden) loss of consciousness due to a lack of oxygen to the brain (i.e., fainting) and resulting in an inability to stay in an upright position. Patients usually recover their orientation quickly, but injuries (e.g., abrasions, lacerations) often result from falling to the ground.

synovial fluid joint fluid.

syringe method method of venipuncture whereby a syringe is used to collect blood that is then transferred to collection tubes.

systemic circuit part of the cardiovascular system that carries blood to the tissues of the body.

therapeutic drug monitoring (TDM) testing procedures to evaluate drug levels in a patient's blood. This is valuable for drug dosage and to monitor the patient for a variety of other factors (clinical effectiveness, toxicity, etc.).

therapeutic phlebotomy removal of blood for therapeutic reasons (i.e., in conditions where there is an excessive production of blood cells).

thermolabile constituents that degrade if exposed to warm temperatures.

thrombi blood clots formed somewhere within the cardiovascular system; they may occlude a vessel or attach to the wall of a vessel.

timed specimen a test is ordered to be drawn at a particular time.

tissue (interstitial) fluid fluids found in between and around tissues that are not blood.

tourniquet a soft rubber strip typically about 1 inch wide and 15 to 18 inches long used on the arm to help find a site for venipuncture. The ends are stretched around a patient's arm about 3 inches above the venipuncture area. The tightening of the tourniquet causes venous filling in the veins and enables better visualization and feel of the prominent veins in the area.

transmission-based precautions categories of precautionary measures based on the route of transmission of disease. Three types of transmission-based precautions are airborne, droplet, and contact precautions.

transverse plane imaginary line running crosswise, or horizontally, on the body, dividing the body into upper and lower sections.

trough a term used for therapeutic drug monitoring to describe the blood sample that is taken just prior to the next dose, or when the drug is at a low concentration in the patient's serum (i.e., the "trough" level).

turbid cloudy or milky in appearance.

urinary system body system referring to processes enabling the production and elimination of urine. Consists of kidneys, ureters, bladder, and urethra.

vacuum (evacuated) tube color-coded specimen collection tube that contains a vacuum so as to aspirate blood when a needle enters a patient's vein. The tubes are part of a blood collection method that also requires a double-pointed needle and a special plastic holder (adapter). One end of the double-pointed needle enters the vein, the other pierces the top of the tube, and the vacuum aspirates the blood into the tube. Tubes may contain anticoagulants.

vascular a network of blood vessels that includes veins, arteries, and capillaries.

vasoconstriction rapid constriction of the blood vessels to decrease blood flow to the area.

veins blood vessels that carry blood toward the heart after oxygen has been delivered to the tissues.

vena cavae largest veins of the body.

ventral surface region of the body characterized by the front (or anterior) area and including the thoracic, abdominal, and pelvic cavities.

ventricles two of the four chambers of the heart.

venules minute veins that flow into larger veins.

visceral (nonstriated, smooth, involuntary) muscles muscles that line the walls of internal structures (e.g., veins and arteries).

virology study of viruses.

volume space occupied by a liquid and usually measured in liters or milliliters.

whistle blowing disclosure of a legal wrongdoing by an employee of the same organization (e.g., an illegal action is reported by an employee to appropriate authorities such as a governmental agency or accreditation agency). Employees who speak out to reveal illegal actions may fear reprisals that could jeopardize their safety or their job. Thus, numerous laws are in place to protect employees who report legitimate wrongdoings.

white blood cells (WBCs or leukocytes) blood cells that provide for defense against infectious agents.

winged infusion system also called a butterfly set or scalp needle set, the system can be used for difficult venipunctures due to small or fragile veins. The needle is typically smaller, and it has a thin tubing with a Luer adapter at the end so that it can be used on a syringe or an evacuated tube system during venipuncture.

work practice controls practices that diminish the likelihood of exposure to hazards by altering the manner in which the work is performed (e.g., prohibiting the recapping of needles with a two-handed approach).

zone of comfort area of space surrounding a person/patient that is considered "private or personal"; if a stranger (or phlebotomist) gets too close to the individual (i.e., beyond the zone of comfort), the person/patient may begin to feel uncomfortable.

Index